Language Research in Post-Traumatic Stress

This collection brings together different perspectives on post-traumatic stress, considering its causes, its impact on different groups, and ways forward toward equipping speech-language clinicians, educators, and scholars to better understand and support the individuals and communities with which they work.

The volume defines post-traumatic stress, unpacking its causes and how they might be mitigated. The 11 chapters critically reflect on the wide-ranging effects traumatic stress has on the brain, communication, language, literacy, and life skills of different groups, including children, adolescents, adults, refugees, and victims of racialized violence. This book also includes examples of interventions demonstrated to be effective with affected individuals. The range of perspectives highlights the importance of culturally responsive and trauma-informed practices and the need for language and literacy professionals to engage in transdisciplinary practice in order to develop more effective supports for those experiencing post-traumatic stress. Looking ahead, the volume discusses recommendations for curriculum content, clinical practice, and changes to policy toward ensuring all people with post-traumatic stress are able to fully participate in daily life.

This book will be of interest to students and scholars in speech-language sciences, social work, occupational therapy, and clinical psychology, as well as clinicians and educators in these areas.

Yvette D. Hyter is an ASHA Fellow, has received ASHA Honors, is a Professor Emerita of Speech, Language and Hearing Sciences at Western Michigan University, USA, and is the Owner of Language & Literacy Practices, LLC, in Kalamazoo, Michigan, USA.

Routledge Research in Speech-Language Pathology
Series editor: Louise Cummings

Routledge Research in Speech-Language Pathology looks beyond traditional areas of study within the discipline to showcase topics historically underserved in research on communication disorders, highlighting fresh perspectives on issues of key importance in speech-language pathology. The series offers comprehensive treatments of communication disorders and the work of speech-language pathology with an eye toward pushing the field forward, critically examining challenges in addressing disparities in speech-language pathology and exploring the latest developments in related disciplines with implications for the future of research on communication disorders. Volumes in this series will be of particular interest to students, scholars, and clinicians in speech-language pathology, speech and language therapy, and clinical linguistics, as well as related fields such as special education, psychology, neurology, psychiatry, social work, and nursing.

Language Case Files in Neurological Disorders
Louise Cummings

COVID-19 and Speech-Language Pathology
Louise Cummings

Communication and Sensory Loss
Global Perspectives
Edited by Kathryn Crowe

Language Research in Post-Traumatic Stress
Edited by Yvette D. Hyter

For more information about this series, please visit: https://www.routledge.com/Routledge-Research-on-Speech-Language-Pathology/book-series/RRSLP

Language Research
in Post-Traumatic Stress

Edited by Yvette D. Hyter

Routledge
Taylor & Francis Group

NEW YORK AND LONDON

First published 2024
by Routledge
605 Third Avenue, New York, NY 10158

and by Routledge
4 Park Square, Milton Park, Abingdon, Oxon, OX14 4RN

Routledge is an imprint of the Taylor & Francis Group, an informa business
© 2024 selection and editorial matter, Yvette D. Hyter; individual chapters, the contributors

Library of Congress Cataloging-in-Publication Data
Names: Hyter, Yvette D., editor.
Title: Language research in post-traumatic stress /
edited by Yvette D. Hyter.
Other titles: Routledge research in speech-language pathology
Description: New York: Routledge, 2024. |
Series: Routledge research in speech-language pathology |
Includes bibliographical references and index. |
Identifiers: LCCN 2023059030 | ISBN 9781032125855 (hardback) |
ISBN 9781032125862 (paperback) | ISBN 9781003225270 (ebook)
Subjects: MESH: Stress Disorders, Post-Traumatic | Language
Therapy—methods | Speech Therapy—methods
Classification: LCC RC552.P67 L353 2024 | NLM WM 172.5 |
DDC 616.85/21—dc23/eng/20240228
LC record available at https://lccn.loc.gov/2023059030

ISBN: 9781032125855 (hbk)
ISBN: 9781032125862 (pbk)
ISBN: 9781003225270 (ebk)

DOI: 10.4324/9781003225270

Typeset in Sabon
by codeMantra

Contents

List of Contributors   *vii*
Acknowledgments   *xi*
Preface   *xii*

1 Introduction to Language Research in Post-Traumatic Stress   1
   YVETTE D. HYTER

PART I
**Post-Traumatic Stress: Considerations, Concepts,
and Consequences within Language Research**   9

2 Racialized Stress and Trauma in Black Communities:
   Lessons for Speech and Language Professionals   11
   PAUL ARCHIBALD AND LAJUANA ARCHIBALD

3 Post-Traumatic Stress, Autobiographical Memory, and
   Cultural Neuroscience: Implications for Migrants
   and Refugees   37
   CAROL WESTBY

4 Post-Traumatic Stress, the Brain, and Social Pragmatic
   Communication   68
   YVETTE D. HYTER

5 Neurodevelopmental Impact of Post-Traumatic Stress   91
   MICHELLE A. SUAREZ AND CARA MASSELINK

6   The Impact of Post-Traumatic Stress on
     Cognitive-Communication in Multilingual Children
     and Adults   115
     SULARE TELFORD ROSE AND JENNIFER RAE MYERS

PART II
Post-Traumatic Stress: Considerations Across the
Lifespan for Language Development and Functioning   155

  7   Post-Traumatic Stress: Child Language Development
      and Functioning   157
      NA'AMA YEHUDA

  8   Addressing the Impact of Post-Traumatic Stress
      on Adolescent Language and Identity: An Interdisciplinary
      Approach   180
      GINGER G. COLLINS, JAYNA MUMBAUER-PISANO, AND
      TOBIAS KROLL

  9   Attachment-based Narrative Speech Styles in Adults with
      Post-Traumatic Stress   206
      KARIN RIBER AND EMMA BECK

10   Post-Traumatic Stress Disorder and Cognitive
      Communication Effects   227
      LINDA CAROZZA

11   Language Research in Post-Traumatic Stress: Where Do
      We Go from Here?   255
      YVETTE D. HYTER

      Index   *263*

Contributors

Paul Archibald, DrPH, LCSW-C, is an associate professor and MSW Program Director in the Department of Social Work at the College of Staten Island, City University of New York. He has over a decade of clinical practice and training dedicated to the prevention and treatment of mental and physical health outcomes among persons exposed to trauma and chronic stressors. His current research agenda utilizes an intersectional approach to survey the role of racialized stress and trauma in the contribution of health disparities. He is a firm believer that "it takes a whole community to make a community whole!"

Lajuana Archibald, MS, CCC-SLP, has been a licensed speech-language pathologist for over 20 years. She earned her Bachelor of Science degree in Speech-Language Pathology and Audiology and her Master of Science degree in Speech-Language Pathology. She is currently a New York State-certified speech-language pathologist and a member of the American Speech and Hearing Association. She has worked as an independent contractor for Early Intervention and is currently employed by the NYC Department of Education. She remains committed to shaping the overall development of children with a focus on pervasive developmental disorders, learning disabilities, and speech impairments.

Emma Beck holds a PhD and an MSc in psychology from the University of Copenhagen and an MRes.psych. from the University College London. She has published internationally on attachment security, psychotherapy research, and mentalization-based treatment. She is trained and experienced in conducting the Adult Attachment Interview and Adult Attachment Projective Picture System. She is a clinical, licensed psychologist and psychotherapist with more than ten years of experience working with adults, adolescents, and their parents within psychiatric settings and psychotherapeutic clinics. She has specific expertise in attachment-related trauma, adolescent personality pathology, and complicated grief. She is currently in private practice.

Linda Carozza, PhD, CCC-SLP, FNAP, is a tenured associate professor in the Communication Sciences and Disorders Graduate Program at Pace University in New York City and an ASHA-certified speech-language pathologist. She is also a clinical assistant professor in the Department of Rehabilitation Medicine at NYU Langone Health. Her professional interests are neurogenic communication disorders in adults. She is the author of three books and numerous articles, specializing in quality of life, mentorship, and multicultural issues.

Ginger G. Collins, PhD, CCC-SLP, is a licensed speech-language pathologist specializing in language-based literacy disorders in adolescents. She is a professor in the School of Speech, Language, Hearing, and Occupational Sciences at the University of Montana. Her current research interests involve investigating how school-based speech-language pathologists are preparing students with communication deficits for life after graduation with a particular focus on adverse police-initiated interactions.

Yvette D. Hyter, PhD, CCC-SLP, ASHA Honors, Professor Emerita at Western Michigan University, has worked with children and families with histories of maltreatment for over two decades. She co-directs the *Resiliency Center for Families and Children* and owns *Language & Literacy Practices, LLC*, providing culturally/linguistically and trauma-responsive and globally sustainable consultations and courses for educational agencies. She is a founding member of the *SLHS Equity Action Collective*, whose members established an open-access journal, the *Journal of Critical Studies of Communication and Disability*, and who are transforming scholarship, practice, and policy using critical science, equity, and social justice.

Tobias Kroll, PhD, CCC-SLP, is a licensed speech-language pathologist with a specialization in language and literacy development and qualitative research. He is an associate professor at Texas Tech University Health Sciences Center. His current research interests center on the role of cognitive flexibility in reading comprehension, and the intersection of social communication and identity formation in diverse contexts.

Cara Masselink, PhD, OTRL, ATP, is an associate professor at the Department Occupational Therapy, Western Michigan University. Clinical pediatric experience in early intervention, private practice, and hospitals led her to work with assistive technology. She has a PhD in Interdisciplinary Health Sciences. Her current research focuses on the utilization of appropriate equipment to enable occupational performance, with a specific focus on impacting healthcare policy. She is the Executive Director of the Clinician Task Force, a nonprofit organization of occupational and physical therapists across the United States, that advocates for policy change and best practices for complex seating and wheeled mobility.

Jayna Mumbauer-Pisano, PhD, is an assistant professor in the Department of Counseling at the University of Montana. Her clinical expertise is in counseling children and adolescents through mental health challenges, including anxiety, depression, school refusal, and significant life adjustments. Her research interests include children's mental health literacy, trauma-informed care, and creative interventions in counseling.

Jennifer Rae Myers is the founder and executive director of the RB 'A Way With Words' Foundation, a nonprofit organization that provides free expressive arts and communication health programs to underserved communities. She also co-directs "CulturallySMART," a multicultural awareness and research training fellowship for underrepresented graduate students in communication sciences. She received her BS in Communication Disorders from Bowling Green State University, an MS in Communication Sciences & Disorders, and a PhD in Neuropsychology with a minor in Cognitive Psychology—both from Howard University. Her mission is to create a socially equitable health ecosystem for priority populations in communication health.

Karin Riber, PhD, MSc in Psychology, is a licensed psychologist and specialist in adult clinical psychology and psychotherapy. She has published internationally in attachment, psychotherapy, and refugee trauma. She is trained in the adult attachment interview, is a certified coder of reflective functioning on the AAI, and is specialized in mentalization-based group therapy and compassion-focused therapy. For more than ten years, Dr. Riber has worked as a clinical psychologist in the mental health services with PTSD, complex refugee trauma, and psychopathology. She is currently at The Danish National Centre for Grief, working with complicated grief and intervention with bereaved young adults and the elderly.

Michelle Suarez, PhD, OTRL, is an associate professor in the Department of Occupational Therapy at Western Michigan University (WMU; Kalamazoo). She is a co-director of the Resiliency Center for Families and Children and has spearheaded efforts for trauma treatment at the university. She has initiated caregiver coaching for mothers in opioid recovery and their infants born with neonatal abstinence syndrome and for foster and adoptive parents caring for children with severe regulation challenges. She is a member of the Brain Research and Interdisciplinary Neuroscience Lab (WMU) and is on the editorial board for *The Open Journal of Occupational Therapy*.

With expertise in child language development and multilingualism, **Sulare Telford Rose**, PhD, CCC-SLP, brings a unique perspective to her research, shaped by her experiences as a Black, South American, Caribbean immigrant. Her work focuses on the languages and cultures of origin within African American, Caribbean, and Latinx communities. She is an assistant professor of speech-language pathology at the University of the District of Columbia and a founding member of the university's bilingual certification program. Additionally, she serves as the Professional Development Manager for the American Speech-Language-Hearing Association's Special Interest Group on Global Issues in Communication Sciences and Related Disorders.

Carol Westby, PhD, CCC-SLP, is a consultant for Bilingual Multicultural Services in Albuquerque, NM, and holds an affiliated appointment in Communication Disorders at Brigham Young University in Provo, UT. She is a fellow of the American-Speech-Language-Hearing Association (ASHA), has received the Honors of ASHA and the Kleffner Lifetime Clinical Achievement Award, and holds Board Certification in Child Language and Language Disorders. She has received the Distinguished Alumnus Award from Geneva College and the University of Iowa's Department of Speech Pathology and Audiology and the ASHA Award for Contributions to Multicultural Affairs.

Na'ama Yehuda, MSc, is a speech-language pathologist and a clinician for 35 years. She specializes in developmental trauma and complex clinical presentations. She was elected to and served in professional organizations in communication disorders (ISHLA) and in mental health (ISSTD), volunteers, consults and publishes internationally (including award-winning book on trauma and communication), and she is dedicated to interdisciplinary collaboration. Na'ama has written numerous articles about trauma, language, and dissociation. Her book, *Communicating Trauma: Clinical Presentations and Interventions with Traumatized Children*, is published in both English and Spanish.

Acknowledgments

I met Dr. Louise Cummings (virtually) several years ago when she invited me to write a chapter in her book on *Research in Clinical Pragmatics, Series: Perspectives in Pragmatics, Philosophy, & Psychology, Vol. 11.* Several years later, she encouraged me to write a proposal for a book on language and trauma, and this text, *Language Research in Post-traumatic Stress*, was conceptualized. Thank you, Louise, for your encouragement and support throughout the development and production of this volume.

I want to acknowledge the work that each author in this volume does with individuals and families who have experienced post-traumatic stress. This work can be difficult but also very rewarding. Each author has made a valuable contribution to the literature through their contribution to this volume.

I appreciate the guidance I received from the publishing staff at Routledge/ Taylor & Francis Group. Specifically, I would like to thank Elysse Preposi and Jasmine Erice-Harling for their assistance in bringing this volume to fruition.

Finally, I want to thank my husband, W. F. Santiago-Valles, for his patience, encouragement, and support while I was glued to my computer writing and editing chapters for this text.

Preface

Since the mid-1980s, I have spent a significant number of years caring for children with trauma histories and their families. My first encounter with children who had exposure to complex trauma, the type of trauma that takes place within the caregiving system, was in a transdisciplinary (although this terminology was not used then) preschool setting while working alongside a special education teacher, play therapist, and teacher's aide. Trauma was not a word used widely at that time, and certainly not in speech, language, and hearing sciences. As I think back to that time, I now know that the children and families on my caseload all those years ago were exposed to overwhelming events – sometimes at home, or through systems, or in places of work and schooling – that left them feeling helpless, hopeless, and a profound sense of loss. I also realized the rewarding magic of a transdisciplinary approach to supporting children and their families with trauma histories, so much so that I spent the next 16 years of my career trying to replicate that interaction in my speech-language practice. In 2000, collaboration with a social worker, occupational therapist, pediatrician, and counselor led to the creation of a center that specialized in providing comprehensive, integrated, and contextualized assessments for children and families with trauma histories. I worked there for 20 years, and now, I am co-director of a resiliency center that supports individuals and families with complex needs, such as those who have experienced trauma, have a disability or neurodevelopmental disorders, or addiction.

As a speech-language clinician, educator, and scholar, I know that it is imperative for members of this profession to understand trauma, its impact on the brain, and the many ways it changes and complicates communication, language, and literacy abilities. The literature in this topical area in speech-language and hearing is quite thin, yet there is growing interest. This interest grew exponentially during the COVID-19 pandemic when every human was experiencing more stress than usual.

For Such a Time as This

In 2019 and 2020, the world changed because of a global pandemic. As a result of the measures taken to keep everyone safe, isolation increased, children did not attend school in person, and many adults began working remotely. These changes resulted in job and economic insecurity, food scarcity, increased anxiety, and devastating losses resulting from many deaths caused by COVID-19. Most families experienced profound loss, and unfortunately, these losses were disproportionately represented in impoverished communities and communities of color. In addition to the global pandemic, armed conflicts, wars, and mass shootings and their consequences have strained mental health. Additionally, complex trauma and systemic trauma (caused by exploitation, exclusion, repression, and dispossession) persist. Worldwide, the World Health Organization[1] estimates that there are over 1 billion children affected by maltreatment (physical, sexual, emotional abuse, neglect), human trafficking, and bullying every year. This text is needed for such a time as this.

The Current Need

There is significant information available that defines trauma, explains its impact on the brain, and mentions its psychological and physiological effects. What is sorely lacking in the extant literature on speech-language and hearing is how toxic stress, trauma, and post-traumatic stress can affect communication, language, and literacy – abilities that are essential for engaging in social interactions, academic success, and functioning effectively in daily life. The goal of this text is to continue to address the dearth of information on trauma, specifically to examine *Language Research in Post-traumatic Stress*. Individuals and families who have experienced post-traumatic stress have complicated needs requiring collaboration among multiple disciplines and an interdisciplinary (at the least) or transdisciplinary approach (at best). Psychologists, psychiatrists, social workers, and medical personnel often collaborate in many organizations focused on trauma. However, the speech-language clinician, scholar, and educator are often absent from those conversations and collaborations, but we *must* be present. Communication is an essential ingredient in the success of post-traumatic intervention and resilience.

In this text, the writings of 15 authors from various disciplines and expertise have been curated across 11 chapters. These authors are from speech-language-hearing sciences, counseling, education, occupational therapy, psychology, and social work. In their chapters, each author speaks to the impact that post-traumatic stress can have on communication, language, or literacy and provides information on the latest assessment and intervention approaches to support children, adolescents, and adults experiencing post-traumatic stress or post-traumatic stress disorder. This text will be a steady companion for supporting the communication, language, and literacy of those who have experienced or are experiencing post-traumatic stress.

Note

1 https://www.who.int/news-room/fact-sheets/detail/violence-against-children#:
~:text=Globally%2C%20it%20is%20estimated%20that,lifelong%20health%20
and%20well%2Dbeing.

1 Introduction to Language Research in Post-Traumatic Stress[1]

Yvette D. Hyter[2]

1.1 "Gabe"

September 3rd, Gabe's 10th birthday, was the height of his week. There had been no screaming or crying in his house, and most importantly, his mom's boyfriend didn't hit her or him. Gabe went to bed feeling hopeful that this night would be different than the rest, but as usual, he couldn't sleep. He never slept soundly; he spent his nights mostly listening to what was happening outside of his room. In his half-sleep state, he heard sirens, and his heart started racing and beating harder and harder. Then came the heavy footsteps of the police coming into his house. From his bedroom, Gabe then heard what sounded like screaming, crying, and muffled voices, and finally, the pop of a gun. He knew that sound all too well because his mom's boyfriend often shot his gun in the backyard at night. (Once, the boyfriend shot the gun in the house, and the bullet just missed Gabe's mother but didn't hit her, thankfully.) Gabe's breathing was heavy, but he tried to breathe quieter but couldn't. Gabe hears his mom crying now, louder than he had ever heard. He ran, without thinking, he ran as fast as he could. He ran past his mom's boyfriend on the floor, through all the blood on the floor, past his mom, past the policemen, and out of the policeman's grasp. It was as if Gabe had the speed and strength that far surpassed his typical physical capabilities, and then he felt that hot searing pain of a bullet going through his leg. When in the hospital later, the police asked him what happened in his house, Gabe remembered the emotions, the fear, the running, and the bullet, but could not remember all of the details that led up to him getting shot by the police.

1.2 Post-Traumatic Stress

Post-traumatic stress (PTS) and post-traumatic stress disorder (PTSD) are public health threats, contributing to the "global disease burden" as they

DOI: 10.4324/9781003225270-1

affect billions of people around the world (Hoppen & Morina, 2019, p. 2). PTS may result from myriad direct and indirect causes including, but not limited to, maltreatment (i.e., abuse and neglect), community violence, racialized violence, forcible displacement, medical trauma, and the experience of war. At the time of this writing, it is estimated that only within the last year, 1 billion children in the world have experienced maltreatment (WHO, 2022) and over 400 million children are suffering from the consequences of war (UNICEF, 2023).

Post-traumatic stress affects the brain and is caused by exposure to a traumatic event or events (APA, 2013), resulting in extreme fear, helplessness, or overwhelm (van der Kolk, 2015; Yehuda, 2016). Post-traumatic stress caused by a range of experiences can result in emotional, cognitive, mental, neurological, and physiological responses mediated by cultural experiences (Chiao et al., 2010; Harris, 2018; Westby, 2018). The impact of post-traumatic stress on these systems can have consequences for all areas of child and adolescent development, academic success, and adult functioning. For people experiencing post-traumatic stress disorder, their bodies remember and react to the trauma(s) (Harris, 2018; van der Kolk, 2015). This reaction, or stress response, may manifest as fight (confronting), flight (running away), freeze (becoming motionless), appease (placating others), and/or dissociative (disconnecting) behaviors (Haines, 2019). These trauma responses can affect a person's ability to learn, pay attention, inhibit responses, remember events about one's life, and recount stories for example.

Post-traumatic stress often causes compromised functioning across all areas of development, impeding opportunities for successful participation in schooling and activities of daily living. According to the DSM-5, PTSD requires exposure to a "traumatic or stressful event" that results in:

a re-experiencing symptoms (e.g., intrusive symptoms such as unwanted memories, nightmares, or flashbacks),
b avoidance (e.g., avoiding the location of where the traumatic experience took place),
c negative thoughts (e.g., negative thoughts about oneself or the world; difficulty remembering some parts of the traumatic experience), and
d trauma-related arousal (e.g., risky behavior, hypervigilance, heightened startle reaction). These symptoms must last for more than one month; must impact functioning; and cannot be due to medication, substances, or another illness (US Department of Veteran's Affairs, 2023).

PTSD is differentiated from post-traumatic stress (PTS) in the literature. Post-traumatic stress is our body's *typical* response to stress – it activates the body's stress response of fight, flight, or freeze. PTS may cause our heart to race, and our hands to become sweaty; we may feel anxious or have bad dreams about the experience(s). We also may have difficulty recalling all the details about the event or experience. Often, PTS symptoms will improve on their own within one month or so, unlike the symptoms of PTSD. Gabe, the child described at the beginning of this chapter, may be experiencing PTS but due to the consistent nature of his traumatic experiences, he may also develop PTSD.

1.3   Introducing Language Research in Post-Traumatic Stress

Due to the many areas of concern associated with post-traumatic stress disorder, professionals in the health and human service and education sectors, like speech-language professionals, occupational therapists, social workers, medical personnel, clinical psychologists, and educators, are often the first to encounter and provide support to people experiencing post-traumatic stress. This text, *Language Research in Post-Traumatic Stress*, is an essential text that includes various perspectives on post-traumatic stress and post-traumatic stress disorder; provides guidance on neurodevelopmental impacts of post-traumatic stress and how post-traumatic stress affects various groups – children, adolescents, adults, refugees, and victims of racialized violence; provides current research on the relationships between post-traumatic stress and language functioning, autobiographical memory, and cultural neuroscience; and provides guidance about assessment and intervention.

Speech-language professionals (SLPs), educators, and healthcare workers, counselors, other service professionals are often on the front lines in terms of providing support to individuals with post-traumatic stress and their families. Due to the impact of post-traumatic stress on cognitive skills and social pragmatic communication, individuals with post-traumatic stress are often referred to speech-language professionals (SLPs) for assessments and services (Hyter, 2012, 2020; Hyter et al., 2003; Westby, 2007; Yehuda, 2016). Although SLPs are one of the first groups that support individuals and families with post-traumatic stress, the extant speech-language literature about the scope of post-traumatic stress, its effect on various linguistic and communication systems, and discussions about the most effective assessment and intervention practices are significantly limited in SLP literature. This dearth of information on how to effectively assess and intervene with individuals and families with trauma histories is the primary motivation for this text.

The aims of the book are to:

1 Define post-traumatic stress, explain its various causes, and how these causes can be mitigated and/or eliminated.

2 Explain the wide-ranging effects that traumatic stress has on one's communication, language, and literacy development, incorporating information on the whole being (e.g., biological, psychological, social, and educational effects).
3 Demonstrate that it is essential for language and literacy professionals to engage in transdisciplinary interprofessional practices to acquire accurate information about an affected person's strengths and challenges and to develop effective supports for such individuals, their families, and communities. In this regard, an aim is to equip SLPs, educators, and other health providers with the knowledge and skills required to understand, assess, and support the growing number of children, adolescents, and adults experiencing post-traumatic stress.
4 Explain the importance of culturally responsive trauma-informed practices.
5 Provide examples of assessments that can provide accurate information about a person's strengths and challenges.
6 Provide examples of interventions with demonstrated evidence for being effective with children, adolescents, and adults affected by post-traumatic stress and provide information about ways to support resiliency.

There are two parts to this text. The first part, *Post-Traumatic Stress: Considerations, Concepts, and Consequences within Language Research*, includes Chapters 2–6 that concentrate on (a) the impact of post-traumatic stress on social groups – communities of color, migrants and refugees, and speakers of multiple languages, and (b) the neurodevelopmental capacities of sensory modulation, emotional regulation, social cognition, executive functions, and pragmatic language.

1.3.1   Part 1: Post-Traumatic Stress: Considerations, Concepts, and Consequences within Language Research

More specifically, in Chapter 2, "Post-traumatic stress, racialized stress, and trauma," Paul Archibald and Lajuana Archibald examine how racialized stress caused by systemic trauma in the form of stereotypes, biases, systemic forms of exclusion, and inequities within the social structures impact people's daily existence. Included in their treatment of this topic is a discussion of the disproportional impact that COVID-19 had (and continues to have) on Black and Brown communities, and the inequities "caused by pervasive racist policies and practices that promote an unequal distribution of social-economic resources" (p. 12) that impact mental health contributing to traumatization. The authors define racism, discuss the relationship between racism and trauma in Black communities, provide support for identifying trauma in Black persons, and identify the societal drivers of racial inequities. The authors end the chapter by providing a list of adverse experience and trauma screeners, and two case studies related to speech and language.

In Chapter 3, "Post-traumatic stress, autobiographical memory, and cultural neuroscience: Implications for migrants and refugees," Carol Westby underscores the relationship between post-traumatic stress and autobiographical memories, the memories that we have about our own lives and histories. Westby addresses post-traumatic stress and autobiographical memory as they converge in migrants and refugees, who are likely to have experienced trauma before they leave their home countries, during their movement across borders, and once settled in a new country. Post-traumatic stress fragments autobiographical memories, which Westby explains has three different levels – knowledge of "lifetime periods, general events, and event-specific knowledge" (p. 42). Autobiographical memory is of significance because it helps one process their experiences and contributes to resilience and healing.

Yvette D. Hyter focuses on the impact that trauma has on the interactive and cognitive underpinnings of communication in Chapter 4, "Post-traumatic Stress and Social Pragmatic Communication." In this chapter, Hyter uses a conceptual cognitive model (Hyter, 2012, 2017) to explain the impact that toxic stress has on the brain and components of social pragmatic communication. These components include social cognition, such as Theory of Mind and perspective taking; cognitive skills such as executive functions and memory; and pragmatic language (discourse management, presupposition skills, and communicative functions).

Michelle Suarez and Cara Masselink address the "cost" of post-traumatic stress on children in Chapter 5, "Neurodevelopmental Impact of Post-Traumatic Stress." They focus on the effects of post-traumatic stress on the brain, sensory modulation, and emotional regulation in children. Suarez and Masselink begin with a discussion of the impact that trauma has on the brain and then discuss the impact on sensory and emotional regulation and executive functions. Included in the chapter is information on assessment and intervention options for supporting sensory processing and regulation.

In Chapter 6, "Impact of Post-Traumatic Stress on Cognitive-Communication in Multilingual Children and Adult," Sulare Telford Rose and Jennifer Myers discuss the impact of trauma on cognitive communication abilities of children and adults who are multilingual. Telford Rose and Myers address the impact of PTS on multilingualism, which can cause delays in one's first or second language. They also include a discussion of the importance of supporting translanguaging and understanding raciolinguistics with working with immigrants and refugees, deaf and hard of hearing populations, and African American language speakers. The authors provide some guidelines for trauma-informed care when engaged in practice/collaboration with multilingual individuals and introduce their multilingual UPLIFT approach to trauma-informed care.

1.3.2   *Part 2: Post-Traumatic Stress: Considerations across the Lifespan for Language and Communication*

The second part of the text, *Post-traumatic stress: Considerations across the lifespan for language and communication*, includes Chapters 7–10. Chapter 7, "Post-traumatic stress: Child language development and functioning," written by Na'ama Yehuda, focuses on the ways that trauma impacts language development and production. Yehuda begins the chapter by defining communication, describing how language development and learning occurs, and the ways that trauma disrupts language meaning and structure. She ends the chapter by providing assessment and intervention suggestions.

Ginger G. Collins, Jayna Mumbauer-Pisano, and Tobias Kroll in Chapter 8, "Addressing the impact of post-traumatic stress on adolescent language and identity: An interdisciplinary approach," explain the impact that trauma exposure has on adolescent language and identity development. After providing some demographics about the number of adolescents that experience trauma in a year and explaining the cognitive and language development in adolescents, they discuss the impact that trauma has on adolescent development. They state that "unfortunately more than any other developmental stage, adolescence is associated with increased risk of trauma exposure, which often disrupts identity development" (p. 185). They end the chapter by presenting some trauma-informed approaches to supporting adolescents with trauma histories, and a case study that exemplifies the issues addressed in the chapter.

In Chapter 9, "Post-traumatic stress and attachment-based narrative speech styles in adults," Karin Riber and Emma Beck write about how attachment theory explains the characteristics of complex post-traumatic stress disorder, and how these characteristics show up in the narratives of adults with trauma histories. Two case studies are provided illustrating how trauma impacted these adults' narrative production and functioning. The authors end with an explanation of a mentalization-based approach, which has implications for communicating with adults who have complex trauma.

Linda Carozza focuses on the impact of post-traumatic stress on veterans and other vulnerable people in Chapter 10, "PTSD and cognitive communication effects." In this chapter, Carozza discusses the needs of adults with PTSD and includes suggested assessment and intervention strategies.

Carozza includes current research on interventions that can mitigate the effects of PTSD.

The final chapter of the text, Chapter 11, "Conclusions and unanswered questions," by Yvette D. Hyter is a summary of the findings presented in each chapter and reviews the remaining questions posed by the authors to develop a research agenda and outline a plan that can be used not only to support individuals with post-traumatic stress but also to begin to think of ways to eliminate it.

Notes

1 At Language & Literacy Practices, LLC in Kalamazoo, Michigan in Kalamazoo.
2 The name of this child and some of the circumstances have been changed to protect their identity.

References

American Psychiatric Association (2013). *Diagnostic and statistical manual of mental disorders* (5th ed.). Retrieved from https://dsm.psychiatryonline.org/doi/book/10.1176/appi.books.9780890425596

Chiao, J. Y., Hariri, A. R., Haradam, T., Mano, Y., Sadato, N., Parrish, T. B., & Lidaka, T. (2010). Theory and methods in cultural neuroscience. *Social Cognitive and Affective Neuroscience, 5*(2), 356–361. Retrieved from https://academic.oup.com/scan/article/5/2-3/356/1665044

Haines, S. K. (2019). *The politics of trauma: Somatics, healing and social justice.* North Atlantic Books.

Harris, N. B. (2018). *The deepest well: Healing the long-term effects of childhood adversity.* Boston, MD: Houghton Mifflin Harcourt.

Hoppen, T., & Morina, N. (2019). The prevalence of PTSD and major depression in the global population of adult war survivors: A meta-analytically informed estimate in absolute numbers. *European Journal of Psychotraumatology, 10,* 1578637. https://doi.org/10.1080/20008198.2019.1578637

Hyter, Y. D. (2012). Complex trauma and prenatal alcohol exposure: Clinical implications. *Perspectives of the ASHA Special Interest Groups, 13*(2), 32–42. https://doi.org/10.1044/sbi13.2.32

Hyter, Y. D. (2017). Pragmatic assessment and intervention in children. In L. Cummings (Ed.), *Research in clinical pragmatics* (pp. 493–526). Springer International.

Hyter, Y. D. (2020). Language, social pragmatic communication, and childhood trauma. In D. Scott (Ed.), *Cases on communication disorders in culturally diverse populations* (pp. 54–88). Hershey, PA: IGI Publisher.

Hyter, Y. D., Henry, J., Atchison, B., Sloane, M., Black-Pond, C., & Shangraw, K. (2003, November 1). Children affected by trauma and alcohol exposure. *The ASHA Leader, 8*(21), https://doi.org/10/1044/leader.FTR2.08212003.6

UNICEF (2023). *Children in war and conflict*. Retrieved from https://www.unicefusa. org/what-unicef-does/emergency-response/conflict#:~:text=Over%20400 %20million%20children%20live,separated%20from%20parents%20and%20 caregivers

US Department of Veteran's Affairs (2023). PTSD: *National center for PTSD*. Retrieved from https://www.ptsd.va.gov/professional/treat/essentials/dsm5_ptsd. asp

van der Kolk, B. (2015). *The body keeps the score: Brain, mind, and body in the healing of trauma*. New York: Penguin Books.

Westby, C. E. (2007). Child maltreatment: A global issue. *Language, Speech and Hearing Services in Schools, 38*(2), 140–148. https://doi.org/10.1044/ 0161-1461(2007/014

Westby, C. E. (2018). Adverse childhood experiences: What speech-language pathologists need to know. *Word of Mouth, 30*(1), 1–4. Retrieved from https:// journals.sagepub.com/doi/full/10.1177/1048395018796520

World Health Organization (2022, November 29). *Violence against children*. Retrieved from https://www.who.int/news-room/fact-sheets/detail/violence-against-children#:~:text=Globally%2C%20it%20is%20estimated%20that, the%20past%20year%20(1)

Yehuda, N. (2016). *Communicating trauma: Clinical presentations and interventions with traumatized children*. New York: Routledge.

Part I

Post-Traumatic Stress

Considerations, Concepts,
and Consequences within
Language Research

2 Racialized Stress and Trauma in Black Communities

Lessons for Speech and Language Professionals

Paul Archibald and Lajuana Archibald

2.1 Introduction

The need to understand racialized stress and trauma in Black communities has become more evident as we have been forced to face the *super-pandemic* caused by the collision of the coronavirus disease 2019 (COVID-19) and structural racism. Horesh and Brown (2020) contend that although a large proportion of persons exposed to COVID-19 stress and effects will possess resiliency to its effects, there will be a proportion of those who are more susceptible to symptoms related to post-traumatic stress disorder (PTSD). Some of those most at risk for exposure to PTSD may be those who fall into the high-risk category for more adverse effects of COVID-19 and experience racism (Archibald, 2021; Holden et al., 2022). Research suggests that the disproportionate health effects of COVID-19 in non-Hispanic Black children have mirrored the patterns observed in non-Hispanic Black adults and are influenced by racism. For instance, non-Hispanic Black children reportedly had lower rates of COVID-19 testing, were significantly more likely to be infected by COVID-19, and were more likely to be hospitalized for symptoms related to COVID-19 (Bailey et al., 2021). Simultaneously, research has revealed the impact of trauma on non-Hispanic Black children (Pumariega et al., 2022). Non-Hispanic Black children tend to experience more adverse events than non-Hispanic White children (Maguire-Jack et al., 2020). This includes greater exposure to multiple types of violence during their lifetime (López et al., 2017). When reviewing the trajectories of post-traumatic stress following natural disasters, Lai and colleagues (2021) provided evidence indicating prolonged adverse mental health effects of post-traumatic stress symptoms among non-Hispanic Black children. In addition, as we are grappling with the increase in school shootings, a study reported that non-Hispanic Black children aged 2–17 experienced greater symptoms of anxiety and worry after sniper shootings when compared to their non-Hispanic White counterparts (Becker-Blease et al., 2008).

DOI: 10.4324/9781003225270-3

This brief overview of the prevalence and impact of COVID-19 stress and trauma on non-Hispanic Black children provides the backdrop of the critical nature of investigating and understanding ways to prevent the exacerbation of these occurrences when providing speech-language services. It is evident that the COVID-19 pandemic unearthed the deep-rooted and unsurprising inequities in the United States. The inequities are caused by pervasive racist policies and practices that promote an unequal distribution of socioeconomic resources (e.g., education, employment, income, housing, and residential neighborhood) and ultimately power among communities based on race, place, gender, socioeconomic status, and other factors. The American Speech-Language-Hearing Association (ASHA, 2020) developed a Position Statement that stated:

> ASHA explicitly condemns systemic racism and oppression, and the violent acts that took the lives most recently of Ahmaud Arbery, Breonna Taylor, and George Floyd—and so many before them. We support our Black audiologists, speech-language pathologists, related professionals, and students, as well as Black clients/patients/students and their families. We stand with these individuals in supporting their communities, protecting their families, and fighting for their children's opportunities. We stand with our members who are distressed, saddened, angry, and calling for change. We commit to rooting out the systemic inequities that exist in our communities—within our professions, our schools and universities, and workplaces. Most ASHA members provide services in education and health care settings, institutions with pervasive histories of systemic racial discrimination in the United States. This is a time for evaluating our individual and collective contributions to maintaining the status quo and our responsibility to change it. We must identify meaningful solutions that address the challenges facing Black people to enable every person to be heard, to feel safe, and to thrive.
>
> (Paragraphs 1–2)

This Position Statement demonstrates an understanding that the speech-language profession is not outside of racialized social systems; especially when working with Black children. ASHA (2020) stated that they envision a future where "inclusive policies and practices are in place within the Association and throughout the discipline, to ensure that there is a diversity of perspective that informs professional practice and decision-making." This includes "increasing the diversity of the membership and increasing members' cultural competence" (ASHA, 2020). Therefore, when working with Black children, speech-language professional services must consider the racialized social system that determines the conditions and circumstances in which Black children are born, grow up, live, work and age (Bonilla-Silva, 1997; WHO, 2019).

This chapter will describe how racialized inequities inherent in the United States are not solely a political or social issue but impact mental health, specifically, trauma symptomatology. We use Bonilla-Silva's (1997) framework of racialized systems to provide some explanations for the disproportionate stress and trauma in Black communities that ultimately impacts the non-Hispanic Black children that speech-language professionals encounter. Two case examples will be presented to illustrate the impact of the racialized social system on speech-language assessment and treatment among Black children and their families and speech-language professionals. We will provide a roadmap for the development of a trauma-responsive and healing-centered processes when working with Black children and their families. We provoke a call to service for speech-language professionals to develop a culturally relevant trauma-responsive and healing-centered approach to their service delivery. This approach *realizes* that trauma in Black communities is pervasive, and healing is obtainable; *recognizes* the signs and symptoms in Black children; *responds* by fully integrating knowledge about historical and contemporary racial trauma into speech and language policies, procedures, and practices; and *resists re-traumatizing* Black children and their families.

2.2   Historical Context of Racism in the Stress and Trauma Profile of Black People

2.2.1 *Racism Conceptualized*

There are numerous conceptualizations of racism in the literature. However, race is not rooted in biology but is a sociopolitical, economic, and cultural construct that has developed through time and context (Barrett and Roediger, 2012). In Ta-Nehisi Coates' book, *Between the World and Me*, he writes in the form of a letter from a father to a son and coined the phrase "race is the child of racism, not the father" (p. 7). In this context, if race is the child and not the father, then race was birthed from racism. In developing a biopsychosocial model of racism, Clark and colleagues (1999) identified that these conceptualizations could be cataloged into two categories: attitudinal or behavioral. Attitudinal racism refers to attitudes and beliefs that are held about a group of people while behavioral racism is the action taken to block a group of people from equal and equitable access to resources. All of these are based on the phenotypic characteristics or ethnic affiliation of the targeted group. Echoing the premise of that conceptualization, racism is also understood through Ostrom's (1969) adapted socio-psychological ABC model of attitude and behavior. The ABC model of attitudinal and behavioral racism proposes three components that are manifested by the racist perpetrator on the targeted group based on their ethnic affiliation or phenotypic characteristics. A represents the *affective* component, which is prejudicial feelings toward a group of people. B is the *behavioral* component, representing the discriminatory acts toward a group of people. C encompasses the *cognitive* component, incorporating the stereotypes or beliefs about a group of people. Stereotypes (C – cognition) rationalize prejudice (A – beliefs) leading to discrimination (B – behavior) (Dovidio and Gaertner, 1996). However, Bonilla-Silva (1997) argued that racism should be viewed beyond an ideology and more in terms of racialized social systems that are hierarchically structured and based on racial categories that are socially constructed to benefit one group over another. This racialization framework takes into consideration the initial or historical social formation and intent of the racial categories that inform the contemporary racial hierarchical structure. Racial phenomena such as stereotypes, prejudices, and discrimination then become crystalized over the course of social systems' existence producing racial inequities—that ultimately affect health outcomes. Several theoretical frameworks and studies have been developed to explain the effects of racialized systems on health among Black adults. Gabbidon and Peterson (2006) coined the *living while black* phenomenon, which posits that the social cost of being Black in the United States influences health status. Geronimus and colleagues (2006) theorized the *weathering hypothesis* which states that Black adults' exposure to socioeconomic and sociodemographic inequalities and racism subjects them to a higher allostatic load—defined as the accumulated physiological burden of adaptation to chronic stress (McEwen, 1998).

2.2.2 Tracing Racism's Relationship with Stress and Trauma in the Black Population

The United States Black population's racialized stress and trauma can be traced back to the *middle passage*, the human trafficking transport from Africa to the New World. This continued through what was called the *seasoning process*, named by the white plantation owners as the initiation into the New World slavery (Buxton, 1840). It has been estimated that approximately 12.5 percent of slaves died in the middle passage, 4.5 percent died on the shore while waiting to be sold, and one-third died during the seasoning process while attempting to adjust to the New World. This accounted for an average mortality rate of 50 percent (Klein et al., 2001). Legalized slavery in the United States officially lasted from 1619 to 1865, nearly 250 years, and with it a system of oppression, marginalization, and suffering. Keep in mind that although slavery was abolished in 1865, there was one exception that still exists today: "Neither slavery nor involuntary servitude, except as a punishment for crime whereof the party shall have been duly convicted, shall exist within the United States, or any place subject to their jurisdiction" (United States Constitution, Amendment XIII, Section 1). Also, human trafficking, where men, women, and children are enslaved into labor and commercial sexual exploitation, is considered modern-day slavery in the United States (Clawson et al., 2009).

Unfortunately, this system of oppression and marginalization that was birthed in slavery was continued for another 100 years under the Jim Crow Laws which legalized discrimination and then lingered 40 plus years during the integration/desegregation process. The traumatic impact of enslavement, Jim Crow, and integration/desegregation have been shown to persist across generations with long-lasting effects that permeate in the lives of Black people living in the United States (Akbar, 1996). Recent discoveries in the field of epigenetics have demonstrated that the effects of trauma can be transferred on a molecular level from one generation to the next (Westby, this volume; Yehuda et al., 2016). However, Crawford and colleagues (2003) argue that the traumatic effects of slavery are a much more complex trauma mechanism that can also be transmitted via social levels within the family, community, and society.

2.2.3   Recognizing the Signs and Symptoms of Trauma in Black Adults

The trauma symptomatology that stems from the traumatic effects of slavery and the post-slavery events seem to be associated with what is termed "*racial trauma*." Racial trauma is the emotional or psychological injury sustained in response to an experience of a direct or indirect racist event (Pieterse, 2018). Racial trauma is also cumulative and occurs in individuals who share a specific group identity and affiliation such as a nationality, religious affiliation, or ethnicity. It can affect those who have never experienced the traumatic event. The children and descendants exhibit signs and symptoms of trauma. In this context, racial trauma becomes an intergenerational or historical trauma that produces long-term distress among communities (Evans-Campbell, 2008). Due to its poor scientific understanding, the legitimacy of the clinical diagnosis of racial trauma is not widely accepted (Williams et al., 2019). People seem to be more ready to accept the effects of racial trauma based on work that originated in the 1960s to explain the collective distress described by some of the Jewish Holocaust survivors, termed, "*survivor syndrome*." (Sadavoy, 1997). They identified that they presented with the following symptoms: denial, depersonalization, isolation, somatization, memory loss, agitation, anxiety, guilt, depression, intrusive thoughts, nightmares, psychic numbing, and survivor guilt.

Dr. Degruy (2005), in her theory of Post-Traumatic Slave Syndrome (PTSS), identifies several ways that racial trauma manifests. One is *vacant esteem*, where an individual may experience insufficient development in multiple domains along with feelings of hopelessness, depression, and a general self-destructive outlook. Second is *marked propensity for anger and violence*, where an individual may experience extreme feelings of suspicion and perceived negative motivations of others. This is also where an individual engages in violence against self, property, and others. Third is *racist socialization and internalized racism*, where an individual engages in learned helplessness, literacy deprivation, distorted self-concept, and antipathy or aversion for the following: (1) members of one's own identified cultural/ethnic group; (2) mores and customs associated with one's own identified cultural/ethnic heritage; and (3) physical characteristics of one's own identified cultural/ethnic group.

Racial trauma may also be expressed as follows:

1   The exposed individual may present with intrusion symptoms where the traumatic event is persistently re-experienced by unwanted upsetting memories, nightmares, flashbacks, emotional distress after exposure to traumatic reminders, and physical reactivity after exposure to traumatic reminders. This may occur when an individual starts to experience persistent nightmares about some of the events of historical or contemporary racial violence (e.g., lynching, police brutality, separation from family).

2   The exposed individual may experience avoidance symptoms where an individual avoids trauma-related thoughts or feelings or trauma-related external reminders. This may occur when an individual avoids places that adorn the confederate flag because it is a trauma-related stimulus associated with lynching or avoids malls and stores because of racial profiling.

3   The exposed individual may experience negative thoughts or feelings that are exacerbated by the trauma, where an individual may not be able to recall key features of the trauma; has overly negative thoughts and assumptions about self or the world; engages in exaggerated blame of self or others for causing the trauma; presents with negative affect, decreased interest in activities, feelings of isolation; and has difficulties experiencing positive affect. This may occur in Black communities where an individual has negative thoughts about having origins in Africa.

4   The exposed individual may experience alterations in arousal and reactivity where an individual is frequently irritable or aggressive, engages in risky or destructive behavior, is hypervigilant, has a heightened startle

reaction, has difficulty concentrating, and has difficulty sleeping. This may occur when an individual is aggressive toward their own community members who they subconsciously blame for not addressing the trauma.

The symptoms of racial trauma are similar to PTSD described in the Diagnostic and Statistical Manual of Mental Disorders, 5th Edition (DSM-5) for PTSD (American Psychiatric Association, 2013), although it also has very unique presentations. PTSD is a mental illness included as one of the trauma- and stressor-related disorders in the DSM-5 and is characterized by symptoms of intrusion, avoidance, negative alterations in cognition and mood, and changes in arousal and reactivity after direct or indirect exposure to a traumatic event. Racial trauma is characterized by similar symptoms. However, it occurs after ongoing individual and collective exposure and re-exposure to real, perceived, or vicarious racial stereotypes, prejudices, discrimination, and violence coupled with the denial of these harms by societies (Comas-Diaz et al., 2019).

Williams and her colleagues (2018a) at the University of Connecticut have provided a good argument for the inclusion of racial trauma in the Criterion A events of PTSD in the DSM-5. Currently, Criterion A in the DSM-5 limits a traumatic event to direct exposure, witnessing exposure, indirect exposure by learning that a relative or close friend was exposed to a trauma or vicarious trauma exposure during the course of work duties related to death, threatened death, actual or threatened serious injury, or actual or threatened sexual violence (American Psychiatric Association, 2013). However, Williams and her colleagues (2018b) propose that one may use the International Classification of Diseases 10th Edition (ICD-10) criteria to generate a PTSD diagnosis for persons exposed to racial trauma since it is not as restrictive as the DSM-5. The DSM-5 requires that the trauma exposure must be experienced by an individual in the following ways: (1) directly experiences the traumatic event; (2) witnesses the traumatic event in person; (3) learns that the traumatic event occurred to a close family member or close friend (with the actual or threatened death being either violent or accidental); or experiences first-hand repeated or extreme exposure to aversive details of the traumatic event (not through media, pictures, television, or movies unless work-related; American Psychiatric Association, 2013). This limits the scope by which most racial trauma exposures can be captured during a clinical assessment. However, the ICD-10 does not impose those limitations (see comparisons in Table 2.1). The ICD-10 simply requires that there is a delayed or protracted response to an acute or chronic stressful event or situation that is deemed threatening or catastrophic and has the potential to cause long-term distress in most individuals (World Health Organization, 1993).

Table 2.1 PTSD Criteria in DSM-5 and ICD-10

DSM-5 criteria	Symptoms required	ICD-10 criteria	Symptoms required

A Exposure to actual or threatened death, serious injury, or sexual violence
B Persistent re-experiencing
C Persistent avoidance
D Persistent numbing
E Persistent hyperarousal
F Duration of at least 1 month
G Clinically significant distress/impairment
H Not attributable to effects of substances or medications
	1 of 4
	1 of 5
	1 of 2
	2 of 7
	2 of 6
		A Exposure to a stressful event or situation of exceptionally threatening or catastrophic nature likely to cause pervasive distress in almost anyone
		B Persistent re-experiencing
		C Avoidance
		D Either (1) or (2) below:
		
		  1 Inability to recall important aspects of the stressor
		  2 Persistent hyperarousal
		
		E Criteria B, C, and D must all be met within 6 months of the stressful event
			2 of 5

Sources: American Psychiatric Association (2013); World Health Organization (1993).

2.2.4   *The Social, Structural, and Clinical Drivers of Racial Inequities in Stress and Trauma in the Lives of Black People*

The trauma exposure that impacts PTSD symptoms occurs throughout the life course in Black communities (Pearlin et al., 2005). The seminal Adverse Childhood Experiences (ACEs) study found a direct link between childhood trauma and well-being throughout an individual's lifespan (Fellitti et al., 1998). However, the unique historical and contemporary context of Black people in the United States underscores the need to expand the ACEs to include traumatic community and cultural experiences (Degruy, 2005; Cronholm et al., 2015; Dhaliwal, 2015). Thus, when attempting to understand the PTSD disparity in Black communities, exposure to trauma in childhood (e.g., incarcerated family member), community (e.g., crime-ridden neighborhood), and culture (e.g., racism) have been shown to contribute to the higher prevalence and poor outcomes of PTSD in Black people (Degruy, 2005; Cronholm et al., 2015; Dhaliwal, 2015;

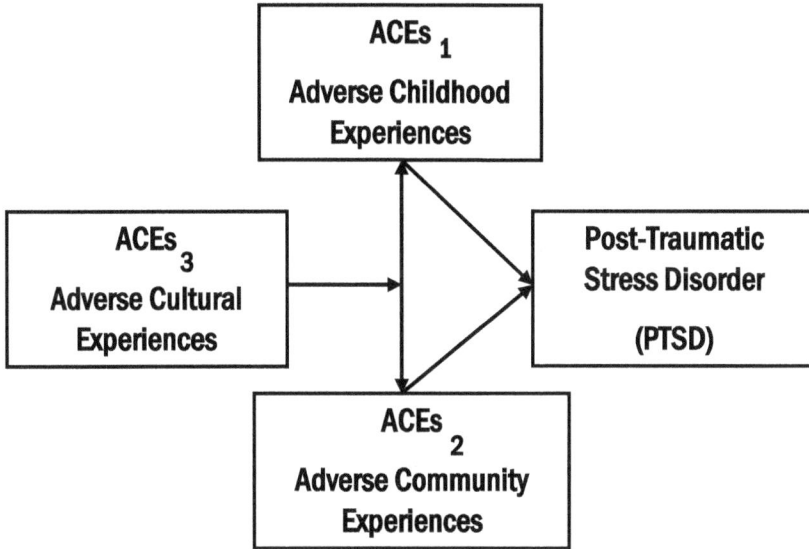

Figure 2.1 Triple ACEs Effect.
Source: Archibald (2021)

Paradies, 2015; Sibraya, 2019). Figure 2.1 depicts a framework coined the *triple ACEs effect* and proposes that the prevalence of PTSD in the Black population extends beyond *adverse childhood experiences* to include *adverse community experiences* and *adverse cultural experiences* linked to PTSD (Paradies, 2015; Berenz et al., 2017; Yousseff, 2017; Archibald, 2021). The adverse cultural experiences affect how Black people experience their childhood and community, ultimately influencing symptoms of PTSD.

Adverse childhood experiences refer to adult memories of traumatic experiences that occurred in a person's life prior to age 18 (Fellitti et al., 1998). They include exposure to physical, emotional, or sexual abuse, domestic violence toward a parent, behavioral health issue of a household member, incarceration of a household member, divorce or separation of a parent, and lack of basic necessities. Slopen and colleagues (2016) found that Black children were exposed to greater adverse childhood experiences than their White counterparts. *Adverse community experiences* refer to the systemic inequities that are present in a person's community (Pinder-hughes et al., 2015). Examples include lack of affordable and safe housing, segregated neighborhoods, community violence, and unkempt built environment. Black neighborhoods caused by residential racial segregation are plagued with increased poverty and higher community violence (Logan and Oakley, 2017; Santilli et al., 2017).

Adverse cultural experiences are defined as chronic exposures to historical and contemporary systemic racial injustices (i.e., racism, discrimination, racial microaggressions) targeted to a specific ethnic group. For instance, in this racialized social system, racism is disproportionately experienced by Black adults. Lee and colleagues (2019) replicated Boutwell and colleagues' (2017) study examining the prevalence of racism in the United States and found a larger difference from their estimates. Boutwell and colleagues (2017) estimated that the racism prevalence rate was 31.88 percent for Blacks and 23.53 for whites. However, Lee and colleagues (2019) found a range of 69.45 percent and 73.62 percent for Blacks and 29.61 percent and 34.48 percent for whites were more accurate estimates. This is important because research has shown that Black people experienced significantly more episodes of discrimination associated with PTSD (Chou et al., 2012). That would mean that the differential experiences of racism among Black adults when compared to other ethnic groups may provide some explanations for the etiology of PTSD among the Black population. Among a sample of 806 participants living in low-income predominantly Black neighborhoods, any person who reported experiencing any discrimination was significantly more likely to meet the criteria for PTSD (Brooks et al., 2020). Sibrava and colleagues (2019) found that in their sample of Black people, PTSD remission rate over five years of follow-up was 0.35, and it was significantly associated with the reported frequency of experiences with discrimination. Paradies and colleagues (2015) evaluated data from 293 studies published between 1983 and 2013 and found an extensive association of self-reported racism with negative mental health outcomes. More than twenty percent of the studies reported an association with psychological distress and 4.8% with PTSD. Negative mental health outcomes had the largest mean-weighted effect size when compared to positive mental health, physical health, and general health, with PTSD demonstrating the largest effect size.

2.3   Screening Tools for Triple ACEs Effect

A successful speech-language treatment process that is trauma responsive using cultural lens includes an assessment of the risks that serve as recovery challenges to their Black students, such as exposure to racism. We propose starting with integrating the Substance Abuse and Mental Health Services Administration's (2014) six key principles of trauma-informed approach into the speech-language treatment process. Table 2.2 provides a sample of how the trauma-informed approach could be included in the speech-language service delivery model and co-designed with students and

Table 2.2 Trauma-Responsive Approach to Speech-Language Service Delivery

Trauma-informed care principles	Description	Application to speech-language service delivery
Safety	Having the structure in place ensures physical, psychological, social, moral/spiritual, and cultural safety in the environment and allows for children who are different than you to feel included and protected within the understanding of their historical and current experiences.	Codesign the speech-language process with children and their families allowing them to define safety and determine if it is achieved.
Trustworthiness and Transparency	Make authenticity a characteristic valued highly within the environment. Do this by recognizing the influence of own background on responses to cultural differences while maintaining confidentiality.	All discussions and decisions about children and their families are made in their presence using regular, open, honest, and direct communications.
Peer support	Create an environment that allows for children with lived experiences to support and connect with each other in large and small group settings. This includes images that look like them who are available to model self-care through their personal practices.	Included in the speech-language agenda should be time for children and their families with similar lived experiences to connect and provide support to each other.
Collaboration and mutuality	Hiring a culturally diverse staff that reflects the children and the families being served. Make sure to conduct trainings and have signage and instructional literature in cultural language and norms of children and the families being served.	During the speech-language treatment process, children and their families set and determine when collaboration and mutuality goals are met.
Empowerment, voice, and choice	Children and their families that are served are given an opportunity and empowered to tell their stories in their own words, understanding that they bring value and wisdom to the environment.	Children and their families are fully integrated into their speech-language intervention process and given a voice for self-advocacy.

(*Continued*)

Table 2.2 (Continued)

Trauma-informed care principles	Description	Application to speech-language service delivery
Cultural, historical, intergenerational, and gender issues	Room is made for the expression of practices in ways that honor the unique cultural, historical, intergenerational, and gender backgrounds of the children and families served.	Speech-language professional recognizes the unique historical, cultural, intergenerational, and gender issues sometimes bound up with trauma that may affect the speech-language treatment process.

Source: Adapted from Substance Abuse and Mental Health Services Administration (2014).

their families. The first principle, *safety*, requires that speech-language professionals (SLPs) collaborate with students and their families. During this co-designing process, students and their families are empowered to define what physical, psychological, social, moral/spiritual, and cultural safety is and how it can be achieved and maintained.

The second principle, *trustworthiness and transparency*, encourages SLPs to value highly an authentic character that recognizes the influences of their own background on responses to cultural differences. If achieved, the speech-language treatment becomes a process where the SLP is comfortable with making all decisions and communications about students and their families in their presence. The third principle, *peer support*, promotes a way for students and their families who share common experiences, engage each other during the speech-language treatment process, build relationships, and share strengths and support. It must be noted here that the SLP allows authentic relationships to be formed among students and their families with similar racial backgrounds, and shared experiences are explored and not assumed. The fourth principle, *collaboration and mutuality*, is the main ingredient of the codesign process for this trauma-informed speech-language treatment process. Having a collaborative process allows students and their families to partner with SLPs to level out the power dynamics that oftentimes plague the speech-language treatment process. Trauma and hurt occur in relationships that do not allow for shared power and decision-making. Healing and resilience become possible in relationships that allow for meaningful shared power and decision-making. The fifth principle, *empowerment, voice, and choice*, creates an atmosphere where the strengths and individual experiences of students and their families are recognized and used as a springboard for their speech-language treatment success.

The sixth principle, *cultural, historical, intergenerational, and gender issues*, focuses the SLP on addressing any historical or contemporary cultural or gender stereotypes and biases. This is the area where the SLP recognizes the multiple exposures of historical and contemporary racialized experiences in the lives of Black students and their families. A full integration of this principle creates an easier transition to a culturally relevant, trauma-responsive, and healing-centered speech-language treatment process. This can be done using the 4-part Safety, Emotions, Loss, and Future (SELF) Conversations to encourage Black students and their families to explore their strengths and opportunities for change (Bloom et al., 2010). During the SELF conversations, SLPs discuss how traumatic racial experiences can affect students and their families. In the first conversation, the different types of **Safety** are identified (physical, psychological, social, moral/spiritual, cultural) by allowing students and their families to draw examples from their community and life, listening nonjudgmentally, openly, and empathetically. In the second conversation, **Emotional** responses are discussed and how they tie into speech and language, validating struggles and successes. In the third conversation, personal, general, or community examples of different types of **Losses** that occurred due to traumatic events are discussed, working toward solutions. The fourth conversation allows the students and their families to discuss **Future** goals for their speech and language treatment, self, using humility and self-disclosure to encourage students and their families to share.

Additionally, there are several tools that can assist with screening for the triple ACEs effect (adverse childhood, community, and cultural experiences). We recommend the following screening tools that have been widely used by pediatricians and mental health and public health practitioners.

2.3.1   *Pediatric ACEs and Related Life-Events Screener (PEARLS)*

The Pediatric ACEs and Related Life-events Screener (PEARLS) is a screening tool that was developed to assess ACEs and other social determinants of health events that are considered risk factors for toxic stress among children and adolescents ages 0–19 (Koita et al., 2018). There are three versions of the screening tool that are specific to the participant's age and the person reporting the data: (1) PEARLS child tool, for ages 0–11, to be completed by a parent/caregiver; (2) PEARLS adolescent tool, for ages 12–19, to be completed by a parent/caregiver; and (3) PEARLS for adolescent self-report tool, for ages 12–19, to be completed by the adolescent. Information about this tool can be found at https://www.acesaware.org/learn-about-screening/screening-tools/.

2.3.2   *Primary Care PTSD Screen for DSM-5 (PC-PTSD-5)*

The PC-PTSD-5 is a Five-item screen for symptoms of PTSD (Prins et al., 2015). This screening tool can be adapted to screen for racial trauma by adding a racial trauma example. The measuring tool starts by asking individuals about exposure to trauma: Sometimes, things happen to people that are unusually or especially frightening, horrible, or traumatic. For example:

- a serious accident or fire
- a physical or sexual assault or abuse
- an earthquake or flood
- a war
- seeing someone be killed or seriously injured
- having a loved one die through homicide or suicide.

To screen for racial trauma, you can add an example such as, "being unfairly treated because of your race." If an individual indicates that they have had any lifetime exposure to any of the examples presented, they are instructed to respond to five additional yes/no questions about how that trauma exposure has affected them over the past month.

2.3.3   *Trauma Symptoms Discrimination Scale (TSDS)*

The TSDS was designed to evaluate anxiety-related symptoms of race-based trauma (Williams et al., 2018a). This measure contains 21 items to assess the extent of distress resulting from discriminatory experiences. Rated on a scale from 1 ("never") to 4 ("often"), the total score consists of the sum of the patient's ratings. At the end of each measure, the patient can report the type of discriminatory activity that was experienced (i.e., racial/ethnic, sexual orientation, age, gender, religious, and other).

2.3.5   *UConn Racial/Ethnic Stress and Trauma Survey (UnRESTS)*

The UnRESTS is used to assess racial stress and trauma and help clinicians ask patients difficult questions about their experiences surrounding explicit and obvious racism, vicarious racism experienced by loved ones or by exposure through learning or watching media, and experiences with microaggressions (Williams et al., 2018b). The UnRESTS survey includes questions that can be used to assess the development of ethnoracial identity, a semi-structured interview to probe for a variety of racism-related experiences, and a checklist to determine whether the patient's racial trauma meets DSM-5 criteria.

2.3.6　Community Experiences Questionnaire (CEQ)

A simplified version of the Survey of Exposure to Community Violence, the 25-item Community Experiences Questionnaire (CEQ) measures how often children have been exposed to violence (Schwartz and Proctor, 2000). On a scale from 1 (never) to 4 (lots of times), respondents rate 25 statements to indicate how often they have been exposed to violence. The CEQ has two subscales: the 11-item Exposure Through Victimization Scale ("How many times has somebody hit, punched, or slapped you?"), and the 14-item Witnessing Violence Scale ("How many times have you seen or heard gunshots?"). Researchers calculate Exposure to Community Violence and Exposure Through Victimization scores by averaging respondents' ratings for each subscale.

2.3.7　The Distressed Communities Index (DCI)

The DCI is used to determine an individual's exposure to adverse community and cultural experiences because it provides a measure of economic well-being across communities throughout the United States (https://eig.org/distressed-communities/2022-dci-interactive-map/). It combines seven complementary economic indicators into a single summary statistic that compares a community's standing to its peers. The seven components of the index are: (1) percent of the 25-year-old and older population with a high school diploma or equivalent; (2) percent of habitable housing that is unoccupied; (3) percent of the population aged 25–54 not currently employed; (4) percent of population living under the poverty line; (5) median household income; (6) percent change in the number of jobs available; and (7) percent change in the number of business establishments. Each community's score on the index is equivalent to its percentile rank across all seven measures combined. To calculate the index, each community is ranked on each measure. Then, each community's seven rankings are averaged and weighted equally to create a preliminary score, which is then normalized into a final score that ranges from approaching 0 (most prosperous) to 100 (most distressed).

2.3.8　The Area Deprivation Index (ADI)

The ADI can be used to determine an individual's adverse community experience because it demonstrates the ADI national percentile rankings at the block group level from 1 to 100 (https://www.neighborhoodatlas.medicine.wisc.edu/mapping). The percentiles are constructed by ranking the ADI from low to high for the nation and grouping the block groups/neighborhoods into bins corresponding to each 1% range of the ADI. Group 1 is the lowest ADI and group 100 is the highest ADI. A block group with a ranking of 1 indicates the lowest level of "disadvantage" within the nation and an ADI with a ranking of 100 indicates the highest level of "disadvantage." Similarly, ADIs are also available in deciles from 1 to 10 for each individual state. The state deciles are constructed by ranking the ADI from low to high for each state alone without consideration of national ADIs. Again, group 1 is the lowest ADI (least disadvantaged) and 10 is the highest ADI (most disadvantaged). We present case studies below to demonstrate how the tools that can assist with screening for the triple ACEs effect (adverse childhood, community, and cultural experiences) may be used by SLPs with students and their families.

2.4   Stress- and -Trauma-Related Speech-Language Case Studies

2.4.1   *Case Study 1*

Student A is an 11-year-old Black male attending a 5th grade 12:1:1 class with a classification of Speech and Language Impairment. He receives both counseling and speech and language therapy. According to Student A's primary caretaker (his aunt), he was diagnosed with autism. Student A lived in a housing project in a large urban city in the United States that was identified as a high drug and crime area. Student A's mother experienced substance use disorder (SUD) issues and reportedly did not receive adequate SUD treatment services in the community. Her SUD treatment services were further dampened by COVID-19 pandemic, causing her to move further away from recovery and deeper into relapse. Unfortunately, Student A's mother died of COVID-19. Student A's father had been incarcerated for many years prior to the death of Student A's mother and remained incarcerated at the time of his mother's death. His paternal grandmother attempted to receive custody of him, but she died suddenly (also from COVID-19), causing Student A to live with his aunt and her five other children. Student A's attendance in school and treatment was inconsistent, which affected his progression within his goals. He enjoys drawing and learning about ocean animals. He often shares his drawing with his peers and teachers. He presents with pragmatic language difficulties and difficulty responding to questions presented. Articulation delays, low vocal volume, difficulty processing information, and difficulty answering questions when presented with short stories are evident as well.

At first glance, the SLP would rightfully focus on the speech and language impairment issues. However, this case is riddled with trauma exposures that range from general to racial. If a complete assessment of Student A's case is not completed to include the triple-ACEs trauma exposures (adverse childhood, community, and cultural experiences), the assessment will be incomplete, and speech and language treatment success may be stifled. One can see that there have been some exposures to adverse childhood (e.g., father's incarceration and mothers' substance use), community (e.g., drugs and crime in community), and cultural and racial (e.g., mother's poor SUD treatment, multiple COVID-19 deaths) experiences. Hence, consultation and collaboration with mental health professionals and educators would strengthen the success of this treatment process. Having the family complete the PEARLS to assess for adverse childhood experiences and other social determinants of health events that place Student A at risk for stress and trauma would be a great first step. The family should also complete the CEQ, since they have reported neighborhood exposure to drugs and crime. This could help us determine the level of victimization exposure as well as witnessing violence that may influence progress in treatment. Then using Student A's addresses (when residing with mom, paternal grandmother, and aunt) to determine distressed community and area deprivation indices, which would provide some much-needed information on what resources could be beneficial for Student A and family. The results of the assessment can then be used to codesign an appropriate treatment process with the family. This process recognizes their whole experience and would benefit the progress of the speech and language treatment process.

2.4.2 Case Study 2

Student B is a six-year-old Black 1st grade student who is attending an Integrated Co-Teaching (ICT) classroom with a classification of Speech or Language Impairment. Initially, Student B lived with his mother in a socioeconomically disadvantaged neighborhood and attended a low-performing elementary school. He was frequently targeted by his White teachers for his difficulties in self-regulating his behaviors in response to either internal or external stimuli. They seemingly did not take the time to investigate his living situation. There were more positive experiences with Black teachers. Student B's mother is reportedly diagnosed with a serious mental illness and is not able to care for her son. There have been multiple episodes of

Student B witnessing his mother being racially profiled for her poor emotional regulation, and she was identified as "an angry Black woman" by the professionals who worked with her. Her mental health issues were not realized by the people she encountered. Currently, Student B is residing with his maternal grandmother causing him to transfer to another school. His maternal grandmother reports her struggle with not receiving the resources that she needs to help her grandson and multiple exposures to racial microaggressions that are causing her distress. Reportedly, his attendance and lateness has been poor, negatively impacting his academic progress. Although Student B enjoys speaking to his teachers and peers, talking about his favorite movies, and responding to questions presented, his overall speech intelligibility is very poor, especially at the sentence and conversational level. He presents with several phonological processes including gliding of liquids (i.e., lamp-->wamp), final consonant deletion (i.e., boat-->bow), and consonant cluster reduction (i.e., skip--->kip). In addition, Student B presents with distortions/substitutions (i.e., /ch/--> /sh/, /j/--> /z/) which negatively impact his overall speech intelligibility. Consequently, Student B's ability to encode and decode is limited as he has difficulty with his speech sound productions.

Student B presents with speech and language impairment that requires immediate attention. The SLP assigned to this case would focus their attention on the phonological process and speech needs. However, ignoring the triple-ACEs trauma exposure in this case would dramatically influence the results of the treatment process. From the information provided, Student B is exposed to adverse childhood (i.e., mother with mental health diagnosis), community (i.e., socioeconomically disadvantaged neighborhood, attending low-performing elementary school), and cultural and racial (targeted by his White teachers, witnessing his mother's profiling experiences, maternal grandmother's exposure to racial microaggressions).

To assist Student B and his family with a successful treatment process, we should start with an interprofessional treatment collaboration between SLPs, educators, and mental health professionals and utilize the PEARLS to screen for adverse childhood experiences, other ACEs, and other risk factors for stress and trauma. Due to Student B's age, we would use the PEARLS child tool, for ages 0–11, which would be completed by the maternal grandmother. We also recommend completing the PC-PTSD-5 with Student B's maternal grandmother since she reported her exposure to multiple racial microaggressions. She may also help determine if she recognized any racial trauma exposure to Student B. If there is any indication of lifetime exposure to any of the examples presented and there are affirmative responses to the exposure having a major effect in their lives, the UnRESTS should be administered. The structured interview process of the UnRESTS would help us assess further the racial stress and trauma that may be plaguing this family and influencing the speech and language progress of Student B. We would also use Student B's current address at his maternal grandmother's home as well as his previous address while living with his mother to determine the level of exposure to community distress and deprivation. This process demonstrates to Student B and his family that we are willing to codesign the speech-language treatment process with them. In so doing, we may increase the treatment engagement and overall success of the treatment process.

2.5 Call to Action

We recommend that speech-language professionals use the information in this chapter to inform the development of diversity, equity, inclusion, and belonging (DEIB) initiatives that move away from cultural competency trainings and toward cultural humility trainings. Cultural humility is a life-long self-reflection process for learning about another's culture while simultaneously examining one's own beliefs and cultural identities (Tervalon and Murray-Garcia, 1998). This becomes important because it is not just about increasing levels of diversity, equity, and inclusion, but allowing people to have a sense of belonging. Belonging is more than just feeling included. In a healthy and thriving society, "belonging means that your well-being is considered and your ability to design and give meaning to its structures and institutions is realized" (Powell, 2012, p. 5). Hence, the cultural humility process allows for exposure not only to increased diversity, equity, and inclusion but also to increased sense of belonging for racialized and marginalized people. This allows racialized and marginalized communities to be safe to actively participate in all aspects of society. The support for moving away from cultural competency trainings is rooted in its basic philosophical underpinnings that are counter to the idea of DEIB. For instance, culture, especially one that is not yours, is not something that you can master. What we can instead strive for is an increase in our cultural humility awareness. When SLPs add cultural humility to their treatment approach, sociocultural differences are seen through the lens of the self. This self-first concept emphasizes intersectionality by understanding one's own implicit biases, thereby dismantling the power dynamics in the treatment process. Cultural humility allows SLPs to cultivate self-awareness and self-reflection signifying a willingness to learn to address and dismantle inequitable and unjust policies and practices while increasing equitable intercultural interactions. This is done by the use of less-controlling and less authoritative treatment and communication styles. As SLPs learn to cultivate cultural humility, they will enter into the treatment relationships with students and their families in an open and curious way. It must be noted here that although we have an expectation that SLPS are open and curious about their students and families, we are more interested in their self-directed openness and curiosity. This self-directed openness and curiosity allow SLPs to engage in an ongoing process of examining where there might be shortcomings in their perception about students and their families "race and culture."

This may be accomplished by incorporating the HUMBLE Model as a tool to set DEIB cultural humility benchmarks and gauge progress (Table 2.3):

SLPs can use the H.U.M.B.L.E. model to identify ways to become humbler while continuing to work and collaborate with students and their families. This model allows SLPs to explore their own culture to gain insight into their own perceptions of race and culture and how that translates into racialization, marginalization, and oppression. The following questions can be used, by SLPs, as a guide to increase the cultural humility of the students and families being served:

• Where do I come from?
• What were some of the barriers that were faced when attempting to achieve goals?
• Who were those people who helped me?

Table 2.3 Cultural Humility

Cultural humility
H – Humble about the assumptions made about knowing the world from Black communities' perspective
U – Understand how speech-language profession's background and culture impact speech-language treatment services provided to Black communities
M – Motivate speech-language profession to learn more about the background, culture, health beliefs and practices, as well as the unique points of view of Black families and communities
B – Begin to incorporate knowledge about Black families and communities into speech-language treatment plans
L – Life-long learning commitment to the background, culture, health beliefs and practices, as well as the unique points of view of Black families and communities
E – Emphasize respect and negotiate speech-language treatment plans with Black families and communities.

Source: Adapted from Borkan et al. (2008, p. 364).

What would have happened if I did not receive help from these people?

When did I not receive the help that I needed?

What aspects of my background/family/culture have influenced the SLP that I am today?

2.6   Conclusion

This chapter highlights how racialized inequities impact the mental health of the Black students and families that SLPs encounter, which could ultimately affect speech and language treatment outcomes. The pervasiveness of racism requires that SLPs account for the implications of society's culture of inequity within their treatment practices. To negate the impact of racial trauma leads to a disregard for the experiences of Black students and their families and denies their full humanness. Purposely revising or ignoring the experiences of Black students and their families re-traumatizes them and is contrary to providing a culturally relevant trauma-responsive environment. In this current racialized political climate coupled with the COVID-19 pandemic, it would be incumbent for the ASHA to consider and emphasize a culturally responsive trauma-informed approach within the profession. Black communities are disproportionately affected by both the racialized political system and the COVID-19 pandemic. A culturally responsive trauma-informed approach to speech-language treatment service delivery could assist Black students and their families with maneuvering through the intersection of race and education and personal values that may conflict during this time of profound racial divide in the United States. This can be done by simply considering whether questions about potential past/current racial trauma exposures are included in intake processes. It does not stop there because there should be consideration for the possible triggers and/or positive solutions that are reported by students and their families that they have used to cope. This demonstrates that you truly see the whole student and their families. By engaging in curiosity about our students and their families, we show that we want to know their "story" and to use it as a part of their treatment process. In considering a culturally responsive trauma-informed approach within speech-language treatment service delivery, SLPs would acknowledge the challenges faced by many Black students and their families when navigating their authentic racial identity while also adapting to the ever-changing landscape of the educational system. This, in turn, reduces the re-traumatization of Black students and their families, moving them toward healing and resilience and greater engagement and success in the speech and language treatment process.

References

Akbar, N. (1996). *Breaking the chains of psychological slavery*. Mind Productions & Associates.

American Psychiatric Association (2013). *Diagnostic and statistical manual of mental disorders, text revision (5th ed.)*. Arlington, VA: Author.

American Speech-Language-Hearing Association (2020). *Response to racism* [Position Statement]. Retrieved from https://www.asha.org/policy/response-to-racism/

Archibald, P. (2021). Factors influencing the relationship between work-related stress and posttraumatic stress disorder among working Black adults in the United States. *Yale Journal of Biology and Medicine, 94*(3), 383–394.

Area Deprivation Index. Retrieved from https://www.neighborhoodatlas.medicine.wisc.edu/mapping

Bailey, L. C., Razzaghi, H., Burrows, E. K., Bunnell, H. T., Camacho, P., Christakis, D. A., Eckrich, D., Kitzmiller, M., Lin, S. M., Magnusen, B. C., Newland, J., Pajor, N. M., Ranade, D., Rao, S., Sofela, O., Zahner, J., Bruno, C., & Forrest, C. B. (2021). Assessment of 135,794 pediatric patients tested for severe acute respiratory syndrome coronavirus 2 across the United States. *JAMA Pediatrics, 175*(2), 176–184. https://doi.org/10.1001/jamapediatrics.2020.5052

Barrett, J. E., & Roediger, D. (2012). How white people became white. In P. S. Rothenberg (Ed.), *White privilege. Essential readings on the other side of racism* (pp. 39–44). New York, NY: Worth Publishers.

Becker-Blease, K. A., Finkelhor, D., & Turner, H. (2008). Media exposure predicts children's reactions to crime and terrorism. *Journal of Trauma & Dissociation, 9*(2), 225–248. https://doi.org/10.1080/15299730802048652

Berenz, E. C., Roberson-Nay, R., Latendresse, S. J., Mezuk, B., Gardner, C. O., Amstadter, A. B., & York, T. P. (2017). Posttraumatic stress disorder and alcohol dependence: Epidemiology and order of onset. *Psychological Trauma: Theory, Research, Practice, and Policy, 9*(4), 485–492.

Bloom, S. L., Foderaro, J. F., & Ryan, R. (2010). *SELF: A trauma-informed psychoeducational group curriculum*. Retrieved from http://sanctuaryweb.com/Products/SELFGroupTraining.aspx

Bonilla-Silva, E. (1997). Rethinking racism: Toward a structural interpretation. *American Sociological Review, 62*(3), 465–480. https://doi.org/10.2307/2657316

Borkan, J., Culhane-Pera, K., & Goldman, R. (2008). Towards cultural humility in healthcare for culturally diverse Rhode Island. *Medicine & Health, 91*(12), 361–364.

Boutwell, B. B., Nedelec, J. L., Winegard, B., Shackelford, T., Beaver, K. M., Vaughn, M., Barnes, J. C., & Wright, J. P. (2017). The prevalence of discrimination across racial groups in contemporary America: Results from a nationally representative sample of adults. *PloS One, 12*(8), e0183356. https://doi.org/10.1371/journal.pone.0183356

Brooks Holliday, S., Dubowitz, T., Haas, A., Ghosh-Dastidar, B., DeSantis, A., & Troxel, W. M. (2020). The association between discrimination and PTSD in African Americans: Exploring the role of gender. *Ethnicity & Health, 25*(5), 717–731. https://doi.org/10.1080/13557858.2018.1444150

Buxton, T. F. (1840). *The African slave trade and its remedy.* S.W. Benedict.

Chou, T., Asnaani, A., & Hofmann, S. G. (2012). Perception of racial discrimination and psychopathology across three U.S. ethnic minority groups. *Cultural Diversity & Ethnic Minority Psychology, 18*(1), 74–81. https://doi.org/10.1037/a0025432

Clark, R., Anderson, N. B., Clark, V. R., & Williams, D. R. (1999). Racism as a stressor for African Americans: A biopsychosocial model. *American Psychologist, 54*(10), 805–816.

Coates, T. (2015). *Between the world and me.* Spiegel and Grau.

Comas-Díaz, L., Hall, G. N., & Neville, H. A. (2019). Racial trauma: Theory, research, and healing: Introduction to the special issue. *The American Psychologist, 74*(1), 1–5. https://doi.org/10.1037/amp0000442

Crawford, J., Nobles, W. W., & DeGruy, J. D. (2003). Reparations and health care for African Americans: Repairing the damage from the legacy of slavery. In R. Windbush (Ed.), *Should America pay? Slavery and the raging debate on reparations* (pp. 251–281). Harper Collins.

Cronholm, P. F., Forke, C. M., Wade, R., Bair-Merritt, M. H., Davis, M., Harkins-Schwarz, M., Pachter, L. M., & Fein, J. A. (2015). Adverse childhood experiences: Expanding the concept of adversity. *American Journal of Preventive Medicine, 49*(3), 354–361.

Dhaliwal, K. [Chart]. (2015). *Trauma and social location.* RYSE Center Richmond, CA, Retrieved from http://www.acesconnection.com/blog/adding-layers-to-the-aces-pyramidwhat-do-you-think.

DeGruy, J. (2005). *Post traumatic slave syndrome: America's legacy of enduring injury and healing.* Joy DeGruy Publications Inc.

Distress Community IndexHolden, T. M., Simon, M. A., Arnold, D. T., Halloway, V., & Gerardin, J. (2022). Structural racism and COVID-19 response: Higher risk of exposure drives disparate COVID-19 deaths among Black and Hispanic/Latinx residents of Illinois, USA. *BMC Public Health, 22*(1), 312. https://doi.org/10.1186/s12889-022-12698-9

Horesh, D., & Brown, A. D. (2020). Traumatic stress in the age of COVID-19: A call to close critical gaps and adapt to new realities. *Psychological Trauma: Theory, Research, Practice, and Policy, 12*(4), 331–335.

Klein, H. S., Engerman, S. L., Haines, R., & Shlomowitz, R. (2001). Transoceanic mortality: The slave trade in comparative perspective. *William Mary Quartely, 58*(1), 93–117.

Koita, K., Long, D., Hessler, D., Benson, M., Daley, K., Bucci, M., Thakur, N., & Burke Harris, N. (2018). Development and implementation of a pediatric adverse childhood experiences (ACEs) and other determinants of health questionnaire in the pediatric medical home: A pilot study. *PLOS One, 13*(12), e0208088. 10.1371/journal.pone.0208088

Lai, B. S., La Greca, A. M., Brincks, A., Colgan, C. A., D'Amico, M. P., Lowe, S., & Kelley, M. L. (2021). Trajectories of posttraumatic stress in youths after natural disasters. *JAMA Network Open, 4*(2), e2036682. https://doi.org/10.1001/jamanetworkopen.2020.36682

Lee, R. T., Perez, A. D., Boykin, C. M., & Mendoza-Denton, R. (2019). On the prevalence of racial discrimination in the United States. *PloS One, 14*(1), E0210698. https://doi.org/10.1371/journal.pone.0210698

Logan, J. R., & Oakley, D. (2017). Black lives and policing: The larger context of ghettoization. *Journal of Urban Affairs, 39*(8), 1031–1046. https://doi.org/10.1080/07352166.2017.1328977

López, C. M., Andrews, A. R., Chisolm, A. M., de Arellano, M. A., Saunders, B., & Kilpatrick, D. G. (2017). Racial/ethnic differences in trauma exposure and mental health disorders in adolescents. *Cultural Diversity & Ethnic Minority Psychology, 23*(3), 382–387. https://doi.org/10.1037/cdp0000126

Maguire-Jack, K., Lanier, P., & Lombardi, B. (2020). Investigating racial differences in clusters of adverse childhood experiences. *The American Journal of Orthopsychiatry, 90*(1), 106–114. https://doi.org/10.1037/ort0000405

McEwen, B. S. (1998). Protective and damaging effects of stress mediators. *New England Journal of Medicine, 338*(3), 171–179. https://doi.org/10.1056/nejm199801153380307

Ostrom, T. M. (1969). The relationship between the affective, behavioral, and cognitive components of attitude. *Journal of Experimental Social Psychology, 5*(1), 12–30.

Paradies, Y., Ben, J., Denson, N., Elias, A., Priest, N., Pieterse, A., Gupta, A., Kelaher, M., & Gee, G. (2015). Racism as a determinant of health: A systematic review and meta-analysis. *PloS One, 10*(9), e0138511. https://doi.org/10.1371/journal.pone.0138511

Pearlin, L. I., Schieman, S., Fazio, E. M., & Meersman, S. C. (2005). Stress, health, and the life course: Some conceptual perspectives. *Journal of Health and Social Behavior, 46*(2), 205–219.

Pieterse, A. L. (2018). Attending to racial trauma in clinical supervision: Enhancing client and supervisee outcomes. *The Clinical Supervisor, 37*(1), 204–220.

Pinderhughes, H., Davis, R., & Williams, M. (2015). *Adverse Community Experiences and Resilience: A Framework for Addressing and Preventing Community Trauma.* Prevention Institute, Oakland, CA. Retrieved from https://www.preventioninstitute.org/sites/default/files/publications/Adverse%20Community%20Experiences%20and%20Resilience.pdf

Powell, J. A. (2012). Poverty and race through a belongingness lens. *Policy Matters, 1*(5), 1–26. Retrieved from https://www.law.berkeley.edu/files/PolicyMatters_powell_V4.pdf

Prins, A., Ouimette, P., Kimerling, R., Cameron, R. P., Hugelshofer, D. S., Shaw-Hegwer, J., Thrailkill, A., Gusman, F. D., & Sheikh, J. I. (2003). The primary care PTSD screen (PC-PTSD): Development and operating charcteristics. *Primary Care Psychiatry, 9*(1), 9–14. https://doi.org/10.1185/135525703125002360

Pumariega, A. J., Jo, Y., Beck, B., & Rahmani, M. (2022). Trauma and US minority children and youth. *Current Psychiatry Reports, 24*(4), 285–295. https://doi.org/10.1007/s11920-022-01336-1

Sadavoy, J. (1997). Survivors. A review of the late-life effects of prior psychological trauma. *The American Journal of Geriatric Psychiatry, 5*(4), 287–301. https://doi.org/10.1097/00019442-199700540-00004

Santilli, A., O'Connor Duffany, K., Carroll-Scott, A., Thomas, J., Greene, A., Arora, A., Agnoli, A., Gan, G., & Ickovics, J. (2017). Bridging the response to mass shootings and urban violence: Exposure to violence in New Haven,

Connecticut. *American Journal of Public Health, 107*(3), 374–379. https://doi.org/10.2105/AJPH.2016.303613

Schwartz, D., & Proctor, L. J. (2000). Community violence exposure and children's social adjustment in the school peer group: The mediating roles of emotion regulation and social cognition. *Journal of Consulting and Clinical Psychology, 68*(4), 670–683.

Sibrava, N. J., Bjornsson, A. S., Pérez Benítez, A. C. I., Moitra, E., Weisberg, R. B., & Keller, M. B. (2019). Posttraumatic stress disorder in African American and Latinx adults: Clinical course and the role of racial and ethnic discrimination. *The American Psychologist, 74*(1), 101–116. https://doi.org/10.1037/amp0000339

Slopen, N., Shonkoff, J. P., Albert, M. A., Yoshikawa, H., Jacobs, A., Stoltz, R., & Williams, D. R. (2016). Racial disparities in child adversity in the U.S.: Interactions with family immigration history and income. *American Journal of Preventive Medicine, 50*(1), 47–56. https://doi.org/10.1016/j.amepre.2015.06.013

Substance Abuse and Mental Health Services Administration (2014). *Concept of Trauma and Guidance for a Trauma-Informed Care Approach*. U.S. Department of Health and Human Services. Retrieved from https://ncsacw.samhsa.gov/userfiles/files/SAMHSA _Trauma.pdf

Tervalon, M., & Murray-Garcia, J. (1998). Cultural humility versus cultural competence: A critical distinction in defining physician training outcomes in multicultural education. *Journal of Health Care for the Poor and Underserved, 9*(2), 117–125.

United States Constitution, Amendment XIII, Section 1. Retrieved from https://constitution.congress.gov/browse/essay/amdt13-S1-1/ALDE_00000992/

Westby, C. (2023). Post-traumatic stress, autobiographical memory, and cultural neuroscience: Implications for migrants and refugees. In Y. Hyter (Ed.), *Language Research in PTSD* (pp. 37–67). Routledge.

Williams, J. C., Holloway, T. D., & Ross, D. A. (2019). Witnessing modern America: Violence and racial trauma. *Biological Psychiatry, 86*(11), e41–e42. https://doi.org/10.1016/j.biopsych.2019.09.025

Williams, M. T., Kanter, J. W., & Ching, T. (2018a). Anxiety, stress, and trauma symptoms in African Americans: Negative affectivity does not explain the relationship between microaggressions and psychopathology. *Journal of Racial and Ethnic Health Disparities, 5*(5), 919–927. https://doi.org/10.1007/s40615-017-0440-3

Williams, M. T., Metzger, I. W., Leins, C., & DeLapp, C. (2018b). Assessing racial trauma within a DSM–5 framework: The UConn racial/ethnic stress & trauma survey. *Practice Innovations, 3*(4), 242–260.

World Health Organization (1993). *The ICD-10 classification of mental and behavioral disorders: Diagnostic criteria for research*. Geneva: Author.

World Health Organization (2019). *Social Determinants of Health: Key Concepts*. Retrieved from http://www.who.int/social_determinants/thecommission/finalreport/key_concepts/en/index.html

Yehuda, R., Daskalakis, N. P., Bierer, L. M., Bader, H. N., Klengel, T., Holsboer, F., & Binder, E. B. (2016). Holocaust exposure induced intergenerational effects on FKBP5 methylation. *Biological Psychiatry, 80*, 372–380.

Youssef, N. A., Belew, D., Hao, G., Wang, X., Treiber, F. A., Stefanek, M., Yassa, M., Boswell, E., McCall, W. V., & Su, S. (2017). Racial/ethnic differences in the association of childhood adversities with depression and the role of resilience. *Journal of Affective Disorders, 208,* 577–581. https://doi.org/10.1016/j.jad.2016.10.024

3 Post-Traumatic Stress, Autobiographical Memory, and Cultural Neuroscience

Implications for Migrants and Refugees

Carol Westby

3.1 Migrants, Refugees, and Asylum Seekers

Human migration, for any reason – whether forced migrations as a result of fleeing war and genocide or being displaced due to droughts, floods, or earthquakes; or chosen migrations of persons seeking better educational and economic opportunities – is stressful and puts persons at risk for long-term consequences of trauma, involving a variety of physical and mental health conditions and impairments. The individual response to migration traumas is variable and not due only to the physical stresses encountered. Responses to the stressors of migration are affected by cultural values and belief systems and by genetic makeup. Genetic research has shown that certain genetic variations are directly responsible for diseases/ medical conditions (e.g., cystic fibrosis, muscular dystrophy, cleft lip/palate); other genes increase risks for specific diseases or conditions (e.g., cancer, heart disease); and still, other genes are sensitive to environmental variations in social support/interactions. These latter genes mediate responses to environmental traumas. Persons with genetic alleles that are environmentally sensitive are more likely to experience negative physical and mental consequences of traumatic experiences. Researchers in cultural social neuroscience propose that genes and culture have coevolved (gene-culture coevolution theory) (Chiao & Blizinsky, 2010). As cultures change, genes change; and as genes change, cultures change. Migrations often result in disruptions to cultural values, beliefs, and support systems, placing persons at even greater risk of the negative effects of trauma. Countries receiving large numbers of migrants are struggling with providing the necessary and appropriate health care. This chapter describes trauma factors affecting migrants/refugees, the effects of trauma on memory, frameworks for understanding cultural variations in values, beliefs, and communication styles; neurophysiological/neurogenetic relationships

DOI: 10.4324/9781003225270-4

to these behaviors and beliefs; and how this knowledge can be used to design culturally accepted and effective interventions.

For 2023, the United Nations High Commissioner for Refugees (UN-HCR, 2023) reported a record high of 117 million people being forcibly displaced due to conflict and persecution. There is some confusion regarding the terms used to describe people moving from their homelands to other countries:

- Immigrants are persons who come to live permanently in a foreign country. They have not been forced from or pushed out of their own country; it can be a choice. A distinction is made between legal and undocumented immigrants. Legal immigrants have been allowed to come to a country through approved documents; undocumented immigrants have not.
- Refugees have been forced to leave their countries to escape war, persecution, or natural disaster. For most countries, to be considered a refugee, persons must meet the refugee definition in the 1951 Geneva Convention relating to the Status of Refugees. To meet the definition, a person must be outside their country of origin and have a well-founded fear of being persecuted for reasons of race, religion, nationality, membership in a particular social group, or a political opinion.
- An asylum seeker claims to be a refugee but their claim has not been evaluated. This person has asked for protection in another country. They would have applied for asylum on the grounds that returning to their country would lead to persecution on account of race, religion, nationality, or political beliefs. Undocumented noncitizens arriving in the United States from Central America are asylum seekers, but they are not considered refugees because they do not meet the definition of refugees in the Geneva Convention.
- Migrants are persons who move from one place to another, in order to find work or better living conditions. They can return home whenever they wish. They do not qualify for refugee status because they have not been persecuted according to the Geneva Convention.

3.2   Migrant/Refugee Trauma

Refugees/asylum seekers are highly likely to have had traumatic experiences, but migrants and immigrants are also likely to have been exposed to trauma. All are at increased risk for post-traumatic stress disorder, a mental health condition that develops following exposure to a traumatic event. Increasing numbers of refugees/asylum seekers are unaccompanied children (UAC) under 18 years of age. UACs are not in the care of a parent or legal guardian at the time of entry and do not have a family member or legal guardian willing or able to care for them in the arrival country. Different studies have shown rates of post-traumatic stress disorder (PTSD) and major depression in settled refugees to range from 10 to 40% and 5 to 15%, respectively. Children and adolescents often have higher levels, with various investigations revealing rates of PTSD from 50 to 90% and major depression from 6 to 40% (Refugee Health Technical Assistance, n.d.).

In the United States, the diagnosis of PTSD in individuals over six years is based on the presence of criteria listed in the *Diagnostic and Statistical Manual of Mental Disorders-5* (DSM-5; American Psychiatric Association, 2013). The International Classification of Diseases – 11 (ICD-11; World Health Organization, 2018) is used primarily outside the United States for the diagnosis of PTSD. The ICD-11 has two categories for PTSD – PTSD like the DSM-5 PTSD definition; and complex PTSD (CPTSD), which includes the core elements of PTSD plus additional disturbances of self-organization. Table 3.1 shows a comparison of PTSD and complex PTSD. Refugees are at greater risk for complex PTSD.

3.3 Sources of Trauma

3.3.1 Migration Traumas

Refugees/asylum seekers are highly likely to experience stressors at each stage of migration that can contribute to PTSD. The National Child Traumatic Stress Network (NCTSN) describes current stressors in four categories: pre-migration, resettlement stressors, acculturation stressors, and isolation stressors. Table 3.2 gives examples of these stressors. (Note: The

Table 3.1 Comparison of PTSD and Complex PTSD

PTSD	Complex PTSD
• Core elements	• Core elements: PTSD symptoms + disturbances in self-organization (DSO):
→ Re-experiencing the trauma (flashbacks)	→ Affective dysregulation: Difficulty regulating emotions
→ Avoiding reminders of the trauma	→ Disturbances of self-concept: Feelings of shame, guilt, failure
→ Experiencing a heightened sense of threat and arousal	→ Disturbances of interpersonal relationships
• Generally related to a single event or series of events within a short period of time	• Related to a series of traumatic events over time or one prolonged event
• Response focused mainly on the trauma	• Difficulties ripple more widely through lives.

Table 3.2 Migration Stressors

Pre-migration/ migration	Resettlement	Acculturation	Isolation
• War and persecution • Displacement from their home • Flight and migration • Poverty • Family/ community violence	• Financial stressors • Living in an unsafe neighborhood • Lack of adequate housing • Difficulties finding employment • Loss of community support • Lack of access to resources • Transportation difficulties	• Conflicts between children and parents over new and old cultural views • Conflicts with peers related to cultural misunderstandings • The necessity to translate for family members who are not fluent in English • Problems trying to fit in at school • Struggle to form an integrated identity including elements of their new culture and their culture of origin	• Feelings of loneliness and loss of social support network • Discrimination • Experiences of harassment from peers, adults, or law enforcement • Experiences with others who do not trust the refugee child and family • Feelings of not fitting in with others • Loss of social status

Source: Based on content from the NCTSN website.

NCTSN has a web-based resource, *Refugee and Immigrant Core Stressors Toolkit,* which service providers can employ to assess the current situation and needs of a particular youth or family in these four categories). Based on the assessment, tailored recommendations for resources and interventions are generated (https://www.nctsn.org/resources-services-core-stressor-assessment-tool). Postmigration trauma may impact learning and cognitive functions significantly more than premigration trauma (Graham et al., 2016).

3.3.2 Parenting Challenges

Exposure to atrocities of war and resulting displacement and resettlement can also affect children's development and adjustment through changes in parenting (Gredeback et al., 2021; Sim, Fazel et al., 2018) as shown in Figure 3.1. As a result of war exposure or traumatic migration experiences, parents face a variety of challenges: economic hardships prevent parents from meeting their children's basic needs; parents experience psychological problems due to their own trauma; and parents may have concerns

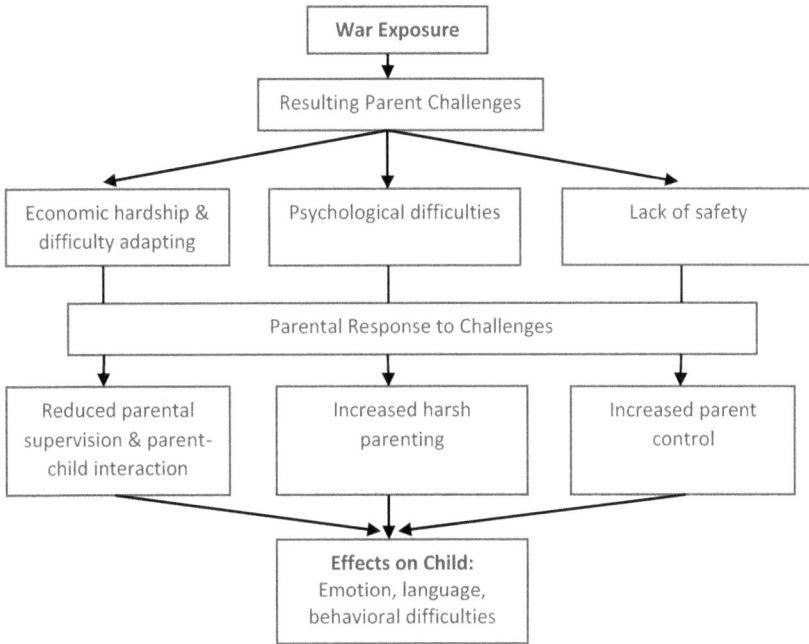

Figure 3.1 Parenting challenges due to trauma.

regarding the continuing lack of safety. In response to these challenges, parents may exhibit reduced parental supervision and parent-child inter-actions; they may exhibit less warmth and more harshness toward their children; and in attempts to keep their children safe, they may become more controlling. Refugee children experience not only trauma from war or disaster experience but also trauma from reduced parental support and attachment. Both types of trauma place children at increased risk for a va-riety of language, learning, behavioral, and mental health problems.

3.4 Effects of Trauma/PTSD on Autobiographical Memory

Trauma and associated PTSD have long been associated with alterations in autobiographical memory (AM); and alterations in AM are associated with PTSD symptoms, such as intrusive memories and flashbacks. Trauma disrupts AM, which is a memory of personally relevant events in one's own life (Watson & Berntsen, 2015). AM entails our memories of the place of the experience (where the event occurred), the when of the expe-rience in terms of both conventional time (e.g., day of the week, month, season) and time in one's own life story (e.g., in what life period the event occurred – preschool, college), and the emotions associated with the experience (Fivush, 2011). AM comprises two different but related types of memory: semantic autobiographical memory and episodic autobiographical memory. Semantic autobiographical memory is a memory for facts about oneself; it ties the memory to a specific time and place. Episodic autobiographical memory is a memory of the sensory and emotional experience. It involves autonoetic consciousness, the phenomenon of self-experiencing the event in reminiscing, termed *mental time travel*. Mental time travel enables one to see oneself in the past and in the future, and in so doing, one is more likely to engage in self-regulatory behaviors in the present as a way to achieve future goals. Thus, trauma affects not only AM but also executive functioning.

There are three levels of autobiographical knowledge: lifetime periods, general events, and event-specific knowledge (Conway & Pleyel-Pierce, 2000). Lifetime periods, such as going to college or working at a particular job, are at the highest level. For some refugees, the migration experience represents a lifetime period because it can last for months or even years. The middle level holds general or categorical events, which are at a more specific level of autobiographical knowledge about repeated events or events that take place over a prolonged period of time, e.g., weekly soccer practice, yearly Thanksgiving at Grandma's, or a summer vacation in the mountains. Event-specific knowledge is vividly detailed information about individual events, often in the form of visual images and sensory-perceptual features, e.g., a day in December 2019 in Nepal, taking a helicopter through a mountain pass to the Annapurna base camp and hiking there in the snow at 14,000 feet.

Persons with depression or PTSD, tend to exhibit over-general autobiographical memories (OGAMs). Their AMs are marked by fewer and less specific details, difficulty in retrieving the AMs they do have, and difficulty reporting their AMs in coherent narratives (Lapidow & Brown, 2015). Adult and child refugees from diverse cultures exhibit similar patterns of OGAMs when asked to recall their experiences (Doost et al., 2014; Graham et al., 2014; Khan et al., 2021). The ability to generate detailed, coherent personal narratives is associated with psychological well-being, self-identity, and self-regulation. Diagnostic criteria for PTSD and CPTSD specifically list difficulties in these areas. Persons who have experienced trauma and PTSD are likely to retrieve memories from the middle level of general events rather than a more specific level. Persons who have experienced multiple adverse childhood experiences (ACEs) or other traumas tend to have fragmented OGAMs not only for traumatic events but also for everyday events (Vanderveren et al., 2017). Deficits in AM result in difficulties in telling organized, coherent personal narratives about experiences (Siegel, 2012). Even when the vocabulary and morpho-syntactic language skills of children who have experienced multiple traumas are within a developmentally appropriate range, the majority of these children exhibit deficits at the discourse or narrative level. If parents have experienced multiple traumas or PTSD, they reminisce with their children in less elaborative and less coherent ways, and as a result, their children exhibit less developed personal narratives (Kelly, 2015). Because AM enables not only travel to the past but also travel to the future, persons with better time travel to the past (retrieval of past personal experiences) have better time travel to the future (the ability to imagine possible events in the future). Future time travel enables planning and goal setting; it is an aspect of executive function. Persons with PTSD have OGAMs not only for past events but also for imagining the future (Sagbakken et al., 2020).

Deficits in AM of persons with PTSD have been associated with misinterpretations of present situations and intrusive memories. Persons with intrusive memories lack the awareness that the memories are something from the past; instead, the memories are experienced as some kind of threat in the present. Schauer & colleagues (2011, 2017) proposed that intrusive memories and incoherent narratives associated with trauma are due to a disconnection of the emotionally arousing aspects of an experience (hot memories; episodic autobiographical emotional content managed by the amygdala) from the spatial and temporal context (cold memories; semantic autobiographical content – where and when the event happened dependent on the functioning of the hippocampus). Because the hot memories are not attached to a time and place, they can appear to be experienced in the present and can be triggered by sensory stimuli in the present situation. The episodic component of AM can be triggered by sounds, smells, and sights. When these episodic memories are triggered but not connected to the semantic knowledge of the time and place, the when and where they occurred, it is as though the event is being experienced in the present – the intrusive memories and flashbacks of PTSD.

3.5   Cultural Considerations in Understanding Trauma

The criterion features of PTSD and CPTSD listed in the DSM-5 and the ICD-11 have been shown to be applicable across cultures (Patel & Hall, 2021), but some cultures have additional symptomatic features associated with trauma and people in many cultures differ in their explanations for the symptoms and how they should be treated (Heim et al., 2022). Most psychological and biological studies have been done on WEIRD people: Western, Educated, Individualistic, Rich, and Democratic (Heinrich et al., 2010). Language/learning and mental health strategies and programs that are acceptable and have proven effective for mainstream persons in developed countries may not be acceptable and effective for persons from developing countries.

The awareness of professionals across educational, social services, and medicine that biology and culture interact (Causadias et al., 2018; Chiao et al., 2016) has given rise to the field of cultural social neuroscience, which is the study of how cultural values, practices, and beliefs shape and are shaped by the mind, brain, and genes. Although people of all cultures are affected by trauma and experience PTSD, genetic and cultural influences affect both the rates and manifestations of PTSD in response to different types of trauma and persons' responses to interventions. If professionals are to adequately diagnose and treat the effects of trauma in culturally diverse populations, they must be aware of cultural neuroscience research. Such knowledge can help them understand cultural differences in human behaviors and how the human brain is shaped by man-made cultural contexts.

3.5.1 Cultural Dimensions

Psychological trauma and PTSD are a cross-cultural universal phenomenon. However, although persons in all cultures around the world are at risk for developing PTSD in response to traumatic events, there is variability in how they interpret and respond to events and how their PTSD is manifested. Consequently, professionals working with migrants/refugees need to develop cultural competence regarding the values, beliefs, and communication styles of the children and families they serve. Awareness of variations in cultural dimensions became well-known through the work of Hofstede (1980) and Hofstede et al. (2010) who derived six dimensions of cultural variability empirically from worldwide surveys. Two of these dimensions typically receive the most attention:

- Individualism/independent – collectivism/interdependent. In individualistic cultures, people´s self-image is defined in terms of "I"; in collective cultures, self-image is defined in terms of "we" (Table 3.3 provides comparisons of the individualistic/collectivistic dimension).
- Power distance (strength of the social hierarchy): High-power distance cultures value inequality with everyone having a rightful place and the hierarchy reflects inequality. Low-power distance cultures, in contrast value equality.

English-speaking countries in the world are members of the WEIRD cultures which typically espouse individualism and low-power distance. Most northern European counties are individualistic; but Norway, Denmark, and Sweden rank low on power distance, whereas France and Belgium rank high on power distance. The country profiles on the Hofstede website

Table 3.3 Individualism versus Collectivism

Component	Individualism	Collectivism
Relationship to others	• Develop early independence • Responsible for self • Loosely linked to others; view self as independent • Tasks more important than relationships • Peers increasingly important	• Learn to depend on others • Responsible for others • Closely linked; view self as part of the group • Relationships more important than tasks • Family most important
Motivation/goals	• Motivated by own preferences, needs, rights • Give priority to own goals over goals of others • Must work to link with others and work to maintain link	• Motivated by the norms of, and duties imposed by, the group • Willing to give priority to group goals over personal goals • Part of a group so don't need to work to maintain relationship
Decision-making	• Make your own decisions • Cognitive skills independent of social skills	• Listen to authority • Cognitive and social skills integrated

(https://www.hofstede-insights.com) represent the most common cultural pattern for the most typical "mainstream" persons within the country. One cannot assume, however, that all citizens of a country hold the same values and beliefs.

These cultural variations affect the ways people remember; think about themselves; perceive, interpret, and reason about situations; and the emotions they prefer and how they regulate and interpret emotions. All of these factors will affect persons' memories of trauma they experienced and how they explain the trauma and their response to it. If service providers are not aware of these cultural variations, they may over- or underdiagnose traumatic stress disorders. Furthermore, the typically recommended Western interventions may be unacceptable or ineffective.

3.5.2 *Influences of Cultural Dimensions*

3.5.2.1 *Culture and Autobiographical Memory*

Autobiographical memory develops as children reminisce with adults in their environment. Cultural orientations to either individualism or collectivism influence parents' goals when reminiscing (Carmiol & Sparks,

2014; Leichtman et al., 2003; Wang, 2014). In response to these different reminiscing styles, children from individualistic cultures learn to relate detailed, coherent, specific narratives of past experiences, referring primarily to their own preferences, behaviors, thoughts, and feelings. They relate the story from their perspective, in the first person. In contrast, children in collective cultures devote more of their focus in their personal stories to the behaviors and feelings of others who were present at the event than to themselves. Their personal narratives are more general than specific and less temporally and causally coherent. Although they may relate their stories in first person, they are also likely to relate the experience in the third person, particularly when they are not the center of the event. They describe the experience as though they were bystanders watching the event (Cohen & Gunz, 2002; Dawson & Bryant, 2016; Martin & Jones, 2012). Narratives told from a third-person perspective are less emotionally arousing than stories told from a first-person perspective, and as a consequence, persons from collective cultures who have experienced trauma are less likely to experience intrusive thoughts, which are associated with highly emotionally arousing events (McIsaac & Eich, 2004).

3.5.2.2   *Culture and Perception*

Orientation to either individualism or collectivism influences a person's perception of situations. Individuals from East Asian cultures, which emphasize interdependence or collectivism, use more monitoring and holistic processing of all the contextual information, while individuals from a Western independent/individualistic culture focus on the most obvious features in a context. For example, individuals from Japan, an Eastern culture, and the United States, a Western culture, were asked to describe what they witnessed after watching a brief video of several fish swimming in an aquarium. Westerners began their descriptions by mentioning the three large fish; in contrast, Easterners twice as often began by mentioning the field (seaweed or other small animals) (Nisbett & Masuda, 2003). Japanese and Canadian children also exhibited this difference in perceptual focus in their drawings (Senzaki et al., 2014). By second grade, Japanese children included more contextual information in their drawings than did Canadian children. Japanese children placed the horizon in their pictures higher, which allowed them more space to include more details. This difference in focus of attention is likely to affect the content of AM.

3.5.2.3   *Culture and Emotions*

Emotional Preferences/Ideal Affect. The individualism/collectivism dimension influences emotions persons prefer or consider ideal and how they regulate their emotions (Tsai & Clobert, 2019). In independent cultures, persons focus on their own emotions; conversely, in East Asian interdependent cultures, persons focus their emotions on others. These differing orientations to either self or others influence the emotions persons report experiencing most frequently. East Asians report experiencing more socially engaging emotions (e.g., friendliness, sympathy, guilt, shame), whereas persons in Western countries more frequently report experiencing socially disengaging emotions (e.g., anger, pride, frustration) (Kitayama et al., 2006).

Orientation to self or others also influences what persons in independent and collective cultures consider to be ideal emotions. Those in independent cultures seek to better themselves by influencing others and their environment. Acting on their environment and influencing others requires increased psychological arousal. Therefore, people in independent cultures tend to value high-arousal positive (HAP) emotions such as excitement and enthusiasm. In contrast, persons in Asian collective cultures focus on adjusting to others by changing their own beliefs, desires, and preferences to be consistent with those around them. This requires that they decrease their action, which reduces their physiological arousal. Persons in collective cultures value low-arousal positive (LAP) emotions such as calm, relaxed, and peaceful (Tamir et al., 2016). Cultural preferences for ideal affect can influence how persons interact with service providers. Sims and colleagues (Sims et al., 2014; Sim, Koopermann-Holm et al., 2018) reported that persons from a Chinese collective culture preferred physicians who displayed their preferred LAP emotions, while European Americans preferred physicians who displayed their preferred HAP emotions. In addition, both the Chinese and European Americans were more likely to follow the recommendations of physicians who displayed their preferred emotions. In contrast to persons in Asian collective cultures who prefer LAP emotions, however, persons in collective Mexican and Latin cultures endorse HAP over LAP emotions (Ruby et al., 2012).

Emotion Regulation. The cultural dimensions of individualism/collectivism and power distance affect expectations regarding emotion regulation (Matsumoto et al., 2008). In individualistic cultures, there is a tendency for people to regulate emotions frequently by reevaluating the situation to change its emotional impact. By reappraising the emotional event, the emotional intensity lessens. In contrast, many persons in collective cultures are concerned that the expression of emotions could negatively affect social relationships, so they more frequently regulate their emotions by suppressing them (Gross & John, 2003; Kim & Sherman, 2007; Miyamoto et al., 2014). Persons in cultures with high power distance are likely to engage in greater emotion suppression; whereas persons in low-power distance cultures have greater emotional autonomy to express their feelings. Adherence to culturally expected forms of emotion regulation influences persons' physiological responses when they are regulating their emotions. Attitudes regarding the expectation to express or suppress emotions influence persons' physiological response when they express emotions. Persons from individualistic cultures are at risk of underestimating the degree of trauma being felt by a person from a collective culture who suppresses emotions.

3.6   Gene-Environment-Culture Interactions

Culture has coevolved with genes. The idea of gene-culture coevolution is that genetic influences shape psychological and behavioral predispositions and cultural influences shape how these predispositions are manifested in social behaviors and psychological outcomes (Sasaki & Kim, 2017). Persons' genetics, as well as their cultural orientations, can influence their response to potentially traumatic situations.

3.6.1   Gene-Environment Interaction

Large-scale genome-wide association studies have shown that PTSD, like many other psychiatric disorders, mental health conditions, and neurodevelopmental disorders, is highly polygenic, meaning it is associated with thousands of genetic variants throughout the genome, each making a small contribution to the disorder (Nievergelt et al., 2019). Individual susceptibility to these conditions is dependent on interactions between genes and environments. Several gene alleles are particularly sensitive to both positive and negative environmental influences, while other genetic variations are not sensitive to environmental influences. Persons with these environmentally sensitive alleles who are reared in adverse environments (experiencing ACEs or traumatic experiences) are at greater risk for behavioral and social-emotional difficulties including anti-social behaviors, reduced empathy, depression, and PTSD (Bakermans-Kranenburg & van IJzendoorn, 2008; Caspi et al., 2002; Gervai et al., 2007; Kim et al., 2010b). Persons with genotypes that are not environmentally sensitive and who are in supportive environments demonstrate greater social skills and empathy and adjust to changes more easily (Lackner et al., 2012). The more environmentally sensitive alleles individuals have, the more they are influenced by their environment, whether positive or negative (Pleuss et al., 2013). Refugee children who carry the genes that are highly sensitive to the environment are at high risk for developing PTSD in response to migration traumas, particularly if they have not experienced adversities in early childhood (Karam et al., 2019). Caregiver-child attachment can mediate the effects of genetic predispositions and the effects of ACEs. Research has shown that children who have experienced war trauma have better mental health if they have had secure attachments (Okello et al., 2014; Punamäki et al., 2018).

3.6.2 Gene-Culture Interaction

Genes influence people's responses to aspects of their environment, and culture influences the manifestation of genes. The expression of some gene alleles varies in societies that differ on individualism-collectivism. The gene expression is dependent on persons' cultural values of individualism or collectivism, not their ethnicity.

3.6.2.1 Mood Disorders

In Western, individualistic cultures, those who have the short allele of the serotonin transporter gene 5-HTTLPR are at greater risk for mood disorders than those who carry the long version of the 5-HTTLPR gene (Munafò et al., 2005). In contrast, persons from Eastern collective nations who carry the short version are at reduced risk for mood disorders. In countries around the world, there is a relationship between the prevalence of mood disorders in relation to the prevalence of the short allele (Chiao & Blizinsky, 2010). The percentage of individuals carrying the short version is greater in China, a highly collective nation, compared to Canada, the United States, and Australia, highly individualistic nations. The collective nations with the highest prevalence of the short allele were also the nations with the lowest prevalence of mood disorders; in contrast, individualistic nations exhibited higher prevalence rates for mood disorders although the short variant of the 5-HTTLPR is less prevalent. Chiao and Blizinsky (2010) suggest that this is an example of gene-culture coevolution – the culture has evolved to protect from the downside of a genetic allele. If a person shifts from a collective to an individualistic orientation, as may occur when they immigrate and acculturate to an individualistic country, they lose the protection of collectivism against mood disorders related to the short allele. Their risk of mood disorders increases.

3.6.2.2 Focus of Attention/Perception

Genes and culture interact to influence one's focus of attention. Some persons from collective cultures with the GG allele of the serotonin receptor gene 5-HTR1A give greater attention to context than to target objects, but persons from individualistic cultures with the GG allele tend to give greater attention to target objects and less attention to context (Kim et al., 2010). Focus of attention can influence autobiographical memory for experiences.

3.6.2.3 Emotion Regulation

Culture interacts with the OXTR rs53576 gene to influence persons' strategies for emotion regulation (Kim et al., 2011). The GG oxytocin receptor polymorphism alleles (OCTR rs53576) influence emotional expression, but in different ways depending on cultural orientation. In a study by Chiao et al. (2009), Koreans with the GG oxytocin alleles exhibited greater suppression of emotional expressions than Koreans with the AA alleles; whereas Americans with the GG oxytocin receptor polymorphism alleles (OCTR) showed greater emotional expression. The Korean-Americans were similar to European-American participants, not to Koreans living in Korea. It appears that these gene-culture interactions are more related to cultural values and beliefs than to ethnicity (Chiao et al., 2009).

3.6.2.4 Support Seeking

The majority of migrants/refugees would benefit from a variety of supports. They are likely to receive and accept economic and educational supports but far less likely to receive social and mental health support or accept social/mental health support when it is offered (Schauer & Schauer, 2010). Support seeking is influenced by both cultural values and genotypes. Asians and Asian Americans in the United States have reported using social support less for coping with stress than European Americans (Taylor et al., 2004). Support-seeking behavior is influenced by whether individuals value cultural goals of promoting themselves or developing social relationships. In individualistic cultures, persons may enlist explicit help or aid from those in their social networks to achieve their personal goals. In collective cultures, the focus of a person's goals may be to promote relationships. In this context, asking one's social network for assistance may risk straining relationships. Therefore, persons with collective values may feel that they have less to gain and more to lose socially by asking others for help. If maintaining relationships is a highly valued goal, then people may prefer to solve their own problems rather than burden their social network. In both American (individualistic) and Korean (collectivistic) cultures, the likelihood of seeking support is mediated by genotype. Americans with the GG OCTR alleles who reported high psychological distress were more likely to seek support than Americans with the AA alleles; in contrast, Koreans with the AA alleles were slightly, but not significantly, more likely to seek support than Koreans with the GG alleles (Kim et al., 2010b).

3.7   Implications of Culture and Trauma Effects for the Asylum Process

The United Nations reports that nearly 117 million people (including 37 million children) will be forcibly displaced by the end of 2023. While many child and adolescent refugees demonstrate tremendous resilience in the aftermath of war and forced migration (Tozer et al., 2017; Vindevogel, 2017), a sizable proportion of this group report high rates of emotional and behavioral difficulties compared with community baseline estimates and matched clinical samples (Betancourt et al., 2017; Graham et al., 2016). The majority of migrants and refugees are moving from areas with collective, high-power distance cultures to countries with individualistic, low-power distance cultures. This changed cultural environment can be an acculturation stressor.

3.7.1 The Interview Process

In the United States, a very small percentage of refugees are granted asylum. Of all asylum seekers to the United States, 75% are rejected. For those from south of the US border 90+% are rejected (TRAC, 2020). The asylum process relies heavily on the refugees' retrieval of autobiographical memories. In Western countries, the asylum process typically requires that the refugees make a claim for asylum by offering an account of their experiences. Applicants for asylum must go through a Credible Fear Interview in which they explain why they believe they are eligible for asylum. They must offer believable accounts that they have suffered persecution in their country of origin related to their race, religion, nationality, or political beliefs, and they must explain why they are afraid to return. The level of specificity in their narratives has been seen as a good way of distinguishing between accurate and inaccurate memories. The more detail a memory has, the more believable and credible the memory is seen to be (Herlihy et al., 2012). General memories are viewed as not credible, false, or exaggerated and are thought to have not been recalled clearly. Border agency personnel frequently base their asylum decision on the level of detail in asylum seekers' claims. The very basis of the asylum claim is an assumption that people can reliably, consistently, and accurately recall autobiographical memories. The common belief is that emotionally charged experiences will be well-remembered. If applicants cannot convincingly describe an event that happened in a specific time and place, then they are likely to be seen as fabricating a story. Although this may be the case, the research on autobiographical memory, which should underpin this guidance, suggests that retrieving an accurate, consistent, and reliable memory when one has experienced trauma is problematic. There is considerable support for the hypothesis that high levels of stress negatively impact eyewitness memory in terms of the proportion of correct identifications and accuracy of eyewitness recall. The literature on the relationship between lack of autobiographical memory specificity and depression and PTSD is well established (see Moore & Zoellner, 2007 for a review). Specifically, those with PTSD, trauma history, and depression have been found to have difficulties in providing specific memories and instead tend to provide overly general memories (Schönfeld et al., 2007).

Another test of the credibility of an asylum claim is the consistency of the applicants' accounts of their experiences. If the individual does not "keep their story straight," then the story is assumed to be fabricated. Lack of consistency in an asylum seeker's account is often a central factor in asylum decisions. However, research suggests that specific and non-trivial trauma memories can be subject to significant distortion, alteration, and discrepancies in refugees (Herlihy et al., 2002; Mollica et al., 2007). Much of the autobiographical memory research suggests that autobiographical memory can contain inconsistencies and inaccuracies, and thus, these features should not be used to deem a memory a false or incredible report. Discrepancies are more likely for peripheral details of traumatic events and for individuals with higher levels of PTSD symptoms, and a longer delay between interviews is associated with more discrepancies.

The majority of refugees are fleeing from countries with collective cultures to countries with predominantly individualistic cultures. The focus and structure of autobiographical memories differ in individualistic and collective cultures. From infancy, persons from individualistic cultures are trained to provide lengthy, autonomous, specific, self-focused, and emotionally elaborate memories that focus on individual experiences, roles, and emotions. In contrast, those from collectivistic cultures tend to focus on collective activities (rather than personal experiences), general routines, and emotionally neutral events (Fivush, 2019; Wang, 2014; Wu et al., 2020) The decision-makers, who are primarily from individualistic cultures, expect lengthy detailed reports of specific experiences from the refugee's perspective. Because of their socialization, the memories produced by refugees do not meet those expectations.

Unaccompanied asylum-seeking children (UASC), ages 12–17 years, are subjected to the adult interview process. As with adults, officials judge the reasonableness of children's asylum claims on the consistency and specific detail of their reported memories. Yet AM is still developing through adolescence (Given-Wilson et al., 2018). Children and most adolescents have not yet achieved the AM development expected for producing coherent, specific personal narratives.

3.7.2 Cultural Misinterpretations

A challenge for Western professionals treating migrants/refugees is that key presentations of psychological responses to trauma, such as distress, depression, anxiety, or PTSD differ greatly across cultures and, consequently, may not be recognized by Western professionals (Hinton & Bui, 2019). Western professionals typically hold individualistic values, whereas most refugees hold collective values. Table 3.4 provides examples of how the effects and response to trauma may differ because of some of

Table 3.4 Cultural Factors in Trauma Response

Trauma effect/response	Individualistic	Collective
Intrusive memories from trauma	Regulate emotion primarily by reappraising situation; expressing emotion leads to well-being, suppressing emotion reduces well-being	May regulate emotion primarily by suppressing emotion; suppressing emotion can promote well-being, expressing emotions reduces well-being
Emotional expression	Prefer use of high-arousal emotions	May prefer the use of low-arousal emotions
Attention bias for encoding memory; may affect memory encoding	Focus on the central, salient object/person in situation; little attention to broader context	Biased to attend to the entire context/background
Interpreting emotions	Rely primarily on the facial cues of the target person to determine persons' feelings'	Rely heavily on information/ cues from other people in the environment of the target person in addition to facial cues of the target person
Autobiographical memory when retrieving memory: Fragmented, incoherent narratives	Specific memories; self-focused memories; memories reported from first-person perspective (1st person perspective heightens emotions)	General memories; other-focused memories; memories reported from both first and third-person perspective (3rd person perspective reduces emotions)
Use of supports	Seek social support from others when stressed	Avoid social support from others when stressed

the cultural variations described in this chapter. If service providers are to reduce sources of miscommunication and misunderstanding with their clients, they must be aware of their own cultural values and beliefs and consider the possible cultural values and beliefs of those they are serving. Miscommunication and misunderstandings may arise because of differences in what persons attend to in contexts, what emotions are valued, how emotions are displayed and regulated, how autobiographical memories are encoded and retrieved, and attitudes about support.

Refugees' divergent conceptualizations and a lack of understanding of Western concepts of health and education in resettlement countries may lead them to fear seeking services, contributing to a delay in treatment (Piwowarczyk et al., 2014; Slewa-Younan et al., 2014). When disabilities or mental health issues are viewed as stigmatizing, refugees may be concerned about being negatively judged or even being ostracized by community members and, as a consequence, they may not seek, or even avoid, services (Bettmann et al., 2015; Shannon et al., 2015). In some communities, beliefs in non-medical explanations of psychological symptoms prevail and therefore help may be sought from spiritual and traditional healers, rather than within the mainstream health and education systems of the host country (Khalifa et al., 2011). Few studies have systematically investigated the ways culture may influence physical and psychological responses to trauma and interpretation of these responses; and even fewer interventions have been specifically developed around cultural content (Hinton & Patel, 2018). Programs provided to refugees often rely on clinicians' cultural competence.

3.8   Assessment Frameworks

The National Child Traumatic Stress Network (NCTSN; https://www. nctsn.org/) provides guidelines for persons working with refugee children. An important first step is that providers attend to cultural considerations. When assessing a child's history, service providers should ask about the child's background, past school experience, trauma history, and current stressors (See Table 3.1). When interviewing caregivers, ask about specific behaviors of the child that might be concerning for caregivers. This can facilitate a culturally appropriate way to discuss learning and behavioral symptoms. Ask about, and respect, the caregiver's or child's interpretation of the symptoms and concerns. You might ask, "Why do you think your child is behaving this way?" or "You know your child best. Do you have any concerns?" To assess if symptoms are culturally specific, you might ask, "Do you know anyone else who has these same problems?"

Questioning in this way enables the interviewer to elicit the family's explanatory model – that is, the way in which they understand the child's behaviors, including ideas about causation and methods for working with the child (Kleinman, 1980). Understanding the family's interpretation of the child's behaviors and providing treatment congruent with their explanatory model is a key ingredient in culturally adapted treatment (Dinos et al., 2017). The *Diagnostic Statistical Manual 5* (American Psychiatric Association, 2013) provides a framework for a Cultural Formulation Interview (CFI) that focuses on four cultural dimensions: definition of the problem; perceptions of cause, context, and support; factors affecting self-coping and past help-seeking; and factors affecting current help-seeking. Lewis-Fernandez et al. (2016) have provided supplemental interview formats, including ones for use with children and adolescents, immigrants and refugees, and one to explore aspects of cultural identity related to national, ethnic, and racial background, language, and migration.

These interviews enable service providers to understand a person's perspective on their situation and to discover their *idioms of distress*. The term, *idioms of distress*, refers to culture-specific expressions, symbols of emotional suffering, or culturally acceptable ways for individuals to communicate distress within specific contexts (Im et al., 2017; Patel & Hall, 2021). These idioms are ways that persons describe or explain their trauma and symptoms, such as PTSD, to others in their community in ways that enable communal understanding and acceptance. By understanding a client's or family's idioms of distress regarding the trauma they have experienced, service providers are better able to select appropriate treatment approaches in collaboration with the client and family, so as to enhance the client's engagement in treatment, to improve the therapeutic bond, and to promote positive expectancy. As part of the intervention, service providers often need to employ *explanatory model bridging*, in which they help a family understand how the proposed interventions will address their concerns (Hinton & Patel, 2018).

3.9   Interventions

3.9.1 Foundations

Child and adolescent migrants/refugees may require interventions to address language, cognitive, and academic needs, in addition to mental health needs. Children and adults who have a history of ACEs and trauma are at risk for telling less coherent personal narratives with less detail, reflecting less organized, less detailed autobiographical memories (AM). These language delays/disorders and effects of trauma in children contribute to delays and impairments in theory of mind (ToM), resulting in ongoing deficits in affective ToM characterized by difficulty accurately recognizing emotions and linking emotions to contextual situations (Sullivan et al., 2008). As a result of these ToM deficits, persons who have experienced maltreatment and trauma misinterpret experiences are likely to interpret threat in situations where threat no longer exists. These misinterpretations are then encoded inaccurately into AM which further contributes to PTSD symptoms.

3.9.2 Trauma-Focused Interventions

Three types of interventions have evidence for reducing the frequency and intensity of symptoms of PTSD/CPTD in children and adults, – eye movement desensitization and reprocessing (EMDR; Banoğlu & Korkmazlar, 2022), trauma-focused cognitive behavior therapy (TF-CBT, Chipalo, 2021), and narrative exposure therapy (NET; Neuner et al., 2018; Ruf et al., 2010). Speech-language professionals can have a special role in narrative exposure therapy. The basic theory behind narrative exposure therapy (NET) is that by talking through traumatic events in chronological order, one can slowly and methodically repair negative associations and responses. The focus of NET is on reconstructing the fragmented autobiographical memories of traumatic experiences into coherent narrations of specific events by reconnecting episodic memories (the sensory and emotional aspects of the experience) with the semantic memories (the temporal and spatial context of the experience). If the semantic and episodic components of the traumatic memory are reconnected, the frequency and the severity of the PTSD symptoms decrease in adults and children (Lely et al., 2019; Peltonen & Kangaslampi, 2019).

NET and KIDNET (a version for children) have been extensively researched, and they have been shown to be effective in reducing the frequency and severity of PTSD symptoms. KIDNET is reportedly one of the most promising and best-studied treatment approaches for war-affected children with PTSD and has generally caused a clinically significant improvement in treated children (Wilker et al., 2020). Treatment studies have demonstrated that KIDNET can be effectively delivered not only by mental health professionals but also by teachers and lay-workers who have received training (Robjant & Fazel, 2010).

Persons receiving NET/KIDNET therapy learn to tell the story of their lives coherently, both the good and bad parts. Because the primary component of KIDNET is developing children's ability to tell coherent personal stories, speech-language professionals (SLPs) can play an important role in this treatment. KIDNET has been used with children aged seven and older with a variety of learning and developmental impairments (Fazel et al., 2020). Typical KIDNET interventions are 8–12 weeks long, but children with language/learning impairments, including deficits in narrative skills and deficits in knowledge of basic emotions and self-regulation strategies, will likely require more time to develop the necessary skills to achieve the most benefit from KIDNET.

Schauer et al. (2017) provide a detailed description of the KIDNET steps. In KIDNET, the clinician and the child create a timeline of the child's life and then elaborate on the events. At the end of therapy, children receive a written narrative of their lives. The clinician will need to interview children's caregivers to know the events to include. The core component of KIDNET is to assign each traumatic and important event in the child's life to a corresponding spatial and temporal context. The child is assisted in putting both positive and negative life events on a biographic timeline. A piece of rope or ribbon is put on the floor or on a table. One end of the rope represents "birth," the unfolded line represents the course of life, and the other end of the ribbon, which is rolled up or has three dots on it indicates the future yet to come. The clinician assists the child in placing flowers along the ribbon to represent positive experiences (e.g., moments of joy, achievements) and then stones to represent negative experiences (moments of fear, horror, sadness, loss). Two addition symbols can be placed on the ribbon to represent experiences: sticks for active involvement in aggressive acts (acts of violence or aggression, e.g., fights, delinquency, combat) and candles for life moments when the child experienced a loss. (see Figure 3.2). The clinician explains the significance of the symbols using child-appropriate labels and descriptions. To facilitate the child's organization of the story, clinicians might teach story grammar components, using icons to help the child know what information to include. Attention is given to the time, place, and emotions associated with the events. In so doing, children integrate the sensory/emotional/perceptual aspects of their episodic autobiographical memory with the time and place of their semantic autobiographical memory. Traumatic events are explored slowly, with questioning of multiple sensory, cognitive, emotional, and physiological information and with active linking to the "cold" memory with contextual information that, due to the high physiological arousal levels, was poorly encoded at the time of the trauma. Questions can be used to facilitate memory retrieval for both cold (semantic) and hot (episodic) memory components.

If educators and speech-language professionals have not had NET/KID-NET training or training in trauma-focused interventions, they should be cautious about asking children to narrate highly emotional traumatic experiences because they are likely not to have the necessary strategies to adequately support children in this task. Remember, however, that children who have experienced trauma are highly likely to exhibit the same types of fragmented narratives when telling past pleasant experiences, even recent pleasant experiences. Educators and speech-language professionals can assist children in learning to tell coherent stories about everyday events and "flower" events in their lives by employing the KIDNET memory retrieval

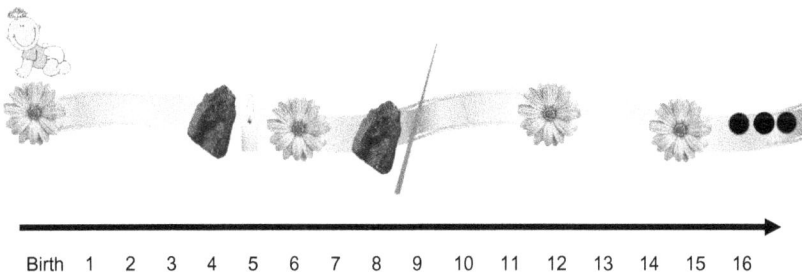

Figure 3.2 KIDNET Timeline ©Carol Westby.

framework. They can begin by reminiscing with children about experiences they have shared with them. Table 3.5 shows KIDNET questions to facilitate retrieval of semantic and episodic autobiographical memories, with an example from a child reminiscing with an adult about a pleasant experience - a trip to a hot-air balloon fiesta. The clinician supports the child in remembering the episodic details of the experience and linking those with the semantic details of time, place, and chronology (Table 3.5).

NET/KIDNET is proving effective with children and adults from diverse cultures (e.g., Afghanistan, Iraq, Korea, Rwanda, Somalia, Syria [Neuner et al., 2008; Nose et al., 2017; Park et al., 2020]). Although there are cultural variations in the expression of PTSD symptoms, trauma reactions are universal phenomena because they result from neurobiological processes to threat and stress. Neuner and colleagues (Neuner et al., 2018), developers of NET, explain they believe that NET/KIDNET is effective across cultures because all cultures have stories. They maintain that hearing and sharing personal histories is a cultural practice that helps survivors of trauma cope with life events and fosters interpersonal closeness.

The importance of personal stories is reflected in the novel, *Ceremony*, by Leslie Marmon Silko (1977), an indigenous author. Silko introduces her novel with the statement, *I will tell you something about stories. They*

Table 3.5 KIDNET Framework for Remembering

Cold memory/context: semantic memories for time/place		
Space	Where did it happen?	Balloon Fiesta Park, Albuquerque, NM
Time	When did it happen?	1st Saturday October/fall; early morning
Chronology	What happened? What happened next?	Went to balloon fiesta; Watched balloons inflate; ate donuts; got in basket; took off; flew; landed

Hot memory: episodic memories for emotions and sensory experiences		
Sensory	What did you see, touch, taste, hear, smell?	Sound of fan/burner; heat from burner; loud sound when burner cord pulled; cars/trees looked so small
Cognitive	What did you think?	Where will we go? How does the pilot drive the balloon? How will we get down?
Emotional	How did you feel?	Scared/worried; excited; happy
Physiological	How did your body react?	Shakey

aren't just entertainment. Don't be fooled. They are all we have, you see all we have to fight off illness and death. You don't have anything if you don't have stories (Silko, 1977, p. 2). The main character in her story, Tayo, a Native American, has returned from World War II suffering from "battle fatigue" (PTSD). It is through participating in the ceremonies of his culture (ritual reenactments of the myths/stories of his culture) that Tayo is ultimately healed. While diagnostic instruments need to be carefully adapted for each language, only minor modifications in the NET procedure are required when this approach is implemented across cultures. The NET/KIDNET approach recognizes that each trauma survivor holds a wide variety of values and attitudes, and comes from differing economic and educational backgrounds. In NET/KIDNET, the client generates their story as they have experienced it; and the clinician does not attempt to interpret the stories from a Western perspective (Schnyder et al., 2016). When employing NET/KIDNET, clinicians can demonstrate a genuine interest in the values, beliefs, and experiences of children and families.

3.10   Conclusion

The Pew Research Center projects that, by 2050, more than one-third of the nation's schoolchildren younger than 17 will either be immigrants themselves or the children of at least one parent who is an immigrant. Given these demographics, schools will need to rethink classroom strategies, family engagement practices, and how to best navigate cultural divides. School personnel need to be aware of the potential long-term effects of the trauma experiences associated with migration and resettlement. Migrant and refugee children are at risk for both under- and over-identification of learning problems and social/emotional difficulties.

Appropriate assessment is essential so that the children's and adolescents' needs are adequately addressed. Trauma-sensitive schools can be particularly beneficial for these students. "A trauma-sensitive school is a safe and supportive community that enables both students and adult to feel safe, build caring relationships with one another, regulate their feelings and behavior, as well as learn" (Alexander, 2019, p. 65). Increasingly, schools and school districts are becoming trauma sensitive by equipping all staff to: understand and recognize child stressors, provide trauma-sensitive responses and supports, understand the challengers of relocation and acculturation, be sensitive to family stressors, and identify children at risk, and understand views regarding mental health (National Association of School Psychologists, 2015). Trauma-sensitive schools provide a hierarchy of tiered services from school-wide services designed to recognize trauma and build resilience in all students, to small group sessions to target skills, to individual mental health sessions. If school personnel are to interpret students' behaviors appropriately and respond in helpful ways, they must develop cultural competence, having an understanding of the students' and their families' cultural values and belief systems and how these systems influence students' responses to trauma and intended support systems.

Although teachers and speech-language pathologists typically do not have the training to assist students in the emotional recounting of their trauma stories, they can facilitate students' development of the vocabulary and narrative content, and narrative organization to recount pleasant events they have experienced recently in school, the community, or with their families. In this way, they provide the foundations students can use to share their life stories coherently, and in so doing, they can begin to heal from the trauma.

References

Alexander, J. (2019). *Building trauma-sensitive schools*. Brookes.

American Psychiatric Association. (2013). *Diagnostic and statistical manual of mental disorders* (5th ed.). American Psychiatric Association.

Bakermans-Kranenburg, M. J., & van IJzendoorn, M. H. (2008). Oxytocin receptor (OXTR) and serotonin transporter (5-HTT) genes associated with observed parenting. *Social Cognitive Affective Neuroscience, 3*(2), 128–134. https://doi.org/10.1093/scan/nsn004

Banoğlu, K., & Korkmazlar, U. (2022). Efficacy of the eye movement desensitization and reprocessing group protocol with children in reducing posttraumatic stress disorder in refugee children. *European Journal of Trauma & Dissociation, 6*(1), 100241. https://doi.org/10.1016/j.ejtd.2021.100241

Betancourt, T. S., Newnham, E. A., Birman, D., Lee, R., Ellis, H., & Layne, C. M. (2017). Comparing trauma exposure, mental health needs, and service utilization across clinical samples of refugee, immigrant, and U.S.-origin children. *Journal of Trauma and Trauma Stress, 30*(3), 209–218. https://doi.org/10.1002/jts.22186

Bettmann, J. E., Penney, D., Clarkson Freeman, P., & Lecy, N. (2015). Somali refugees' perceptions of mental illness. *Social Work in Health Care, 54*(8), 738–757. https://doi.org/10.1080/00981389.2015.1046578

Carmiol, A. M., & Sparks, A. (2014). Narrative development across cultural contexts: Finding the pragmatic in parent-child reminiscing. In D. Matthews (Ed.), *Pragmatic development in first language acquisition* (pp. 279–293). John Benjamín. https://doi.org/10.1075/tilar.10

Caspi, A., McClay, J., Moffitt, T. E., Mill, J., Martin, J., Craig, I. W., Taylor, A., & Poulton, R. (2002). Role of genotype in the cycle of violence in maltreated children. *Science, 297*, 851–854. https://doi.org/10.1126/science.1072290

Causadias, J. M., Telzer, E. H., & Gonzales, N. A. (2018). *Handbook of culture and biology*. John Wiley & Sons. https://doi.org/10.1002/9781119181361

Chiao, J. Y., & Blizinsky, K. D. (2010). Culture–gene coevolution of individualism–collectivism and the serotonin transporter gene. *Proceedings of the Royal Society B: Biological Sciences, 277*, 529–537. https://doi.org/10.1098/rspb.2009.1650

Chiao, J. Y., Cheon, B. K., Pornpattanangkul, N., Mrazek, A. J., & Blizinsky, K. S. (2009). Neural basis of individualistic and collectivistic views of self. *Human Brain Mapping, 30*, 2813–2820. https://doi.org/10.1002/hbm.20707

Chiao, J. Y., Li, S., Seligman, R., & Turner, R. (2016). *The Oxford handbook of cultural neuroscience.* Oxford. https://doi.org/10.1093/oxfordhb/9780199357376.001.0001

Chipalo, E. (2021). Is trauma-focus cognitive behavioral therapy (TF-CBT) effect in reducing trauma symptoms among traumatized refugee children? A systematic review. *Journal of Child and Adolescent Trauma, 14*, 545–558. https://doi.org/10.1007/s40653-021-00370-0

Cohen, D., & Gunz, A. (2002). As seen by the other...: Perspectives on the self in the memories and emotional perceptions of easterners and westerners. *Psychological Science, 13*(1), 55–59. https://doi.org/10.1111/1467–9280.00409

Conway, M., & Pleydell-Pearce, C. (2000). The construction of autobiographical memories in 757 the self-memory system. *Psychological Review, 107*(2), 261–288.

Dawson, K. S., & Bryant, R. A. (2016). Children's vantage point of recalling traumatic events. *PLoS One, 11*(9), e0162030. https://doi.org/10.1371/journal.pone.0162030

Dinos, S., Ascoli, M., Owiti, J. A., & Bhui, K. (2017). Assessing explanatory models and health beliefs: An essential but overlooked competency for clinicians. *British Journal of Psychological Advances, 23*, 106–114 https://doi.org/10.1192/apt.bp.114.013680

Doost, H. T. N., Yule, W., Kalantari, N. M., Rezvani, S. R., Dyregrov, T., & Jobson, L. (2014). Reduced autobiographical memory specificity in bereaved Afghan adolescents. *Memory, 22*(6), 700–709. https://doi.org/10.1080/09658211.2013.817590

Fazel, M., Stratford, H. J., Rowsell, E., Chan, C., Griffiths, H., & Robjant, K. (2020). Five applications of narrative exposure therapy for children and adolescents presenting with post-traumatic stress disorders. *Frontiers in Psychology, 11*(19). https://doi.org/10.3389/fpsyt.2020.00019

Fivush, R. (2011). The development of autobiographical memory. *Annual Review of Psychology, 2*, 559–582. https://doi.org/10.1146/annurev.psych.121208.131702

Fivush, R. (2019). *Family narrative and the development of autobiographical memory: Social and cultural perspectives on autobiographical memory.* Routledge.

Gervai, J., Novak, A., Lakatos, K., Toth, I. D., Ronai, Z., Nebidam, Z., Sasvari-Szekely, M., Bureau, J., Bronfman, E., & Yons-Ruth, K. (2007). Infant genotype may moderate sensitivity to maternal affective communications: Attachment disorganization, quality of care, and the DRD4 polymorphism. *Social Neuroscience, 2*, 307–319. https://doi.org/10.1080/17470910701391893

Given-Wilson, Z., Hodes, M., & Herlihy, J. (2018). A review of adolescent autobiographical memory and the implications for assessment of unaccompanied minors' refugee determinations. *Clinical Child Psychiatry, 23*(2), 209–222.

Graham, B., Herlihy, J., & Brewin, C. (2014). Overgeneral memory in asylum seekers and refugees. *Journal of Behavioral Therapy and Experimental Psychiatry, 45*, 375–380.

Graham, H. R., Minhas, R. S., & Paxton, G. (2016). Learning problems in children of refugees: A systematic review. *Pediatrics, 37*(6), e20153994. https://doi.org/10.1542/peds.2015-3994

Gredeback, G., Haas, S., Hall, J., Pollack, S., Karakus, D. C., & Lindskog, M. (2018). Social cognition in refugee children: An experimental cross-sectional study of emotional processing with Syrian families with Syrian families in Turkish communities, *Royal Society Open Science, 8*, 210362. https://doi.org/10.1098/rros.210362

Gross, J. J., & John, O. P. (2003). Individual differences in two emotion regulation processes: Implications for affect, relationships, and wellbeing. *Journal of Personality and Social Psychology, 85*, 348–362. https://doi.org/10.1037/0022-3514.85.2.348

Heim, E., Karatzias, T., & Maercker, A. (2022). Cultural concepts of distress and complex PTSD: Future directions for research and treatment. *Clinical Psychology Review, 93*, 102143. https://doi.org/10.1016/j.cpr.2022.102143

Herlihy, J., Jobson, L., & Turner, A. (2012). Just tell us what happened to you: Autobiographical memory and seeking asylum. *Applied Cognitive Psychology, 26*, 661–676.

Herlihy, J., Scragg, P., & Turner, S. (2002). Discrepancies in autobiographical memories: Implications for the assessment of asylum seekers: Repeated interviews study. *British Medical Journal, 324*, 324–327.

Hinton, D., & Bui, E. (2019). Cultural considerations in anxiety and related disorders. In B. Olatunji (Ed.), *The Cambridge handbook of anxiety and related disorders* (pp. 394–418). Cambridge: Cambridge University Press. https://doi.org/10.1017/9781108140416.015

Hinton, D. E., & Patel, A. (2018). Culturally sensitive CBT for Refugees: Key dimensions: Theory, research and clinical practice. In N. Morina & A. Nickerson (eds.), *Mental health of refugee and conflict-affected populations*. Springer. https://doi.org/10.1007/978-3-319-97046-2_10

Hofstede, G. (1980). *Culture's consequences: International differences in work-related values*. Beverly Hills, CA: Sage.

Hofstede, G., Hofstede, G. J., & Mickov, M. (2010). *Cultures and organizations: Software of the mind*. McGraw-Hill.

Im, H., Ferwguson, A., & Hunter, M. (2017). Cultural translation of refugee trauma: Cultural idioms of distress among Somali refugees in displacement. *Transcultural Psychiatry, 44*(5–6), 626–652.

Kelly, K. R. (2015). Insecure attachment representations and child personal narrative structure: Implications for delayed discourse in preschool-age children. *Attachment & Human Development, 17*(5), 448–471.

Khalifa, N., Hardie, T., Latif, S., Jamil, I., & Walker, D.-M. (2011). Beliefs about Jinn, black magic and the evil eye among Muslims: Age gender and first language influences. *International Journal of Culture and Mental Health, 4*, https://doi.org/10.1080/17542863.2010.503051

Khan, S., Kuhn, S. K., & Haque, S. (2021). A systematic review of autobiographical memory and mental health research on refugees and asylum seekers. *Frontiers in Psychology, 12*, 658700. https://doi.org/10.3389/fpsyt.2021.658700

Kim, H. S., & Sasaki, J. Y. (2012). Emotion regulation: The interplay of culture and genes. *Social and Personality Psychology Compass, 6*, 865–877. https://doi.org/10.1111/spc3.12003

Kim, H. S., & Sherman, D. K. (2007). "Express yourself": Culture and the effect of self-expression on choice. *Journal of Personality and Social Psychology, 92*, 1–11. https://doi.org/10.1037/0022–3514.92.1.1

Kim, H. S., Sherman, D. K., Mojaverian, T., Sasaki, J. Y., Park, J., Suh, E. M., & Taylor, S. E. (2011). Gene-culture interaction: Oxytocin receptor polymorphism (OXTR) and emotion regulation. *Social Psychological and Personality Science, 2*, 665–672. https://doi.org/10.1177/1948550611405854

Kim, H. S., Sherman, D. K., Taylor, S. E., Sasaki, J. Y., Chu, T. Q., Ryu, C., Suh, E. M., & Xu, J. (2010). Culture, serotonin receptor polymorphism and locus of attention. *Social Cognitive Affective Neuroscience, 5*(2–3), 212–218. https://doi.org/10.1093/scan/nsp040

Kitayama, S., Mesquita, B., & Karasawa, M. (2006). Cultural affordances and emotional experience: Socially engaging and disengaging emotions in Japan and the United States. *Journal of Personality and Social Psychology, 91*, 890–903. https://doi.org/10.1037/0022–3514.91.5.890

Kleinman, A. (1980). *Patients and healers in the context of culture: An exploration of the borderland between anthropology, medicine, and psychiatry.* University of California Press.

Lackner, C., Sabbagh, M. A., Hallinan, E., Liu, X., & Holden, J. A. (2012). Dopamine receptor D4 gene variation predicts preschoolers' developing theory of mind. *Developmental Science, 15*, 272–280. https://doi.org/10.1111/j.1467–7687.2011.01124.x

Lapidow, E. S., & Brown, A. D. (2015). Autobiographical memories and PTSD. In C. R. Martin, V. R. Preedy, & V. B. Patel (Eds.), *Comprehensive guide to post-traumatic stress disorder* (pp. 131–146). Springer. https://doi.org/10.1007/978-3-319-08613-2_117-1

Leichtman, M. D., Wang, Q., & Pillemer, D. B. (2003). Cultural variations in interdependence and autobiographical memory. In R. Fivush & C. A. Haden (Eds.), *Autobiographical memory and the construction of a narrative sef* (pp. 73–97). Erlbaum.

Lely, J. C. G., Smid, G. E., Jongedijk, R. A., Knipscheer, J. W., & Kleber, R. J. (2019). The effectiveness of narrative exposure therapy: A review, meta-analysis and meta-regression analysis. *European Journal of Psychotraumatology, 10*, 1550344. https://doi.org/10.1080/20008198.2018.1550344

Lewis-Fernández, R., Aggarwal, N. K., Hinton, L., Hinton, D. E., & Kirmayer, L. J. (2016). *DM-5 Handbook on the cultural formulation interview.* American Psychiatric Association.

Martin, M., & Jones (2012). Individualism and the field viewpoint: Cultural influences on memory perspective. *Consciousness and Cognition, 21*, 1498–1503. https://doi.org/10.1016/j.concog.2012.04.009

Matsumoto, D., Yoo, S. H., Nakagawa, S., & 37 Members of the multinational study of cultural display rules (2008). Culture, emotion, regulation, and adjustment. *Journal of Personality and Social Psychology, 94*, 925–937. https://doi.org/10.1037/0022–3514.94.6.925

McIsaac, H. K., & Eich, E. (2004). Vantage point in traumatic memory. *Psychological Science, 15*(4), 248–253. ISI:000220383500006. PMID: 15043642

Miyamoto, Y., Ma, X., & Petermann, A. G. (2014). Cultural differences in hedonic emotion regulation after a negative event. *Emotion, 14*(4), 804–815. https://doi.org/10.1037/a0036257

Mollica, R. F., Caridad, K. R., & Massagli, M. P. (2007). Longitudinal study of posttraumatic stress disorder, depression, and changes in traumatic memories over time in Bosnian refugees. *The Journal of Nervous and Mental Disease, 195*(7), 572–579.

Moore, S. A., & Zoellner, L. A. (2007). Overgeneral autobiographical memory and traumatic events: An evaluative review. *Psychological Bulletin, 133*, 419–437.

Munafò, M. R., Clark, T., & Flint, J. (2005). Does measurement instrument moderate the association between the serotonin transporter gene and anxiety-related personality traits? A meta-analysis. *Molecular Psychiatry, 10*, 415–419. https://doi.org/10.1038/sj.mp.4001627

National Association of School Psychologists. (2015). *Supporting refugee children and youth: Tips for educators.* Retrieved from https://www.nasponline.org/resources

Neuner, F., Elbert, T., & Schauer, M. (2018). Narrative exposure therapy (NET) as a treatment for traumatized refugees and post-conflict populations. In N. Morina & A. Nickerson (Eds.), *Mental health of refugee and conflict-affected populations.* Springer Nature. https://doi.org/10.1007/978-3-319-97046-2_9

Neuner, F., Onyut, P. L., Ertl, V., Odenwald, M., Schauer, E., & Elbert, T. (2008). Treatment of posttraumatic stress disorder by trained lay counselors in an African refugee settlement: A randomized controlled trial. *Journal of Consulting and Clinical Psychology, 76*(4), 686–694. https://doi.org/10.1037/0022-006X.76.4.686

Nievergelt, C. M., & the Psychiatric Genomics Consortium (2019). International meta-analysis of PTSD genome-wide association studies identifies sex- and ancestry specific genetic risk loci. *Nature Communications, 10*, 4558. https://doi.org/10.1038/s41467-019-12576-w

Nisbett, R. E., & Masuda, T. (2003). Culture and point of view. *Proceedings of the National Academy of Sciences, 100*, 11163–11170. https://doi.org/10.1073/pnas.1934527100

Nose, M., Ballette, F., Bighelli, I., Turrini, G., Purgato, M., Tol, W., Priebe, S., & Barbul, C. (2017). Psychosocial interventions for post-traumatic stress disorder in refugees and asylum seekers resettled in high-income countries: Systematic review and meta-analysis. *PLoS ONE, 12*(2), e0171030. https://doi.org/10.1371/journal.pone.0171030

Okello, J., Nakimuli-Mpungu, E., Musisi, S., Broekaert, E., & Derluyn, I. (2014). The association between attachment and mental health symptoms among school-going adolescents in northern Uganda: The moderating role of war-related trauma. *PLoS ONE, 9*(3), e88494. https://doi.org/10.1371/journal.pone.0088494

Park, J. K., Park, J., Elbert, T., & Kim, S. J. (2020). Effects of narrative exposure therapy on posttraumatic stress disorder, depression, and insomnia in traumatized North Korean refugee youth. *Journal of Traumatic Stress.* https://doi.org/10.1002/jts.22492

Patel, A. R., & Hall, B. J. (2021). Beyond the DSM-5 diagnosis: A cross-cultural approach to assessing trauma reactions. *Focus on Psychiatry, 19*(2), 197–203.

Peltonen, K., & Kangaslampi, S. (2019). Treating children and adolescents with multiple traumas: A randomized clinical trial of narrative exposure therapy. *European Journal of Psychotraumatology, 10*, 1558708. https://doi.org/10.1080/2 0008198.2018.1558708

Piwowarczyk, L., Bishop, H., Yusuf, A., Mudymba, F., & Raj, A. (2014). Congolese and Somali beliefs about mental health services. *Journal of Nervous and Mental Disease, 202*(3), 209–216. https://doi.org/10.1097/NMD.0000000000000087

Punamäki, R., Qouta, S. R., & Peltonen, K. (2018). Family systems approach to attachment relations, war trauma, and mental health among Palestinian children and parents. *European Journal of Psychotraumatology, 8*, 1439649. https://doi.org/10.1080/20008198.2018.1439649

Refugee Health Technical Assistance (no date). Mental health. Retrieved from https://refugeehealthta.org/physical-mental-health/mental-health/

Robjant, K., & Fazel, M. (2010). The emerging evidence for narrative exposure therapy: A review. *Clinical Psychology Review, 30*(8), 1030–1039. https://doi.org/10.1016/j.cpr.2010.07.004

Ruby, M. B., Falk, C. F., Hine, S. J., Villa, C., & Silberstein, O. (2012). Not all collectivisms are equal: Opposing preferences for idea affect between East Asians and Mexicans. *Emotions, 12*, 1206–1209. https://doi.org/10.1037/a0029118

Ruf, M., Schauer, M., Neuner, F., Catani, C., Schauer, E., & Elbert, T. (2010). Narrative exposure therapy for 7-to 16-year-olds: A randomized controlled trial with traumatized refugee children. *Journal of Traumatic Stress, 23*(4), 437–445. https://doi.org/10.1002/jts.20548

Sagbakken, M., Bregard, I. M., & Varvin, S. (2020). The past, the present, and the future: A qualitative study exploring how refugees' experience of time influences their mental health and well-being. *Frontiers in Sociology, 5*, 46. https://doi.org/10.3389/fsoc.2020.00046

Sasaki, J. Y., & Kim, H. S. (2017). Nature, nurture, and their interplay: A review of cultural neuroscience. *Journal of Cross-Cultural Psychology, 48*(1), 4–22. https://doi.org/10.1177/0022022116680481

Schauer, M., Neuner, F., & Elbert, T. (2011). *Narrative exposure therapy: A short term treatment for traumatic stress disorders* (2nd edition). Hogrefe Publishing.

Schauer, M., Neuner, F., & Elbert, T. (2017). Narrative exposure therapy for children and adolescents (KIDNET). In M. A. Landolt, M. Cloitre, & U. Schnyder (Eds.), *Evidence-based treatments for trauma related disorders in children and adolescents* (pp. 227–249). Springer International. https://doi.org/10.1007/978-3-319-46138-0_11

Schauer, M., & Schauer, E. (2010). Trauma-focused public mental-health interventions: A paradigm shift in humanitarian assistance and aid work. In. E. Martz (Ed.), *Trauma rehabilitation after war and conflict* (pp. 389–428). Springer. https://doi.org/10.10007/978-1-4419–5722-116

Schnyder, U., Bryant, R. A., Ehlers, A., Foa, E. B., Hasan, A., Mwiti, G., Kristensen, G. H., Neuner, F., Oe, M., & Yule, W. (2016). Culture-sensitive psychotraumatology. *European Journal of Psychotraumatology, 7*, 31179. https://doi.org/10.3402/ejpt.v7.31179

Schönfeld, S., Ehlers, A., Böllinghaus, I., & Rief, W. (2007). Overgeneral memory and suppression of trauma memories in posttraumatic stress disorder. *Memory, 15,* 339–352.

Senzaki, S., Masuda, T., & Nand, K. (2014). Holistic versus analytic expressions in artworks: Cross-cultural differences and similarities in drawings and collages by Canadian and Japanese school-age children. *Journal of Cross-Cultural Psychology, 45*(8), 1297–1316. https://doi.org/10.1177/0022022114537704

Shannon, P. L., Wieling, E., Simmerlink-McCleary, J., & Becher, H. (2015). Beyond stigma: Barriers to discussing mental health in refugee populations. *Journal of Loss and Trauma, 20*(3), 281–296. https://doi.org/10.1080/15325024.2014.934629

Siegel, D. J. (2012). *The developing mind* (2nd ed). Guilford.

Silko, L. M. (1977). *Ceremony*. Penguin.

Sim, A., Fazel, M., Bowes, L., & Garner, F. (2018). Pathways linking war and displacement to parenting and child adjustment: A qualitative study with Syrian refugees in Lebanon. *Social Science & Medicine, 200,* 19–26.

Sims, T., Koopermann-Holm, B., Young, H., Jiang, D., Fung, H., & Tsai, J. L. (2018). Asian Americans respond less favorably to excitement (vs. calm)-focused physicians compared to European Americans. *Culture Diversity & Ethnic Minority Psychology, 24*(1), 1–14. https://doi.org/10.1037/cdp0000171

Sims, T., Tsai, J. L., Koopermann-Holm, B., Thomas, E., & Goldstein, M. (2014). Choosing a physician depends on how to want to feel: The role of ideal affect in health related decision-making. *Emotion, 14,* 187–192. https://doi.org/10.1037/a0034372

Slewa-Younan, S., Mond, J., Bussion, E., Mohammad, Y., Uribe, M. G. G., Smith, M., Milosevic, D., Lujic, S., & Jorm, A. F. (2014). Mental health literacy of resettled Iraqi refugees in Australia: Knowledge about posttraumatic stress disorder and beliefs about helpfulness of interventions. *BMC Psychiatry, 14,* Article 320. https://doi.org/10.1186/s12888-014-0320-x

Sullivan, M. W., Bennett, D. S., Carpenter, K., & Lewis, M. (2008). Emotion knowledge in young neglected children. *Child Maltreatment, 13*(3), 301–306. https://doi.org/10.1177/1077559507313725

Tamir, M., Schwartz, S. H., Cieciuch, J., Riediger, M., Torres, C., Scollon, C., & Vishkin, A. (2016). Desired emotions across cultures: A value-based account. *Journal of Personality and Social Psychology, 111*(1), 67–82. https://doi.org/10.1037/pspp0000072

Taylor, S. E., Sherman, D. K., Kim, H. S., Jarcho, J., Takagi, K., & Dunagan, M. S. (2004). Culture and social support: Who seeks it and why? *Journal of Personality and Social Psychology, 87*(3), 354–362. https://doi.org/10.1037/0022-3514.87.3.354

Tozer, M., Khawaja, N. G., & Schweitzer, R. (2017). Protective factors contributing to well-being among refugee youth in Australia. *Journal of Psychologists and Counsellors in Schools, 28*(1), 66–83. https://doi.org/10.1017/jgc.2016.31

TRAC. (2022). *TRAC Immigration*. Retrieved from https://trac.syr.edu/immigration/reports/630/

Tsai, J. L., & Clobert, M. (2019). Cultural influences on emotions: Established patterns and emerging trends. In C. Cohen & S. Kitayama (Eds.), *Handbook of cultural psychology* (pp. 292–318). Guilford Press.

United Nations High Commission for Refugees. (2023). *Global Appeal*. Retrieved from https://reporting.unhcr.org/globalappeal2023

Vanderveren, E., Bijttebier, P., & Hermans, D. (2017). The importance of memory specificity and memory coherence for the self: Linking two characteristics of autobiographical memory. *Frontiers in Psychology, 82*, 2250. https://doi.org/10.3389/fpsyg.2017.02250

Vindevogel, S. (2017). Resilience in the context of war: A critical analysis of contemporary conceptions and interventions to promote resilience among war-affected children and their surroundings. *Peace and Conflict: Journal of Peace Psychology, 23*(1), 76–84. https://doi.org/10.1037/pac0000214

Wang, Q. (2014). The cultured self and remembering. In P. J. Bauer & R. Fivush (Eds.), *The Wiley handbook on the development of children's memory* (pp. 605–625). John Wiley.

Watson, L. A., & Bernsten, D. (Eds.) (2015). *Clinical perspectives on autobiographical memory*. Cambridge.

Wilker, S., Catani, C., Wittmann, J., Preusse, M., Schmidt, T., May, T., Ertl, V., Doering, B., Rosner, R., Zindler, A., & Neuner, F. (2020). The efficacy of narrative exposure therapy for children (KIDNET) as a treatment for traumatized young refugees versus treatment as usual: Study protocol for a multi-center randomized controlled trial. *Trials, 21*, 185. https://doi.org/10.1186/s13063-020-4127-4

World Health Organization. (2018). *International classification of diseases for mortality and morbidity statistics* (11th Revision). https://icd.who.int/browse11/l-m/en

Wu, Y., He, Z., & Jobson, L. (2020). Maternal reminiscing and autobiographical memory features of mother-child dyads in a cross-cultural context. *Child Development, 91*(6), 2160–2177.

4 Post-Traumatic Stress, the Brain, and Social Pragmatic Communication

Yvette D. Hyter

4.1 Post-Traumatic Stress

Trauma is the long-term impact of an event (or series of events) or experience(s) that cause one to experience hopelessness, helplessness, feelings of powerlessness, and a profound sense of loss (SAMHSA, 2022; van der Kolk, 2015). It is how a person, in this case a child, internalizes those experiences or events and the long-term effects on the child's self-perception, as well as their perception of their world. van der Kolk (2015) states that "trauma is not just an event that took place sometime in the past; it is also the imprint left by that experience on the mind, brain, and body." (p. 21).

There are different types of traumas– acute trauma, chronic trauma, complex trauma, and systemic trauma (Dass-Brailsford, 2020; Haines, 2019; NCTSN, n.d.; van der Kolk, 2015). Acute trauma occurs as a single or individual event (van der Kolk, 2015). An acute trauma occurs during a one-time or individual event or experience, such as the collapse of one's apartment building. Such an event recently occurred in Miami, Florida, when part of a 12-story beachfront condominium collapsed (NPR, 2023). Other events that can cause acute trauma are events such as a car accident or an assault. Chronic trauma is when there is repeated violence, such as what happens during war, combat, bullying, or domestic violence (Dass-Brailsford, 2020). Currently, several wars are occurring in the world and individuals who are soldiers, as well as individuals living in a war-torn environment, experience chronic trauma. In the U.S. bullying occurs in person and online. The CDC (2023) reports that one in six high school students are cyberbullied in a year, and both cyberbullying and in-person bullying happen more often in middle school than in other grades. About 40% of high school students who are members of the LGBTQIA+ communities are bulled (CDC, 2023). Additionally, neurodivergent children, as well as children with disabilities, are bullied more often than other school-aged children (Kritz, 2022; Long, 2019).

DOI: 10.4324/9781003225270-5

Complex trauma results from continuing exposure to traumatic events within the caregiving system caused by persons living in the child's household and includes such events as maltreatment like abuse and or neglect (NCTSN, n.d.). This type of trauma often impacts the child's ability to form relationships with others, have positive self-perceptions, and frequently negatively impact developmental and academic outcomes if not supported. As of 2021, the Child Maltreatment Report (USDHHS - ACF, 2023) reveals that in the U. S. 600,000 children in 2021 were victims of child maltreatment. The youngest children were victimized at the highest rates, and more girls were victimized than boys. Although abuse occurs across all socioeconomic strata and ethnic and racial groups, children of color are disproportionally represented in the child welfare system. This is true at all levels of the child welfare system in the U. S. (Children's Defense Fund, 2023), and these families are "subject to higher rates of investigation, are at higher risk of confirmed mistreatment and placement into care and receive disparate treatment while in care" (Children's Defense Fund, 2023, Paragraph 4, Lines 3–5).

Systemic trauma is perpetuated by society and includes events and experiences such as racism and other forms of systemic exclusion, forceful displacement (as what happens with individuals who are refugees), impoverishment, and homelessness. Haines (2019) states that

Systemic trauma is the repeated, ongoing violation, exploitation, dismissal or, and/or deprivation of groups of people. States institutes, economic systems and social norms that systematically deny people access to safety mobility, resources, food, education, dignity, positive reflections of themselves, and belonging have a traumatic impact on individuals and groups.

(p. 80)

In many societies today, the causes of systemic traumas are plentiful. Impoverishment, for example, is "about power, not scarcity" (OXFAM, 2023, paragraph 1, line 1). In the U. S. in 2022, the U. S. Census indicated that there were 37.9 million people in the US who were impoverished (Shrider & Creamer, 2023). About 108.4 million people are forcibly displaced from their homes across and within their country's borders (UNHCR, 2023) (Westby, in Chapter 3, expounds on the traumatic nature of becoming an immigrant and refugee forcibly displaced.)

4.1.1 Levels of Stress

Our bodies are designed to help us respond to stress (van der Kolk, 2015), but when that stress becomes toxic, our bodies and brains become overwhelmed and cannot respond in the ways they were designed (Nelson et al., 2020). Stress can be positive, tolerable, or toxic (Burke Harris, 2018; Heramis, 2020) Positive stress is the typical body's response system and is a part of healthy development. Figure 4.1 shows what a typical stress response might look like. One will experience increased heart rate and adrenaline, which enhances one's focus. An example of positive stress is the first time a child is left with a babysitter (Heramis, 2020), or the stress an introvert might feel when going to a party where they do not know anyone.

Tolerable stress is occurring when an event or experience happens that activates the body's alert system on a short-term basis. Once your body senses danger, the brainstem, hypothalamus, and amygdala work together releasing hormones that initiate the fight flight or freeze response. Adrenaline, released from the adrenal glands, is instrumental is helping us prepare for the possibility of needing to fight or run (flight). This hormone increases blood flow to muscles and increases our capacity for breathing. The impact is temporary if there is a support system in place, such as the co-regulation of a caring person (Heramis, 2020).

Toxic stress is sustained activation of a stress response (Nelson et al., 2020). It occurs when the body is stuck in a feedback loop of stress without any relief. For example, Nadine Burke Harris (2018) gives the example of being chased by a bear, and then when you get to safety (your home for example) you find that the bear is living inside your house. In this situation, one would likely be worried all the time, unable to sleep or eat, be hypervigilant about where the bear was and when or whether it would attack. The stress feedback loop (as depicted in Figure 4.1) does not turn off, and one's stress is prolonged, which has significant negative effects on the brain (Burke Harris, 2018; Heramis, 2020; Nelson et al., 2020), and can cause post-traumatic stress disorder. Toxic stress can cause permanent changes in the body, brain, and mind (Murphy et al., 2022).

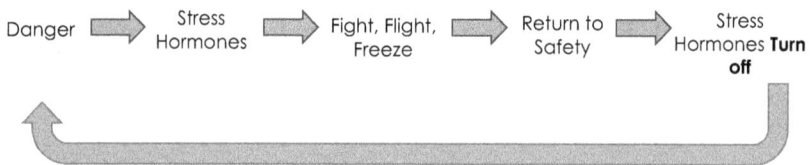

Danger ⇒ Stress Hormones ⇒ Fight, Flight, Freeze ⇒ Return to Safety ⇒ Stress Hormones **Turn off**

Figure 4.1 Schematic of Typical Stress Response.
Source: Hyter (2021)

4.1.2   *Stress and the Brain*

Some structures in the brain are particularly affected by toxic stress. Those structures include the limbic system, including the amygdala mentioned earlier, locus coeruleus, and the prefrontal cortex.

4.1.2.1 *Limbic System*

The limbic system deals with emotions and memory. Burke Harris (2018) label the limbic systems the "fear center" (p. 49) and van der Kolk (2015) indicates it is the "seat of emotions, the monitor of danger, the judge of what is pleasurable or scary, the arbiter of what is or is not important for survival" (p. 56). Two of the primary structures in the limbic system are the amygdala and the hippocampus.

The amygdala, located inside the brain, serves as a siren, alerts us to danger, helps process emotions, and connects those emotions to memories. Additionally, the amygdala has a role in behavioral control and learning. Thy amygdala sends a message to the hypothalamus which activates the hypothalamic-pituitary-adrenal (HPA) axis, which triggers the release of stress hormones (adrenaline; norepinephrine, the adrenaline released in the brain; and eventually cortisol) triggering the fight or flight stress response (Burke Harris, 2018; Harvard Health Publishing, 2020). When a person is experiencing post-traumatic stress disorder or a toxic-stress response, the amygdala is triggered repeatedly, confusing what situations are scary and which ones are safe. In other words, a chronically stressed amygdala sends false signals to the brain (Burke Harris, 2018; Heramis, 2020; van der Kolk, 2015). Consider the following case excerpt.

Angela[1] was a four-year-old attending preschool who had a history of complex trauma. During the time she was in preschool, she was living with her maternal grandmother. She had difficulty making friends – her classmates were afraid of her because she often started hitting and kicking them, but they did not know why. One morning she was sitting alone in the block area building a structure. One of her peers walked behind her on their way to another play area. Angela's body stiffened as her eyes (using her peripheral vision) followed the movement of the other child from one location to the next play center. Angela then stood up walked over to the child who walked behind her and started kicking her.

Angela was stuck in a toxic-stress feedback loop, which caused all activities around her to be perceived as fearful and dangerous. Kicking and hitting classmates was an adaptive behavior – one that she learned to help her survive daily life.

The hippocampus is a structure that is in the temporal lobe of the brain and is significantly involved in learning, emotions, and various types of memory, and in connecting emotions with memories. The hippocampus plays a role in "registering... events, but also their context" (Goode, 2002, p. 3). When the amygdala senses danger it sends a message to the hippocampus to stop writing and storing new memories, and to stop making connections between memories and sensory and emotional information. When the hippocampus is exposed repeatedly to toxic stress, the stress hormones can alter the cells in the hippocampus (Kim et al., 2007; Kim et al., 2015). Post-traumatic stress can prevent people from accessing memories, create intense recollections of the traumatic event(s) or experience(s), as well as fragment one's memory about event sequences (NICABM, 2017).

4.1.2.2 *Locus Coeruleus*

The locus coeruleus is in the pons in the brain. It is the primary area where norepinephrine is synthesized and plays a role in regulating how much norepinephrine is released in the brain (Burke Harris, 2018). It has fibers that project into the hippocampus, cerebellum, and cerebrum, as well as the hypothalamus and amygdala (Morris et al., 2020). The locus coeruleus plays a role in how one responds to stress, as well as plays a role in attention, mood, memory, and decision making (Burke Harris, 2018). The brain that is subjected to toxic stress, can intensify the locus coeruleus, which may release too much norepinephrine, resulting in hyperarousal, anxiety, limited cognitive flexibility, high levels of reactivity to events or experiences (Burke Harris, 2018; Morris et al., 2020). For example, if the locus coeruleus is activated over a long period of time, such as during post-traumatic stress, one could be easily distracted or highly inattentive, overly reactive to stimuli, have limited abilities to set-shift quickly, and their behavior might be disorganized (Burke Harris, 2018; Unsworty & Robinson, 2017).

4.1.2.3 *Prefrontal Cortex*

The prefrontal cortex is often referred to as "the conductor" of the brain (Burke Harris, 2018, p. 68) or the "breaks" of the brain (Sloane, 2018, slides 7–8). The prefrontal cortex governs our executive functions, the ability to make judgments and decisions, to plan, to focus, inhibit responses and engage in cognitive flexibility, as well as to reflect on our behaviors, anticipate how our actions might affect others, and helps us moderate our emotions. Toxic stress can cause diminished prefrontal cortex abilities. Arnsten (2009) states that:

> it is also the brain region that is most sensitive to the detrimental effects of stress exposure. Even quite mild acute uncontrollable stress can cause a rapid and dramatic loss of prefrontal cognitive abilities, and more prolonged stress exposure causes architectural changes in prefrontal dendrites.
>
> (p. 410)

The impact of toxic stress on the brain has significant implications for social pragmatic communication. In the next section of this chapter, social pragmatic communication is discussed, and the parts of the brain impacted by trauma and post-traumatic stress are mapped onto components of social pragmatic communication.

4.2 Social Pragmatic Communication

Social pragmatic communication is the ability to interpret a social situation, as well as interpret others' points of view, and then use language, communicate, and behave in ways that are consistent with, and therefore, effective in that situation (Adams, 2005; Hyter, 2017). Social pragmatic communication requires the support of various cognitive and communicative skills. Hyter (Hyter, 2012, 2017, 2021; Hyter & Sloane, 2013) created a cognitive conceptual model of social pragmatic communication, updated in 2023 (Hyter, 2023), depicted in Figure 4.2. Figure 4.2 shows that social pragmatic communication has been conceptualized as interdependent relationships among social cognition (i.e., theory of mind, perspective-taking, presupposition), cognitive skills (i.e., executive functions, memory), sensory, emotional, and behavioral regulation, and pragmatics (i.e., speech acts, discourse management, and sociolinguistic abilities such as register shifting, reading the context) (Hyter, 2017). Figure 4.3 shows the cognitive conceptual model of social pragmatic communication with corresponding areas of the brain mapped onto it.

4.2.1 Social Cognition

Social cognition is important for effectively engaging in social interactions (De Lillo & Ferguson, 2023; Kanske & Murray, 2019). It is comprised of theory of mind, perspective-taking, and belief attribution, and the use of internal state language (Hyter, 2021). Theory of mind (ToM) is the ability to infer or attribute mental states (thoughts, emotions, beliefs,

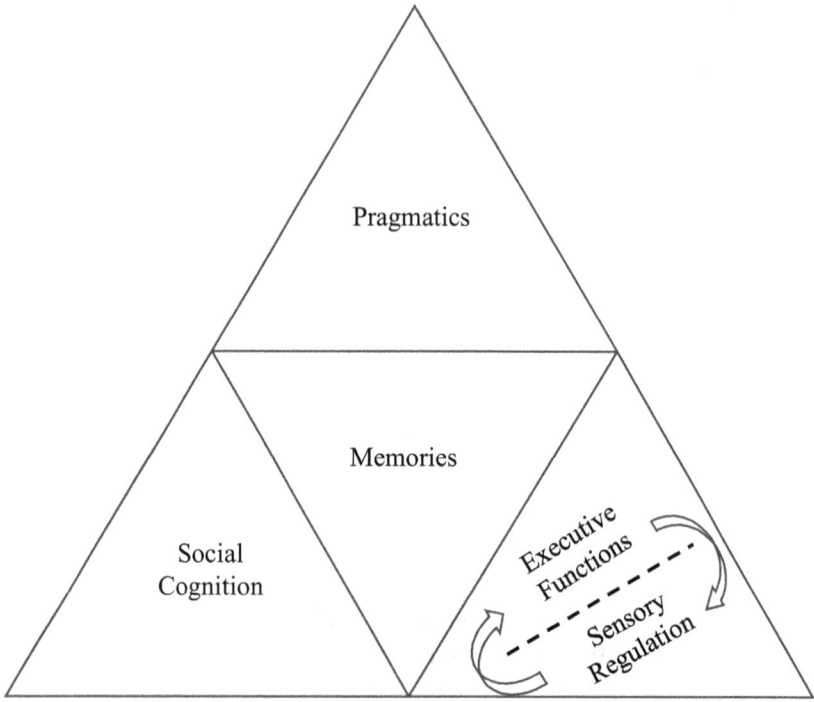

Figure 4.2 Conceptual Model of Social Pragmatic Communication – Version 2.
Source: Hyter (2023)

intentions) to others and to understand them in oneself (Baron-Cohen, 1995; Premack & Woodruff, 1978). ToM has been conceptualized in different ways, but mostly, the focus has been on the cognitive and interpersonal aspects of ToM. The focus has been examining a person's ability to think, recognize, and infer others' mental states (Westby, 2013; Westby & Robinson, 2014). Other aspects, however, are affective ToM, which is the ability to think about and experience emotions, and intrapersonal ToM, the ability to reflect on one's own mental states and emotions (Westby, 2013; Westby & Robinson, 2014).

Perspective-taking is an aspect of ToM and is important for considering others' points of view and is used to generate expectations about one's (as well as others') behaviors (Kanske & Murray, 2019). Using perspective-taking, one can attribute motivations to others' actions. Linguistic perspective-taking is important for understanding written text, plays a role in comprehending and using deixis, and in telling and understanding narratives. Visual perspective-taking is to be able to infer what others can see or hear, for example (Del Sette et al., 2021). Spatial perspective-taking

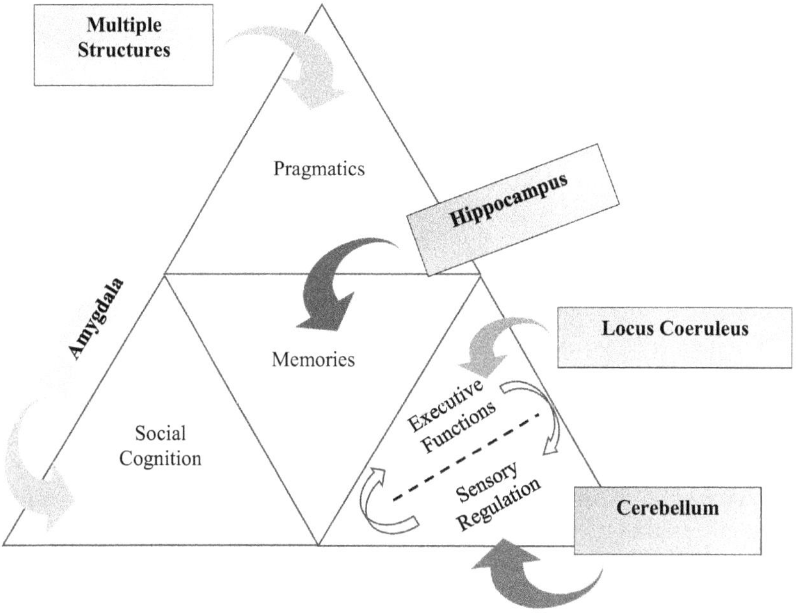

Figure 4.3 Conceptual Model of Social Pragmatic Communication – Version 2 with Brain Structures Mapped on the Conceptual Model.

Source: Hyter (2023)

is imagining how an object or event would seem from the perspective of someone else's spatial (or physical) vantage point (He et al., 2022).

Belief attribution, also related to ToM, allows one to be able to attribute a belief to others, whether the belief is true or false (Perner, 1991). A common activity used to determine if someone can attribute a false belief is a variation of the Sally-Anne task (see Baron-Cohen et al., 1985; Leslie & Frith, 1988). In this task, a character (e.g., Sally) leaves an object, such as a ball, in one location, e.g., in a box, and leaves the room. Then, another character (e.g., Anne) enters the same room, finds the ball in the box, moves it to the closet, and then leaves the room. Sally then returns to get her ball. The test question is "Where will Sally look for her ball?" A person who can attribute false belief to another would say that Sally would look for the ball in the last place she put it, i.e., in the box. In other words, Sally has the false belief that the ball is in the last place it was left. However, the witness (e.g., the person watching this series of events unfold) – the person being administered the task) has information the original character (Sally) does not have and can separate their knowledge from what Sally might think or believe to be true. Whether a child can attribute a belief to others is based on the child's linguistic knowledge, executive functions, and the characteristics of the person to whom they will be attributing a belief. There is evidence in the literature that the traits (e.g., smart, honest, kind, dishonest, and mean) of protagonists influence children's perceptions of their beliefs and knowledge (Lane et al., 2013; Seehagen et al., 2018; Witt et al., 2022). Also, if the protagonist was an adult, young children were less likely to attribute a false belief to that person (Seehagen et al., 2018).

The amygdala plays a significant role in social cognition. The connections between the amygdala and the prefrontal cortex play a role in making inferences about other behaviors, learning, and making decisions (Gangopadhyay et al., 2021). The prefrontal cortex has a role in inhibiting behaviors, thoughts, and cognitive flexibility, but when activation of the amygdala is prolonged due to trauma (toxic stress), it diminishes the activity of the prefrontal cortex (Arnsten, 2009). Trauma interrupts the connection between the amygdala and the prefrontal cortex – the amygdala when triggered. Connections between the amygdala and the hippocampus are connected to memory and helping people interact with others (Meisner et al., 2022). There is also evidence that individuals with trauma histories have difficulty with ToM and with understanding others' perceptions, beliefs, and emotions (Shaw et al., 2004).

In a systematic review of literature, Hyter (2021) found that children with trauma histories experienced more difficulty with interpersonal ToM, perspective-taking and the use of internal state language, e.g. language that describes what someone might be feeling, thinking, or wanting than children without trauma histories. Interpersonal ToM abilities increased with age but at slower rates than children without trauma experiences (Burack et al., 2006; Cicchetti et al., 2003; Hyter, 2021; O'Reilly & Peterson, 2015; Pears & Fisher, 2005; Ramirez et al., 2011).

4.2.2 Cognitive Functions

4.2.2.1 Memory

Memory refers to the ability to convert, store, and access information. Psychology Today (2023) indicates that memory is a "record of experience" (paragraph 1, line 2). Short-term memories are temporary and easily accessible, although they can become long-term memories within the hippocampus (Cowan, 2008). Long-term memory can last for several decades (Cowan, 2008) and refers to information you consciously (explicit memories) or unconsciously (implicit memories) remember. There are different types of long-term memories, and all are negatively affected by post-traumatic stress. NICABM (2017) produced an infographic (see Figure 4.4) explaining trauma's impact on explicit and implicit memories.

Part 3: How Trauma Impacts the Four Different Types of Memory

EXPLICIT MEMORY		IMPLICIT MEMORY	
SEMANTIC MEMORY	EPISODIC MEMORY	PROCEDURAL MEMORY	EMOTIONAL MEMORY
How Trauma Can Affect It	**How Trauma Can Affect It**	**How Trauma Can Affect It**	**How Trauma Can Affect It**
Trauma can prevent information (like words, images, sounds, etc.) from different parts of the brain from combining to make a semantic memory.	Trauma can shutdown episodic memory and fragment the sequence of events.	Trauma can change patterns of procedural memory. For example, a person might tense up and unconsciously alter their posture, which could lead to pain or even numbness.	After trauma, a person may get triggered and experience painful emotions, often without context.
Related Brain Area	**Related Brain Area**	**Related Brain Area**	**Related Brain Area**
The temporal lobe and inferior parietal cortex collect information from different brain areas to create semantic memory.	The hippocampus is responsible for creating and recalling episodic memory.	The striatum is associated with producing procedural memory and creating new habits.	The amygdala plays a key role in supporting memory for emotionally charged experiences.
Temporal lobe Inferior parietal lobe	Hippocampus	Striatum	Amygdala

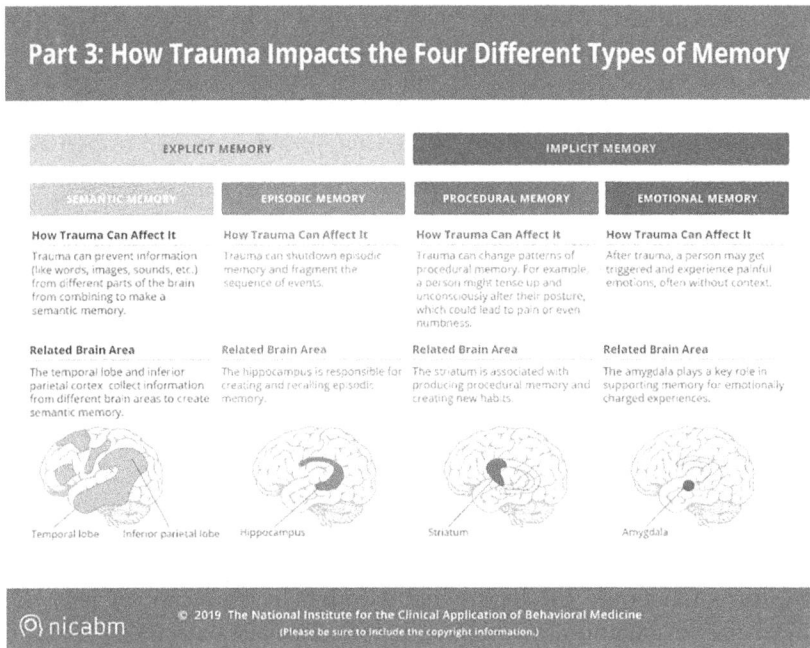

Figure 4.4 NICABM Infographic about the Impact of Trauma on Memory.

As outlined in this infographic, trauma impacts explicit memory comprised of semantic memory and episodic memory. Semantic memory is memory for general facts and information, such as remembering what objects are (e.g., remembering what a book is). Trauma interrupts the brain's ability to combine words and pictures that create semantic memories (NICABM, 2017). Episodic memory (discussed in detail in Westby's Chapter 3) is one's memory of what happened to them (NICABM, 2017). An example of episodic memory, for example, is remembering that you left a rare one-of-a-kind book worth a lot of money on the bus. Trauma "shuts down and fragments the sequence of events/experiences" (NICABM, 2017, second column, third paragraph). Trauma also impacts and implicit memory – memories that are unconscious that one does not need to think about. Emotional and Procedural memories are types of implicit memories. Emotional memory is remembering the emotions experienced during an event. You might feel fear, worry, and anxiety in the book scenario. Trauma can cause one to experience the emotions experienced during a painful event outside of the context of the event. In other words, Procedural memory is remembering how to do something without thinking about it (e.g., riding a bike, swimming, walking). Trauma can cause the development of a reaction (protective/adaptive behaviors, much like Angela presented at the beginning of this chapter), consequently creating a procedural memory of that reaction (Levine, 2015). Trauma is "less likely to be stored as an integrated and/or narrative memory and more likely to be stored as (non-declarative) procedural memory of unconscious conditioned responses of somatic and sensory experience" (Levine, 2015; van der Kolk, 2014; Yehuda, 2016, p. 132).

Hyter's (2021) systematic review of the literature specifically focused on working memory rather than memory in general. Working memory is holding on to information while processing additional information (Diamond, 2013). Some studies reviewed showed that spatial working memory (the memory for where things are in space, such as where you put your shoes or how to get to work) was less well developed in children with histories of maltreatment than those without histories of maltreatment (Augusti & Melinder, 2013).

4.2.2.2 *Executive Functions*

Executive functions (EFs) are cognitive abilities that control behavior, emotion, and cognition, resulting in goal-directed behavior (Nigg, 2017, p. 363). EFs have a significant role in self-regulation, inhibition of behaviors and thoughts, and cognitive flexibility, also called set-shifting (McCloskey et al., 2009). Self-regulation allows one to control one's thinking, feelings, and behavior (Nigg, 2017). Inhibition is the ability to suppress attention, behavior, thoughts, and emotions (Diamond, 2013). Cognitive flexibility/set-shifting refers to being able to quickly modify one's thoughts, behaviors, or actions (Irwin et al., 2019). Hyter's (2021) systematic review of the literature found that negative emotions may have negative influences on EFs (Fay-Stammbach et al., 2017); adolescents with a maltreatment history have lower executive function abilities than their non-maltreated peers (Kavanaugh & Holler, 2014), poorer performance on inhibition but intact set-shifting (Kirke-smith et al., 2014), poorer performance in cognitive flexibility, and difficulty engaging in behaviors that do not result in a negative response (Meszzacappa, 2001). An unexpected finding was that children with only one maltreatment experience performed less well with cognitive flexibility than those with multiple maltreatment experiences (Mothes et al., 2015). There is a relationship between sensory regulation and EFs. Individuals with sensory regulation concerns may experience difficulties with EFs. Please refer to Chapter 5, Suarez and Masselink, for a detailed discussion of the impact of post-traumatic stress on the sensory system.

4.2.3 Pragmatics

Pragmatics has traditionally been used to use language structure and meaning effectively in social contexts (Bates, 1976). Less traditionally, the study of pragmatics has focused on communicators (not only language users) and their cultural and social contexts (Hyter, 2017; Perkins, 2007; Rivers et al., 2012), which includes daily interactions, diverse worldviews, and a history of social practices (Hyter, 2007). Pragmatics includes verbal and nonverbal communicative intentions or communicative functions, discourse management, and sociolinguistic skills.

Communicative intentions or communicative functions, also called speech acts, are the intentions conveyed by a communicator and the impact those intentions have on others (Austin, 1975; Rivers et al., 2012). Speech acts include interpretations of one's intent or meaning-making, the actual intention or meaning being conveyed, and the forms (e.g., words, sentences, gestures, facial expressions) used to convey those intentions. Discourse refers to various types of spoken, written, or signed units of interactions, including conversations, narratives, and expository texts. Pragmatics is particularly impacted by trauma. For example, accounts of personal experiences, or personal narratives, develop early and are often spontaneously produced (Westerveld et al., 2022). Personal narratives help us make sense of and process our experiences, which is an important part of recovery and resilience. When this process is interrupted by traumatic events or experiences, recovery is challenging.

A systematic review of the literature (Hyter, 2021) found that children with maltreatment histories have more difficulty with pragmatics than their non-maltreated counterparts. Specifically, children with maltreatment make comments that are less informative, less descriptive, and less relevant to the conversation at hand; and less frequently refer to people and places in their conversations (Coster et al., 1989). Pesco and O'Neill (2016) examined children with maltreatment and those without using the Language Use Inventory-French, which is a standardized parent questionnaire designed to assess the pragmatic language of children between 18 and 47 months of age. On this measure, children with maltreatment histories performed less well than children without maltreatment histories in word usage, requests for help, attention-getting, asking questions, making comments, using words to communicate, showing a sense of humor, employing presupposition skills and narrative abilities. Ciolino et al. (2020) found narrative cohesion, informativeness, expository text, and communicative intentions were difficult for children with exposure to maltreatment. Difficulties with conversations have implications for making and maintaining friendships. Difficulties with narrative and expository discourse have implications for academic success, reading comprehension, and reporting the trauma one may have experienced.

4.2.4   *Assessment and Intervention for Social Pragmatic Communication*

Assessment and intervention for social pragmatic communication is necessary, but it is also difficult to achieve because of the contextualized and culturally laden nature of social pragmatic communication. Assessment and intervention suggestions are discussed next.

4.2.4.1 *Assessment*

Ciolino et al. (2020) found that children with histories of maltreatment presented with intact language structure and semantics; most children in their study, however, exhibited challenges in social pragmatic communication. Assessment should focus on areas of language and communication that are known to be challenging for individuals with post-traumatic stress, including social cognition, memory, EFs, regulation (sensory, behavioral, and emotional), and pragmatics.

Due to the contextual and cultural nature of social pragmatic communication, assessments should be conducted in situ whenever possible while individuals are engaged in their daily lives in interactions with others who are part of their networks and/or families. Using narrative and expository text as assessment tools is imperative, particularly personal narratives. Narratives can be used to determine the person's strengths and challenges in recounting events, giving explanations, understanding, and conveying their interpretation of others' beliefs, emotions, or thoughts. Children with trauma histories often have difficulty recounting events and connecting events with their causes and consequences (Yehuda, 2016).

In the literature, various assessments have been utilized to evaluate components of social pragmatic communication, although there are not yet any assessments that address all aspects of social pragmatic communication (Hyter, 2017). Hyter (2017) provides a detailed list of standardized norm-referenced assessments, checklists and observation protocols, discourse analysis protocols, and analog tasks. Analog tasks are of particular interest for assessing social pragmatic communication as they are tasks that can be designed to mimic real-life interactions. A brief outline of tools published in the last 25 years are listed below in chronological order.

- *Strong Narrative Assessment Procedure* (SNAP; Strong, 1998) uses narrative retell to assess narrative micro- and macro-structure elements.

- *Test of Narrative Language* (TNL; Gillam & Pearson, 2004) examines narrative comprehension and expression with specific focus on narrative sequence, cohesion, and coherence.
- *Children's Communication Checklist – 2* (CCC-2; Bishop, 2006), is a parent questionnaire that examines speech, language structure, semantics, and discourse, as well as scripted language, nonverbal communication, and social interactions.
- *Index of Narrative Microstructure* (INMIS; Justice et al., 2006) can be used to examine narrative microstructure.
- *Pragmatic Language Skills Inventory* (PLSI, Gillam & Miller, 2006), is a standard protocol completed by parents and/or teachers who observe the child in their daily contexts. The observations focus interpersonal interactions, understanding classroom and/or communicative rules, and classroom interactions.
- *Language Use Inventory* (LUI, O'Neill, 2007), is parent questionnaire that examines language competence in young children as they are used in daily interactions.
- *Narrative Assessment Protocol* (NAP; Pence et al., 2007) can be used by teachers as well as speech-language clinicians to examine the narrative retells produced by children. The analysis focuses on narrative microstructure.
- *Test of Pragmatic Language – 2* (TOPL-2; Phelps-Terasaki & Phelps-Gunn, 2007) examines the context, the audience, topic maintenance, gesture usage, and pragmatic evaluations. The TOPL-2 focuses on the child's ability to cognitively judge how to respond in various situations from another person's perspective.
- *Favorite Game or Sport* (FGS task; Nippold et al., 2005, 2008) is a protocol for assessing expository text.
- *Theory of Mind Inventory* (ToMI; Hutchins et al., 2012) is a parent questionnaire with statements where the response to the statements would reveal the child's ability to engage in ToM. Such a statement is, "My child understands that people can be wrong about what other people want." (Hutchins et al., 2012, p. 333).
- *Narrative Language Measures* (NLM; Petersen & Spencer, 2010) focus on narrative retells and generated personal narratives. Narrative comprehension, micro- and macro-structure are analyzed.
- *Narrative Scoring Scheme* (NSS; Heilmann et al., 2010) has the child provide a narrative retell of a wordless picture book, and that narrative's microstructure is analyzed.
- *Targeted Observation of Pragmatics in Children's Conversation* (TOP-ICC, Adams et al., 2011) is an observation protocol that assesses reciprocity, presupposition, turn-taking, management, and communicative functions used within conversational discourse.

- *Pragmatics Observational Measure* (Cordier et al., 2014) assesses the production and comprehension of verbal and nonverbal communication functions, social emotional attunement, and EFs.

4.2.4.2 Intervention

Interventions are necessary for supporting the social pragmatic communication abilities of individuals with trauma experiences. Any intervention must be culturally responsive, and trauma informed and responsive. And interventions of social pragmatic communication should be naturalistic – occurring within a natural context, such as a classroom or home where children will have opportunities to practice engaging with peers (Stanton-Chapman et al., 2008). To date, however, there are no published evidenced-based interventions specifically designed to support social pragmatic communication of individuals who have post-traumatic stress (Rupert & Bartlett, 2021). Rupert and Bartlett (2021) administered a survey to speech-language clinicians working with children who have trauma experiences. The results of this survey showed that clinicians made adaptations to their practice when they knew a family/child had been exposed to trauma. These adaptations included activities such as being extra careful about whether families would be able to carry out intervention strategies, increased parent education, and the clinicians altered their expectations about how much progress would be made through intervention. With regard to their specific practices, clinicians indicated that they had increased flexibility, made extra efforts to be nurturing and aware of events that could be triggering for the child. What follows is a summary of social pragmatic communication interventions that currently exist for the general population.

- Multicomponent intervention (Stanton-Chapman, 2008) primarily is designed to increase social communication among preschool peers. This intervention was comprised of a planning period, where children were read a storybook that focused on social pragmatic communication strategies, vocabulary, and play themes; a play time where the children were coached by the interventionists; and a section where children reviewed the social pragmatic strategies and vocabulary employed during their play. The results of this study showed that children increased social communication behaviors (responding to questions or peer actions; getting the attention of a peer; maintaining social interaction with a peer) (p. 207). The intervention, however, did not produce a consistent or large effect for all participants.

- Parent-implemented training and coaching (Meadan et al., 2014) was a pilot study that was implemented to determine whether a home-based parent training and coaching program was feasible and effective. This intervention was implemented with parents of children with Down Syndrome. There were multiple stages of the intervention that included baseline, periods of training parents to use certain strategies, followed by modeling and coaching parents to use those strategies (Meadan et al., 2014). The results of this study showed that parents not only learned new teaching strategies but were able to implement them with consistently; and parents reported that their children's social pragmatic communication abilities had improved.
- Social communication intervention program (SCIP; Adams et al., 2012; Adams & Gaile, 2020) is an intervention that is designed for children with autism spectrum disorder where children are trained Speech-language clinicians and focuses on three components (1) language processing (vocabulary development; understanding and producing stories; understanding and producing idiomatic language), (2) pragmatics (knowledge about how to engage in conversations), and (3) social understanding and interpretation (learning to read social signals and engage in reciprocal interactions). Results of studies evaluating the SCIP showed that it was effective in improving social pragmatic skills of children.

4.3   Summary

In this chapter, the impact that trauma can have on the brain and social pragmatic communication was explained. Individuals with post-traumatic stress may have challenges with language structure and content but primarily have difficulties with social pragmatic communication. Analog assessments and those that occur in natural environments are preferable for examining social pragmatic communication strengths and challenges, and several assessment protocols were summarized. Unfortunately, there are not yet any published evidenced-based social pragmatic communication interventions designed for individuals with post-traumatic stress. Some interventions designed for children with autism spectrum disorder, or preschoolers, were summarized and could possibly be able to be adapted to be administered in ways that are trauma responsive.

Note

1 The name and some contextual information were altered to protect the child and their family's privacy and identity.

References

Adams, C., Gaile, J., Lockton, E., & Freed, J. (2011). TOPICCAL applications: Assessing children's conversation skills: Turning a research instrument into a clinical profile. *Speech and Language Therapy in Practice, Spring*, 7–9. Retrieved from https://www.escholar.manchester.ac.uk/api/datastream?publicationPid=uk-ac-man-scw:83594&datastreamId=POST-PEER-REVIEW-PUBLISHERS.PDF

Adams, C., Lockton, E., Freed, J., Gaile, J., Earl, G., McBean, K., Nash, M., Green, J., Vail, A., & Law, J. (2012). The social communication intervention project: A randomized controlled trial of the effectiveness of speech and language therapy for school-age children who have pragmatic and social communication problems with or without autism spectrum disorders. *International Journal of Language and Communication Disorders, 47*(3), 233–244. https://doi.org/10.1111/j.1460-6984.2011.00146.x

Adams, C., & Gaile, J. (2020). Evaluation of a parent preference-based outcome measure after intensive communication intervention for children with social (pragmatic) communication disorder and high-functioning autism spectrum disorder. *Research in Developmental Disabilities, 105*, 103752. https://doi.org/10.1016/j.ridd.2020.103752

Allen, G. (2023, June 15). A Florida condo tower's collapse may have begun on its pool deck. *National Public Radio*. Retrieved from https://www.npr.org/2023/06/15/1182502745/surfside-florida-condominium-collapse-investigation

Arnsten, A. F. T. (2009). Stress signaling pathways impair prefrontal cortex structure and function. *Nature Reviews Neuroscience, 10*(6), 410–422. https://doi.org/10.1038/nrn2648

Augusti, E. M., & Melinder, A. (2013). Maltreatment is associated with specific impairments in executive functions: A pilot study. *Journal of Traumatic Stress, 26*(6), 780–783. https://doi.org/10.1002/jts.21860

Baron-Cohen, S. (1995). *Mindblindness: An essay on autism and theory of mind.* MIT Press.

Baron-Cohen, S., Leslie, A. M., & Frith, U. (1985). Does the autistic child have a "theory of mind"? *Cognition, 21*, 37–46. https://doi.org/10.1016/0010-0277(85)90022-8

Bates, E. (1976). *Language and context.* Academic.

Bishop, D. (2006). *The children's communication checklist-2.* Psychological Corporation.

Bremmer, J. D. (2006). Traumatic stress: Effects on the brain. *Dialogues in Clinical Neuroscience, 8*(4), 445–461. https://doi.org/10.31887/DCNS.200.8.4/jbremmer

Burack, J. A., Flanagan, T., Peled, T., Sutton, H. M., Zygmuntowicz, C., & Manly, J. T. (2006). Social perspective-taking skills in maltreated children and adolescents. *Developmental Psychology, 42*(2), 207–217. https://doi.org/10.1037/0012-1649.42.2.207

Burke Harris, N. (2018). *The deepest well: Hearing the long-term effects of childhood trauma and adversity.* Second Mariner Books.

Center for Disease Control and Prevention (CDC, 2023). *Fast facts: Preventing bullying.* Retrieved from https://www.cdc.gov/violenceprevention/youthviolence/bullyingresearch/fastfact.html

Children's Defense Fund (2023). *The state of America's children 2023: Child welfare.* Retrieved from https://www.childrensdefense.org/the-state-of-americas-children/soac-2023-child-welfare/

Cicchetti, D., Rogosch, F. A., Maughan, A., Toth, S. L., & Bruce, J. (2003). False belief understanding in maltreated children. *Development and Psychopathology, 15*(4), 1067–1091. https://doi.org/10.1017/S0954579403000440

Ciolino, C., Hyter, Y. D., Suarez, M., & Bedrosian, J. (2020). Narrative and other pragmatic language abilities of children with a history of maltreatment. *Perspectives of the ASHA Special Interest Groups.* Advance online publication. https://doi.org/10.1044/2020_PERSP-20-00136

Coster, W. J., Gersten, M. S., Beeghly, M., & Cicchetti, D. (1989). Communicative functioning in maltreated toddlers. *Developmental Psychology, 25*(6), 1020–1029. https://doi.org/10.1037/0012-1649.25.6.1020

Cowan, N. (2008). What are the differences between long-term, short-term, and working memory? *Progress in Brain Research, 169*, 323–338. https://doi.org/10.1016/@0079-6123(07)00020-9

Cummings, L. (2009). *Clinical pragmatics.* Cambridge: Cambridge University Press.

Cummings, L. (2015). *Pragmatic and discourse disorders: A workbook.* Cambridge: Cambridge University Press.

Dass-Brailsford, P. (2020). *Trauma, violence, and abuse with ethnic populations.* Cognella: Academic Publishing.

De Bellis, M. D., Baum, A. S., Keshavan, M. S., Eccard, C. H., Boring, A. M., Jenkins, F. J., & Ryan, N. D. (1999). A.E. Bennett research award: Developmental traumatology: Part I: Biological stress systems. *Biological Psychiatry, 45*(10), 1259–1270. https://doi.org/10.1016/s0006-3223(99)00044-x

Del Sette, P., Bindemann, M., & Ferguson, H. J. (2021). Visual perspective-taking in complex natural scenes. *Journal of Experimental Psychology, 75*(8), 1541–1551. https://doi.org/10.1177/17470218211054474

De Lillo, M., & Ferguson, H. J. (2023). Perspective-taking and social inferences in adolescents, young adults, and older adults. *Journal of Experimental Psychology, 152*(5), 1420–1438. https://doi.org/10.1037/xgc001337

Diamond, A. (2013). Executive functions. *Annual Review of Psychology, 64*(1), 135–168. https://doi.org/10.1146/annurev-psych-113011-143750

Dunn, L., Dunn, L. L., Gangopadhyay, P., Chawla, M., Dal Monte, O., and Chang, S. W. C. (2021). Prefrontal-amygdala circuits in social decision making. *Nature Neuroscience*, 24(1), 5–18. https://doi.org/10.1038/s41593-020-00738-9.

Fay-Stammbach, T., Hawes, D. J., & Meredith, P. (2017). Child maltreatment and emotion socialization: Associations with executive function in the preschool years. *Child Abuse & Neglect, 64*, 1–12. https://doi.org/10.1016/j.chiabu.2016.12.004

Gilliam, J. E., & Miller, L. (2006). *Pragmatic language skills inventory.* Pro Ed.

Gillam, R. B., & Pearson, N. (2004). *Test of narrative language.* Pro Ed.

Haines, S. (2019). *The politics of trauma: Somatics, healing, and social justice.* North Atlantic Books.

Harvard Health Publishing (2023, July 6). *Understanding the stress wwresponse.* Retrieved from https://www.health.harvard.edu/staying-healthy/understanding-the-stress-response

He, C., Chrastil, E. R., & Hegarty, M. (2022). A new psychometric task is measuring spatial perspective taking in ambulatory virtual reality. *Frontiers in Virtual Reality, 3*, 971502. https://doi.org/10.3389/frvir.2022.971502

Heilmann, J., Miller, J. F., Nockerts, A., & Dunaway, C. (2010). Properties of the narrative scoring scheme using narrative retells in young school-age children. *American Journal of Speech-Language Pathology, 19*(2), 154–166. https://doi.org/10.1044/1058-0360(2009/08-0024)

Heramis, L. (2020). *Developing a trauma-informed perspective in school communities: An introduction for educators, school counselors, and administers.* Cognella Academic Publishing.

Hutchins, T. L., Prelock, P. A., & Bonazinga, L. A. (2012). Psychometric evaluation of the theory of mind inventory (ToMI): A study of typically developing children and children with autism spectrum disorder. *Journal of Autism and Developmental Disorders, 42*(3), 327–341. https://doi.org/10.1007/s10803-011-1244-7

Hyter, Y. D. (2007). Pragmatic language assessment: A pragmatics-as-social practice model. *Topics in Language Disorders, 27*(2), 128–145. https://doi.org/10.1097/01.TLD.0000269929.41751.6B

Hyter, Y. D. (2012). Complex trauma and prenatal alcohol exposure: Clinical implications. *SIG 16 Perspectives on School Based Issues, 13*(2), 32–42. https://doi.org/10.1044/sbi13.2.32

Hyter, Y. D. (2017). Pragmatic assessment and intervention in children. In L. Cummings (Ed.), *Research in clinical pragmatics* (pp. 493–526). Springer International Publishing.

Hyter, Y. D. (2021). Childhood maltreatment consequences on social pragmatic communication: A systematic review of the literature. *Perspectives of the ASHA Special Interest Groups, 6*, 262–287. https://doi.org/10.1044/2021_PERSP-20-00222

Hyter, Y. D. (2023). *Conceptual model of social pragmatic communication – Version 2* [Unpublished document]. Language & Literacy Practices.

Hyter, Y. D., & Sloane, M. (2013). *Theoretical model of social pragmatic communication* [Unpublished document]. Western Michigan University.

Irwin, L. N., Kofler, M. J., Soto, E. F., & Groves, B. (2019). Do children with attention-deficit/hyperactivity disorder (ADHD) have set shifting deficits? *Neuropsychology, 33*(4), 470–481. https://doi.org/10.1037/neu0000546

Justice, L., Bowles, R. P., Kaderavek, J. N., Ukrainetz, T. A., Eisenberg, S. L., & Gillam, R. B. (2006). The index of narrative macrostruture: A clinical tool for analyzing school-age children's narrative performances. *American Journal of Speech-Language Pathology, 15*(2), 177–191. https://doi.org/10.1044/1058-0360(2006/017)

Kanske, P., & Murray, R. J. (2019). Understanding others: The neurobiology of social cognition. *Cortex, 121*, A1–A2. https://doi.org/10.1016/j.cortex.2019.11.003

Kavanaugh, B., & Holler, K. (2014). Executive, emotional and language functioning following childhood maltreatment and the influence of pediatric PTSD. *Journal of Child & Adolescent Trauma, 7*(2), 121–130. https://doi.org/10.1007/s40653-014-0014-z

Kirke-Smither, M., Henry, I., & Messer, D. (2014). Executive functioning: Developmental consequences on adolescents with histories of maltreatment. *British*

Journal of Developmental Psychology, 32(3), 305–319. https://doi.org/10.1111/bjdp.12041

Kim, J. J., Lee, H. J., Welday, A. C., Song, E., Cho, J., Sharp, P. E., Jung, M. W., & Blair, H. T. (2007). Stress-induced alterations in hippocampal plasticity, place cells, and spatial memory. *Proceedings of the National Academy of Sciences, 104*, 18297–18302. https://doi.org/10.1073/pnas.0708644104

Kim, E. J., Pellman, B., & Kim, J. J. (2015). Stress effects on the hippocampus: A critical review. *Learning & Memory, 22*(9), 411–416. https://doi.org/10.1101/lm.037291.114

Kritz, F. (2022, April 12). A report on violence against kids with disabilities is sobering – if not surprising. *National Public Radio*. Retrieved from https://www.npr.org/sections/goatsandsoda/2022/04/12/1091679303/a-report-on-violence-against-kids-with-disabilities-is-sobering-if-not-surprisin

Landa, R. J. (2005). Assessment of social communication skills in preschoolers. *Mental Retardation and Developmental Disabilities Research Reviews, 11*(3), 247–252. https://doi.org/10.1002/mrdd.20079

Lane, J. D., Wellman, H. M., & Gelman, S. A. (2013). Informants' traits weigh heavily in young children's trust in testimony and their epistemic inferences. *Child Development, 84*, 1253–1268. https://doi.org/10.1111/cdev.12029

Leslie, A. M., & Frith, U. (1988). Autistic children's understanding of seeing, knowing and believing. *British Journal of Developmental Psychology, 6*(4), 315–324. https://doi.org/10.1111/j.2044-835X.1988.tb01104.x

Levine, P. A. (2015). *Trauma and memory: Brain and body in search for the living past*. North Atlanta Books.

Long, C. (2019, November 25). To prevent bullying of students with autism, training is key. *NEAToday*. Retrieved from https://www.nea.org/nea-today/all-news-articles/prevent-bullying-students-autism-training-key

Maeden, H., Angell, M. E., Stoner, J. B., & Daczewitz, M. E. (2014). Parent implemented social-pragmatic communication intervention: A pilot study. *Focus on Autism and Other Developmental Disabilities, 29*(2), 95–110. https://doi.org/10.1177/1088357613517504

Manso, J. M. M., Baamonde, E. M. G., Alonso, M. B., Romero, J. M. P., & Merino, M. J. G. (2016). Social communication disorders and social cognitive strategies and attitudes victims of child abuse. *Journal of Child Family Studies, 35*(1), 241–150. https://doi.org/10.1007/s10826-015-0192-9

Manso, J. M. M., Sanchez, E. M. G. B., Alonso, M. B., & Barona, E. G. (2010). Pragmatic language development and educational style in neglected children. *Child and Youth Services Review, 32*(7), 1028–2034. https://doi.org/10.1016/j.childyouth.2010.04.008

McCloskey, G., Perkins, L. A., & Van Divner, B. (2009). *Assessment and intervention for executive function difficulties*. Routledge.

Meisner, O. C., Nair, A., & Chang, S. W. C. (2022). Amygdala connectivity and implications for social cognition and disorders. In G. Miceli, P. Bartolomeo & V. Navarro (Eds.), *Handbook of Clinical Neurology, 187,* 381–403. https://doi.org/10.1016/B978-0-12-823493-8.00017-1

Mezzacappa, E. (2001). Child abuse and performance task assessments of executive functions in boys. *The Journal of Child Psychology and Psychiatry, 42*(1), 1041–1048. https://doi.org/10.1111/1469-7610.00803

Morris, L. S., McCall, J. G., Charney, D. S., & Murrough, J. W. (2020). The role of the locus coeruleus in the generation of pathological anxiety. *Brain and neuroscience Advances, 4.* https://doi.org/10.1177/2398212820930321

Mothes, L., Kristensen, C. H., Grassi-Oliveira, R., Fonseca, R. P., de lima Arigimon, I. I., & Irigary, T. Q. (2015). Childhood maltreatment and executive functions in adolescents. *Child and Adolescent Mental Health, 20*(1), 56–62. https://doi.org/10.1111/camh.12068

Murphy, F., Nasa, A., Cullinan, D., Raajakesary, K., Gazzaz, A., Sooknarine, V., Haines, M., Roman, E., Kelly, L., O'Neill, A., Cannon, M., & Roddy, D. W. (2022). Childhood trauma, the HPA Axis and psychiatric illnesses: A targeted literature synthesis. *Frontiers in Psychiatry, 13.* https://doi.org/10.3389/fpsyt.2022.748371

National Child Traumatic Stress Network (NCTSN, n. d.). *Complex trauma.* Retrieved from https://www.nctsn.org/what-is-child-trauma/trauma-types/complex-trauma

NICABM (2017). *How trauma impacts four different types of memory.* Retrieved from https://www.nicabm.com/trauma-how-trauma-can-impact-4-types-of-memory-infographic/?itl=homepageinfographics

Nigg, J. T. (2017). Annual research review: On the relations among self-regulation, self-control, executive functioning, effortful control, cognitive control, impulsivity, risk-taking, and inhibition for developmental psychopathology. *Journal of Child Psychology and Psychiatry and Allied Disciplines, 58*(4), 361–383. https://doi.org/10.1111/jcpp.12675

Nippold, M. A., Hesketh, L., Duthie, J., & Mansfield, T. (2005). Conversational versus expository discourse: A study of syntactic development in children, adolescents, and adults. *Journal of Speech, Language, and Hearing Research, 48*(5), 1048–1064. https://doi.org/10.1044/1092-4388(2005/073)

Nippold, M. A., Mansfield, T. C., Billow, J. L., & Tomblin, J. B. (2008). Expository discourse in adolescents with language impairments: Examining syntactic development. *American Journal of Speech-Language Pathology, 17*(4), 356–366. https://doi.org/10.1044/1058-0360(2008/07-0049)

Nelson, C. A., Scott, R. D., Bhutta, Z. A., Harris, N. B., Danese, A., & Samara, M. (2020). Adversity in childhood is linked to mental and physical health throughout life. *BMJ, 371*, m3048. https://doi.org/10.1136/bmj.m3048

O'Neill, D. K. (2007). The language use inventory for young children: A parent-report measure of pragmatic language development for 18- to 47-month-old children. *Journal of Speech, Language, and Hearing Research, 50*(1), 214–228. https://doi.org/10.1044/1092-4388(2007/017)

O'Reilly, J., & Peterson, C. (2015). Maltreatment and advanced theory of mind development in school-aged children. *Journal of Family Violence, 30*(1), 93–102. https://doi.org/10.1007/s10896-014-9647-9

OXFAM (2023). *Poverty in the USA.* Retrieved from https://www.oxfamamerica.org/explore/countries/united-states/poverty-in-the-us/

Pears, K. S., & Fisher, P. A. (2005). Emotion understanding and theory of mind among maltreated children in foster care: Evidence of deficits. *Development and Psychopathology, 17*(1), 47–65. https://doi.org/10.1017/S0954579405050030

Pence, K., Justice, L. M., & Gosse, C. (2007). *Narrative assessment protocol.* Columbus Preschool Language and Literacy Lab: The Ohio State University.

Perkins, M. (2007). *Pragmatic impairment.* Cambridge University Press.

Perner, J. (1991). *Understanding the representational mind.* Cambridge, MA: MIT Press.

Pesco, D., & O'Neill, D. K. (2016). Assessing early language use by French-speaking Canadian children: Introducing the LUI-French. *Canadian Journal of Speech-Language Pathology and Audiology, 40*, 198–217. https://www.cjslpa.ca/detail.php?ID=1203&lang=en

Petersen, D. B., & Spencer, T. (2010). *The narrative language measures.* Language Dynamics Group.

Phelps-Terasaki, D., & Phelps-Gunn, T. (2007). *Test of pragmatic language* (2nd ed.). Pro-Ed.

Premack, D., & Woodruff, G. (1978). Does the chimpanzee have a theory of mind? *Behavioral and Brain Sciences, 1*(4), 515–526. https://doi.org/10.1017/S0140525X00076512

Prince-Embury, S., & Saklofske, D. H. (2013). Translating resilience theory for application: Introduction. In S. Prince-Embury & D. Saklofske (Eds.), *Resilience in children, adolescents, and adults translating research into practice* (pp. 1–8). Springer.

Psychology Today (2023). *What is memory?* Retrieved from https://www.psychologytoday.com/us/basics/memory

Ramírez, C., Pinzón-Rondón, A. M., & Botero, J. C. (2011). Contextual predictive factors of child sexual abuse: The role of parent–child interaction. *Child Abuse and Neglect, 35*(12), 1022–1031. https://doi.org/10.1016/j.chiabu.2011.10.004

Rivers, K. O., Hyter, Y. D., & DeJarnette, G. (2012). Parsing pragmatics. *The ASHA Leader, 17*(13), 14–17. https://doi.org/10.1044/leader.FTR1.17132012.14

Rupert, A. C., & Bartlett, D. E. (2021). The childhood trauma and attachment gap in speech-language pathology: Practitioners' knowledge, practice, and needs. *American Journal of Speech-Language Pathology, 31*, 287–302. https://doi.org/10.1044/2021_AJSLP-21-00110

Seehagen, S., Dreier, L., & Zmyj, N. (2018). Overrated adults: 4-year-olds' false belief understanding is influenced by the believer's age. *Journal of Experimental Child Psychology, 167*, 328–335. https://doi.org/10.1016/j.jecp.2017.11.007

Shaw, P., Lawrence, E. J., Radbourne, C. et al. (2004). The impact of early and late damage to the human amygdala on 'theory of mind' reasoning. *Brain, 127*, 1535–1548. https://doi.org/10.1093/brain/awh168

Shrider, E. A., & Creamer, J. (2023, September 12). *Poverty in the United States: 2022.* Retrieved from https://www.census.gov/library/publications/2023/demo/p60-280.html#:~:text=The%20official%20poverty%20rate%20in,and%20Table%20A%2D1).

September Substance Abuse and Mental Health Services Agency (SAMHSA) (2022). *Trauma and violence.* Retrieved from https://www.samhsa.gov/trauma-violence

Sloane, M. (2018, March 22). *Understanding the Intersection of Genetics, Prenatal Exposure, & Post-natal Traumatic Stress.* Invited short course taught at the Annual Convention of the Michigan Speech-Language-Hearing Association, Kalamazoo, MI.

Stanton-Chapman, T, L., Kaiser, A. P., Vijay, P., & Chapman, C. (2008). A multicomponent intervention to increase peer-directed communication in head start children. *Journal of Early Intervention, 30*(3), 188–212. https://doi.org/10.1177/1053815108318746

United Nations Refugee Agency (2023). *Key facts and figures.* Retrieved form https://www.unhcr.org/us/?gclid=Cj0KCQiAgK2qBhCHARIsAGACuzmWnC-H04rUk0Qjc0s6zfsxsaGyDnX-i1SyWwVo51KlkRwAqxVosRsaApHhEALw_wcB

Unsworth, N., & Robinson, M. K. (2017). A locus coeruleus-norepinephrine account of individual differences in working memory capacity and attention control. *Psychonomic Bulletin & Review, 24*, 1282–1311. https://doi.org/10.3758/s13423-016-1220-5

U.S. Department of Health & Human Services, Administration for Children and Families, Administration on Children, Youth and Families, Children's Bureau (2023). *Child Maltreatment 2021.* Retrieved from https://www.acf.hhs.gov/cb/data-research/child-maltreatment.

van der Kolk, B. (2015). *The body keeps the score: Brain, mind, and body in the healing of trauma.* Penguin books.

Westby, C. (2013). Evaluating theory of mind development. *Word of Mouth, 24*(3), 12–15. https://doi.org/10.1177/1048395012465600d

Westby, C., & Robinson, L. (2014). A developmental perspective for promoting theory of mind. *Topics in Language Disorders, 34*(4), 362–382. https://doi.org/10.1097/TLD.0000000000000035

Westerveld, M., Lyons, R., Nelson, N. W., Chen, K. M., Claessen, M., Ferman, S., Fernandes, F. D. M., Gillon, G. T., Kawr, K., Kraljevic, J. K., Petinou, K., Theodorou, E., Tumanova, T., Vogandroukas, I., & Westby, C. (2022). Global TALES feasibility study: Personal narratives in 10-year-old children around the world. *PloS One, 17*(8), e0273114. https://doi.org/10.1371/jornal.pone.0273114

Wimmer, H., & Perner, J. (1983). Beliefs about beliefs: Representation and constraining function of wrong beliefs in young children's understanding of deception. *Cognition, 13*(1), 103–128. https://doi.org/10.1016/0010-0277(83)90004-5

Witt, D., Seehagen, S., & Zmyj, N. (2022). The influence of group membership on false-belief attribution in preschool children. *Journal of Experimental Child Psychology, 222*, 105467. https://doi.org/10.1016/j.jecp.2022.105467

5 Neurodevelopmental Impact of Post-Traumatic Stress

Michelle A. Suarez and Cara Masselink

Children are exposed to violence and traumatic events at a concerning rate (Briggs et al., 2021). When children experience stressful events that are brief and transitory, they can recover and even grow from these experiences. However, when the stressor is life threatening and/or occurs within a relationship that is meant to be safe and protective, the impact of this trauma can severely hamper development and functioning (Ayre & Krishnamoorthy, 2020). According to the American Academy of Child and Adolescent Psychiatry (2023), "a child's risk of developing PTSD is related to the seriousness of the trauma, whether the trauma is repeated, the child's proximity to the trauma and his/her relationship to the victim(s)."

Many children who experience trauma develop post trauma stress disorder (PTSD) that can become chronic and debilitating. This chapter focuses on trauma that occurs within the relational system in the form of child maltreatment. The neurodevelopmental impact of these traumatic experiences is examined and resources for evaluation and intervention are provided.

5.1 Child Maltreatment

Child maltreatment encompasses all harmful, or potentially harmful, acts of any caregiver on a person who is younger than 18, even when the intent for harm was not planned or intended (Fortson et al., 2016). Four main types of maltreatment exist: (1) Physical abuse, (2) Sexual abuse, (3) Psychological/emotional abuse, and (4) Neglect; although children who are exposed to traumatic incidents, such as intimate-partner violence, may also experience disruptive psychological or neurological effects (Fortson et al., 2016; Gilbert et al., 2009). Human trafficking is an additional category of maltreatment and awareness of this issue has risen (Children's Bureau, 2022). Maltreatment frequently crosses categories, with many children experiencing at least two types of abuse (Dong et al., 2004). Frequency of exposure to or experience of abuse, as well as the intensity and

DOI: 10.4324/9781003225270-6

consistency at which the abuse occurs, interacts with the child's personal and environmental context (chronological and developmental age, medical status, environment, nutrition, and more) to impact the child's physical and emotional development (Ford et al., 2022; Fortson et al., 2016; Gilbert et al., 2009; Teicher et al., 2016). Severe maltreatment may end with devastating, long-term consequences to the child, even death, and the after-effects of experiencing abuse are invasive and life-long (Gilbert et al., 2009; Zarse et al., 2019).

5.1.1 Developmental Trauma Disorder

Although the Diagnostic and Statistical Manual of Mental Disorders, 5th Ed (DSM-5) does not recognize developmental trauma as a diagnosis, experts in the field vehemently disagree (Bremness & Polzin, 2014; van der Kolk et al., 2009). van der Kolk et al. (2009) proposed that Developmental Trauma Disorder be diagnosed by exposure to trauma with two of the three following: (1) neurological consequences, including the inability to modulate arousal level and sensory input, (2) negative attention and behavior characteristics, or (3) difficulty maintaining healthy relationships. The child must exhibit these characteristics for at least six months and demonstrate impairment in function either in academic, family, or peer relationships, activity with legal consequences, or physical health (van der Kolk et al., 2009).

5.1.2 Trauma and the Brain

The brain is not a static object; rather, it is a dynamic organ that grows and changes in relationship to the environment and interactions around it. When environmental or interactional exposure is negative, threatening, or depraving in nature, the changes in brain structure will likely result in the child exhibiting altered behavior, function, and thinking. The brain's plasticity, or propensity to change due to internal and/or external factors, is exponentially greater at certain vulnerable time points of development (as areas of the brain grow faster at different developmental time points) and vary based on the child's sex (Kelly et al., 2009; Thomason & Marusak, 2017; Tottenham & Sheridan, 2009). Therefore, the total impact of trauma on an individual child's development is difficult to predict, although it is clear that the developmental process disrupts many simple and complex developmental processes (Toth & Manly, 2018).

When trauma occurs, the brain's limbic system reacts protectively in a stress-response process producing an output described as hyperarousal (Atchison, 2007). In the stress-response, the central and peripheral nervous systems activate, releasing the hormone cortisol through the hypothalamic-pituitary-adrenal axis (Atchison, 2007; Thomason & Marusak, 2017). Predictably, vital systems in the body respond to the release of cortisol with increased heart rate, respiration, and blood pressure, and the body's storage of glucose is released to prepare for a fight (Atchison, 2007; Thomason & Marusak, 2017); essentially, the body responds to the threat by prioritizing survival mechanisms. Over time, the child's body learns it is not safe to rest (or transition into a parasympathetic state), but rather, it must stay on alert. This results in the child displaying "hypervigilant" behavior with inattention, decreased focus in their daily activities, and limited initiation and exploration in their environments and relationships (Atchison, 2007).

Furthermore, the stress response that occurs when experiencing maltreatment may impact development of global and specific brain structures. Trauma earlier in life and occurring for longer periods of time may reduce overall brain volume (Hart & Rubia, 2012). More specifically, the development of limbic system structures, the amygdala (also plays a role in social cognition), hippocampus, and pre-frontal cortex, respond negatively, impacting emotional processing (a function of the amygdala) and learning and memory (functions of the hippocampus) (Hart & Rubia, 2012; Thomason, & Marusak, 2017; Tottenham & Sheridan, 2009). Furthermore, evidence suggests that the male brain may be more susceptible to changes due to the impact of stress than the female brain, at least during certain developmental periods (Teicher et al., 2016). The pre-frontal cortex develops later, into adulthood, and governs executive functions including appropriate behavior in professional and social interactions such as motivation, initiation, and other higher-level functions (Hart & Rubia, 2012). The resulting effect on the child's self-regulation and cognitive advancement will be further explained below.

5.1.3   Impact on Regulation

An infant, through processes in the brainstem, largely self-regulates autonomous body functions such as breathing, heart rate, temperature, and respiration, although these vitals demonstrate unique responses when sensory input is provided by a parent or familiar caregiver (Buhler-Wassmann & Hibel, 2021; Ionio et al., 2021; Kommers et al., 2019; Suga et al., 2019; Yoshida et al., 2020). The maturing child's brain and body work to maintain homeostasis to optimize their development, but in infancy this often requires input from a caregiver to respond to challenges occurring beyond the child's ability (Graf et al., 2022). A child's physiological processes respond to caregiver contact; however, so do the child's developing emotional system. Supportive sensory input, such as the act of hugging (tactile and proprioceptive), the child looking at their parent's face (visual input), or hearing their parent talk (auditory), may increase the child's temperature, or slow respirations as the child calms, an act known as "co-regulation." Over time, the developing child takes on more of this responsibility for themselves, progressing to "self-regulate" both physiological and emotional responses to environmental stimuli. Harmful relationships from caregivers disrupt this important process, changing how the child's brain responds to stress, impacting their ability to regulate physiologically and emotionally, and even how their brain thinks and learns through adolescence and into adulthood (Hart & Rubia, 2012).

5.1.3.1 *Physiological Regulation with Sensory Processing*

Sensory processing begins with interoception, the "... overall process of how the nervous system (central and autonomic) senses, interprets, and integrates signals originating from within the body... " (Berntson & Khalsa, 2021, p. 18). When an infant is born, they innately cry when they are hungry and tired, a response from their internal signal of hunger and fatigue. Responsively, caregivers communicate with infants occurs through sensory input, tactile, proprioceptive, vestibular, visual, and auditory input are used to communicate regulatory messages. In this way, infants rely on co-regulation to communicate their own needs and acquire a calm and alert ("just-right") state (Graf et al., 2022). Over time, the central nervous system grows to modulate inhibitory and excitatory messages from internal and external environments, self-seeking just-right level of arousals (Atchison, 2007). It is through these sensory experiences and predictable caregiver responses that the child attachments are formed, the child learns to safely explore, and learning and growth occurs (Atchison, 2007).

As the child learns and grows, their ability to modulate incoming sensory information improves as a result of the practiced patterns performed with consistent caregivers; thus, the need for the support of co-regulation recedes. Sensory modulation, key for self-regulating an effective level of arousal and producing appropriate responses, "... occurs within the central nervous system by balancing both excitatory and inhibitory sensory inputs that arise within one's sensory mechanisms, as well as those that occur external to the body." (Atchison, 2007, p. 110). When modulating sensory input, the child's brain evaluates incoming sensory input and then directs a response to match the expected need. However, when the input requires a greater actual response than expected, an adaptive response is required to maintain appropriate behavior, or the child responds in a maladaptive manner due to an over-responsive or under-responsive nervous system reaction (Atchison, 2007). If parts of the brain that process sensory information have been altered or redirected from maltreatment, this complex process cannot occur in the intended manner. Even after the child is separated from the offender, these nervous system responses are likely to remain as they were conditioned over time. An over-responsive reaction to non-aversive stimuli may result in loud, extreme, or aggressive behavior; alternatively, an under-responsive reaction may look like resistance to following directions, difficulty engaging in tasks, or poor eye contact. Furthermore, the immediate and chronic nervous system reactions to maltreatment change the physiological state of the child. An increased level of arousal is accompanied by increases in heart rate, respiration, and blood pressure, as well as changes in glucose storage as the body prepares to fight or flee (Atchison, 2007). These alterations in body chemistry impact how the child processes sensory information.

Although neurological studies describe changes in the brain due to trauma, few studies have examined the relationship of maltreatment and resulting impact on sensory processing challenges. Based on what has already been described, the state of hyperarousal, or hypervigilance (a constant awareness for threats), limits the child's ability to explore and learn in their environment with appropriate behavior, and modulated responses to environmental stimuli (Atchison, 2007). Even so, anticipating the type of sensory processing challenges a child will experience in relationship with the type of maltreatment grows more difficult; although the multitude of factors (age, sex, caregiver situation, and more) beyond "type of maltreatment" that exists in each unique situation complicates matters.

However, research is emerging. In adolescence, trauma scale scores are directly related to higher scores on the Adolescent/Adult Sensory Profile (AASP; Dunn, 2014), with vision, auditory, and tactile subsections achieving a moderate strength relationship (Jeon & Bae, 2022). Similarly, greater responsivity to visual and tactile information was reported in alternative high school students over those enrolled in standard high school; the alternative high school students also reported greater experiences of physical violence (Jeon & Bae, 2022). The impact of childhood trauma on sensory processing appears to extend into adulthood. Adults diagnosed with depression were investigated and reported under responding to sensory input when they had experienced physical or emotional neglect, emotional abuse, or emotional neglect and emotional abuse (Serafini et al., 2016). Additionally, a history of physical neglect, emotional abuse, and emotional neglect were related to avoiding sensory input (Serafini et al., 2016).

5.1.3.2 *Emotional Regulation*

Impaired emotional regulation exists as a hallmark symptom of the developmental disruption that occurs from experiencing trauma (Ford et al., 2022). In infancy, emotional regulation relies heavily on the unique context the child is in, if familiar or novel, and the engagement available from the primary caregiver (Bridges et al., 1997; Graf et al., 2022). Studies show that fearful responses can be mediated through co-regulation by the smell of the mother entering the infant's system by the olfactory system, suppressing cortisol production and amygdala activity and producing effective regulatory responses (Graf et al., 2022). Although, the converse is also true, the odor of a fearful or agitated parent heightens amygdala activity, thereby impacting an infant's emotional regulation negatively (Graf et al., 2022). When maltreatment occurs, the infant processes and responds to inconsistent input from the parent, heightening amygdala activity and altering neural connectivity (Jenness et al., 2020). The amygdala plays a multi-faceted role in emotional processing, both in identifying and labeling stimuli with significance as well as planning and producing a response (Thomason & Marusak, 2017). Furthermore, the amygdala retains associations made with stimuli to use in future interactions and similar situations (Graf et al., 2022); with trauma, the disrupted function of the amygdala may apply emotions to even non-threatening stimuli (Wilson et al., 2011). Thus, the experience of maltreatment alters both current and future emotional responses, negatively impacting the process of emotional regulation.

The stress from maltreatment, over time, results in an over-responsive limbic system (Teicher et al., 2016). The amygdala accommodates, not only demonstrating a heightened responsivity to negative stimuli, but also a dulled response to positive, rewarding stimuli (Thomason & Marusak, 2017). Studies show that the amygdala physically responds in size dependent on the timing of the trauma – increasing in volume with early maltreatment yet decreasing in volume when maltreatment occurs in adolescence and later in life (Teicher et al., 2016). For the child, often this results in a lower emotional response when receiving awards, difficulty interpreting negative facial expressions and nonverbal emotional cues (important for social cognition), and higher emotional reactivity; furthermore, as they age, the adolescent may develop anxious and depressive symptoms (Hart & Rubia, 2012; Jenness et al., 2020; Thomason & Marusak, 2017).

5.1.3.3   *Executive Functioning and Higher-Level Pre-Frontal Cortex Skills*

Executive functioning skills organize, regulate, and require decision-making and inhibition control (Hart & Rubia, 2012). The complex nature of these skills requires the coordination of higher-level cognitive functions, such as attention and memory, to plan, sequence, think in abstract terms, initiate and monitor actions, and make decisions. This work is largely done in the hippocampus and pre-frontal cortex areas of the brain, which quickly mature during childhood (Gerge, 2020; Wilson et al., 2011). When the experience of maltreatment occurs, the brain responds to the stressful experience by releasing cortisol (Gerge, 2020; Thomason & Marusak, 2017). The cortisol damages the sensitive hippocampus, decreasing it in size (Gerge, 2020).

The impact of trauma on executive functioning skills depends on the duration and frequency of the event(s). Cognitive skill development of children experiencing chronic or frequent maltreatment is impacted by living in a state of hypervigilance, leaving them with difficulty focusing on daily activities due to the constant threat of harm (Atchison, 2007). Furthermore, the changes in the hippocampus resulting from experiencing maltreatment or abuse result in functional deficits for learning, memory, and time awareness, as demonstrated in studies in this area (Ainamani et al., 2021; Gerge, 2020; Hart & Rubia, 2012; Wilson et al., 2011). Visual and auditory attention to task, required for learning a task, decreases (Hart & Rubia, 2012; Thomason & Marusak, 2017), an underlying skill needed to utilize working memory, or the act of holding information in the mind to use while doing a task (Ainamani et al., 2021). During adolescence, growth of self-awareness and reflective skills may bring attention to these deficit areas, impacting the person's mental health further (Wilson et al., 2011).

5.1.4   Functional Implications of Trauma

The functional impact of trauma extends into every area of a child's life. Children who have been maltreated often have lower academic achievement, with studies revealing they may be more likely to receive special education, be retained, and have lower grades than children who have not had these adverse experiences (Jonson-Reid et al., 2004; Romano et al., 2015). This may be related to difficulty with regulation and executive functioning that impacts maintaining a calm-alert state, inhibiting impulses and problem solving that impedes participation at school (Jenness et al., 2021). It appears that this extends into adult life, with a history of maltreatment being linked to disruptions in employment and participation in lower-level vocational positions (Bunting et al., 2018).

Activities of Daily Living are also impacted by trauma. Children often struggle with things like poor hygiene, bladder control, and food issues including food hoarding (Atchison & Morkut, 2017). Sleep is impacted; a systematic review of behavioral sleep disturbance found a robust association between maltreatment and sleep difficulties (Brown et al., 2022). Caregivers report that these children often have nightmares, difficulty falling and staying asleep and experience bedwetting later into childhood (Schonning et al., 2022).

Finally, play, leisure and social participation are frequently affected by adverse experiences (Cohen et al., 2010; Valentino et al., 2006). Many children have delayed play skills, experience bullying or become bullies themselves due to difficulty with building and sustaining relationships (Hodgdon et al., 2016). These children also experience depression, anxiety, and isolation at a much greater rate than peers (Kisley et al., 2018; Kisley, 2020). Overall, exposure to trauma has functional implications that can follow a child throughout adulthood.

5.1.5   Evaluation of Trauma and Impact on Functioning

Since developmental trauma is associated with changes in brain development that impact many areas of functioning, a comprehensive evaluation of the child's strengths and challenges is important for crafting a treatment and support plan for the child (Hyter et al., 2003). This evaluation paints a holistic view of the child through the gathering of many interwoven assessment tools. Areas of evaluation include a description of the child's experiences, assessment of cognitive functioning and strengths and challenges in several developmental areas. Table 5.1 provides a summary of evaluation strategies that match the narrative description that follows. Awareness of cultural, gender identity, and community style diversity is essential to honor the individual needs of children in the context of their family systems, values, history, religious beliefs and other personal aspects that are all an essential part of their identity (Hall, 2020).

5.1.6   Life Experiences

A comprehensive evaluation of a child who has experienced trauma begins with gathering a history so that the child can be understood in the context of their experiences. An ethnographic interview with a caregiver that is very familiar with the child is an ideal way to collect this information. According to Westby et al. (2003), this interview includes five types of descriptive questions that are highlighted in Table 5.2.

In addition to the ethnographic interview, a specific understanding of the child's trauma history is important. The effect of different types of traumas on functioning can vary with the frequency and intensity of the child's experiences (Martinez et al., 2014). Table 5.2 includes several checklists to quantitatively and qualitatively measure the child's exposure to trauma. Insight into the child's experiences, individual characteristics and environmental influences lays the groundwork for the rest of the evaluation.

5.1.7   Cognitive Functioning

Children who have experienced complex trauma often demonstrate lower cognitive functioning on standardized measures of intelligence (Su et al.,

Table 5.1 Comprehensive Evaluation of the Impact of Trauma: Assessment Tools

What is measured	Specific assessments
Life experiences	
History	Ethnographic interview (Westby et al., 2003)
ACES, Trauma checklist	Trauma Symptom Checklist for Children (TSCC) (Briere, 1996)
	Child Behavior Sexual Inventory (Friedrich et al., 1992)
	CTAC Trauma Screening Checklist (Henry et al., 2010)
Cognitive functioning	
IQ	Kaufman Brief Intelligence Test (Kaufman & Kaufman, 1998)
	Wechsler Intelligence Test (WISC-V) (Wechsler, 2014)
Attention	ADHD Rating Scale (DuPaul et al., n.d.)
	Conners Teacher and/or Parent Rating Scales (Connors et al., 1998)
Executive functioning	Behavior Rating Inventory of Executive Function (BRIEFs) (Gioia et al., 2015)
Memory	Children's Memory Scale (Cohen, 1997)
Sensory processing	Sensory Profile 2 (Dunn, 2014)
Neurodevelopment	
Language	Clinical Evaluation of Language Fundamentals, 5th Edition (CELF) (Wiig et al., 2013)
	Bayley Scales of Infant Development (Bayley, 2005)
Pragmatic and social communication	Pragmatic Language Protocol (Hyter & Jackson, 2010)
	Assessment of Pragmatic Language and Social Communication (APLSC) (Hyter & Applegate, 2012)
Visual perception	Beery-Buktenica Developmental Test of Visual-Motor Integration, 6th Edition (VMI) (Beery & Beery, 2010)
	Motor-Free Visual Perception Test 3rd Edition (MVPT-3) (Colarusso & Hammill, 2015)
Motor skills	Quick Neurological Screening Test 3rd Edition (QNST) (Mutti et al., 2018)
	Bayley Scales of Infant Development (Bayley, 2005)
	Peabody Developmental Motor Scales (Folio, 2000)
Mental health	
	Child Dissociative Checklist (CDC) (Putnam, 1990)
	Multidimensional Anxiety Scale for Children (MASC) (March & Parker, 1997)
	Children's Depression Inventory 2 (CDI 2) (Kovacs, 2010)
	Children's Alexithymia Measure (CAM) (Way et al., 2010)
	Adolescent Dissociative Experiences Scale (A-DES) (Armstrong et al., n.d.)
	Resiliency Scales for Children & Adolescents (RSCA) (Prince-Embury, 2006)

(*Continued*)

Table 5.1 (Continued)

What is measured	Specific assessments
Behavior and adaptive functioning	
	Knox Preschool Play Scale (Bledsoe & Shepherd, 1982; Knox, 1974)
	Vineland Adaptive Behavioral Scale Third Edition (Sparrow et al., 2016)
	Child Behavior Checklist (CBCL; Achenbach & Roscorla, 2001)

Table 5.2 Ethnographic Interview Questions

Question type	Question description	Example
Grand tour	Broad question about everyday life	"Tell me about a specific day for your child"
Mini tour	Broad perspective of specific activity	"Tell me about what bedtime is like for your child"
Activity example	Hones in on specific activity	"You mentioned that your child goes from 0–100 without warning. Can you describe the last time this happened?"
Experience	Elicits information about a particular setting or unusual incident	"Tell me about your child's experience on the playground."
Native language	Provides understanding of meaning that interviewee attaches to certain words	"You mentioned that your child is stubborn, if you were going to describe this trait, how would you do so?"

Source: Adapted from Westby (2003).

2019). They also have a greater tendency to struggle with attention, executive functioning, learning, memory, and processing sensory information. Assessment of general intellectual functioning is necessary to interpret other assessment results as well as guiding which areas of development to target when completing domain-specific developmental evaluation (Hyter et al., 2003).

Attention/concentration and executive functioning are the foundation for efficient processing and functional utilization of internal and external stimuli (Goldstein & Naglieri, 2014). Children with developmental trauma struggle with executive functioning, including the ability to inhibit impulses, self-regulate, control behavior, and to problem-solve while working effectively toward goals (Op den Kelder et al., 2018). Measures of attention/concentration and executive functioning illuminate a child's skill in this area to contextualize whether the demonstration of other developmental difficulties is impacted by the child's ability to remain on task.

Early life stress from developmental trauma can impact processing speed and working memory (Kaczmarczyk et al., 2018). In addition, research has shown reduced volume of the hippocampus, which is responsible for learning and memory, in adults who have been maltreated (McCrory et al., 2010). It is important to assess a child's capability to form memory as a foundation for learning and academic performance. Westby's (2023) chapter in this text summarizes the impact of trauma on autobiographical memory.

Finally, sensory processing is impacted by adverse experiences. A study by Atchison in 2007 revealed that children who had experienced trauma demonstrated both hyper and hypo responses to sensation. Ineffectual processing of sensory information can make it difficult to match a behavioral response to the demands of the environment (Miller, 2014). Table 5.2 includes examples of measures to assess the cognitive functions specified above.

5.1.8   Neurodevelopment

In the area of neurodevelopment, it is important to gather information from several areas that are often impacted by trauma. For example, children who have been maltreated often struggle with understanding and expressing ideas using language (Sylvestre et al., 2016). This is particularly true in the area of social pragmatic communication (Hyter, 2021). For example, Ciolino and colleagues (2021) found that children who had experienced trauma had difficulty with the cohesion of a narrative and expository description.

In addition, there is evidence that children who have experienced trauma struggle with the development of motor and visual perceptual skills. For example, Wade and colleagues (2018) found that preschool children who had been maltreated had prevalence of impaired fine and gross motor skills at a rate of five–seven times more than would be expected in the typically developing population. In terms of visual-spatial skills, it is possible that maltreatment causes reduction in the corpus callosum and hemispheric integration is reduced impacting visual-spatial skill development (Davis et al., 2014). Table 5.2 provides several examples of neurodevelopmental assessments that are useful for capturing skill development and deficits for children who have experienced trauma.

5.1.9 Mental Health

Children who have experienced trauma struggle to regulate their affective states. Maltreatment and affect dysregulation have been linked to comorbid mental health diagnosis. For example, one study found that over 50% of adults diagnosed with schizoaffective disorder, bipolar disorder and depression reported a history of childhood maltreatment (Struck et al., 2020). Children who have experienced trauma have higher rates of depression and anxiety disorders (Gardner et al., 2019; Humphreys et al., 2020). It is very important that children who have experienced trauma are screened for mental health disorders so appropriate management can be recommended.

5.1.10 Behavioral and Adaptive Functioning

Adaptive functioning encapsulates the way in which children navigate through their environment, cope with everyday stressors and manage potential conflict with others (Becker-Weidman, 2009). A child's outward behavior is a result of the inner functioning of brain and body and internalizing and externalizing behavior can facilitate or hinder adaptive functioning (Achenbach & Rescorla, 2001). In addition to understanding the cognitive and neurodevelopmental impact of trauma, gathering information about a child's behavior and adaptive functioning can allow for a baseline understanding of the impact of trauma on everyday functioning.

Cultural humility is an essential value that needs to be interwoven into the assessment process (Ranjbar et al., 2020). Incorporating understanding and respect for the cultural heritage of the individual will provide a more genuine and helpful lens from which to frame the individual's experiences. This will allow for the results of the assessment to guide the intervention process in a holistic manner that honors the full repertoire of the individual's life experience.

5.2 Intervention

Treatment for individuals who have experienced trauma focuses on healing the brain that has been damaged by maltreatment (Perry, 2009). The goal of treatment is often to build the individuals capacity for regulation, the formation of healthy relationships and reasoning skills through situational demands. As the brain heals and the individual builds skills, functioning through daily activities can flourish.

Several treatment protocols have proven effective for ameliorating the impact of trauma. Intensive training and in some cases, certification is needed to utilize these protocols with fidelity. However, awareness of protocol components can be useful for understanding the needs and strategies for people who have experienced trauma. The following provides an overview of several key trauma treatments for children who struggle to function due to their history of maltreatment.

5.2.1   Trust Based Relational Intervention

Trust Based Relational Intervention (TBRI[R]), is a trauma responsive intervention that focuses on healing the brain to facilitate more normal development in children who have experienced trauma or generally come from "hard places" (Purvis et al., 2013). The principles of this intervention method can be used in all the settings in which children live, learn, and play. A closer look at the TBRI principles of Connection, Empowerment and Correction provides an introductory overview of this treatment approach.

5.2.1.1   Connection

Early experiences with caregivers provide an infant with the brain template for all future relationships. When the baby cries and an adult comes to be with them and meet their needs, the child learns that people are caring, helpful and trustworthy (Geva & Feldman, 2008). However, when a baby is harmed or their needs are ignored, the child's brain fails to organize in a way that supports the development of regulation and healthy, safe, and stable relationships.

Infant attachment is the emotional relationship between a baby and their caregiver (Howe et al., 1999). Children who experience maltreatment often develop ineffective attachment styles for healthy function within current and future relationships. Table 5.3 provides an overview of Infant Attachment Styles that are often developed as a result of the relationships that the child has experienced.

The ability to connect with another person starts with regulation that is facilitated by a safe person until the child is able to regulate themselves (Geva & Feldman, 2008). The child needs to experience felt-safety and a calm-alert state in order to have the capacity to "be together" with another person. Felt-safety is defined as a deep, profound and basic sense of feeling safe in the environments in which they function (Purvis et al., 2013). In the TBRI model, the caregiver regularly checks in with the child and attunes to the child's current state (Howe et al., 1999; Purvis et al., 2013). Then, TBRI encourages the use of several strategies to help the child with attachment to create a new template for healthy relationships. For example, touch, at the level in which the child is comfortable, is used to help them regulate and connect. For some children, a hug is welcomed. For others, touch is overwhelming and they can only accept warm proximity with a

Table 5.3 Understanding Attachment Style through Caregiver Behavior and Its' Impact on the Child

Style of attachment	Caregiver	Impact on child Child develops to:
Secure	Synchronized harmony between caregiver and child Consistent and predictable response to the child's needs	Explore the world and return to parent for support when needed Integrate and regulate own thoughts and feelings View others and emotionally available and dependable Develop into autonomous beings that can manage their own emotions
Avoidant/dismissive	Caregiver is emotionally less available and can be psychologically distant	Experience wariness or anxiety entering relationships Shut down, ignore or deny emotions Know how to avoid rejection but not how to facilitate connection
Ambivalent	Caregiver is inconsistently sensitive and unpredictable responsive Caregiver response to the child is not contingent on the child's needs or behavior	Experience deep anxiety about lovability Experience separation anxiety with clingy behavior with attempted boundary establishment Demand attention with crying, clinging, or making constant demands
Disorganized	Caregiver is scary, violent or deeply confusing and creates fear in the child	Manifest secure, avoidant or ambivalent attachment when not experiencing fear and distress Experience absence of organized behavioral strategy to gain proximity to caregiver and may appear confused, frozen or apprehensive in presence of caregiver Experience overwhelming distress

Content of the table was adapted from Howe et al. (1999).

caregiver to start. Connection principles are used to build a foundation of relational connection and foster healthy attachment.

5.2.1.2 *Empowerment*

Children who have experienced trauma or maltreatment have fragile nervous systems (Howe et al., 1999). That is why it is particularly important to closely monitor and meet the physical needs of these children to provide them with the foundational capacity to regulate, relate to others, and build skills. Empowerment Principles create conditions that encourage a feeling of safety in order to sooth the sympathetic nervous system so that the child can use their frontal lobe, executive functioning skills (Howe et al., 1999; Purvis et al., 2013).

A first step in using Empowerment Principles is to investigate the root causes of a child's behavior. For example, has the child experienced food insecurity and is fearful about being hungry again? Is the child dehydrated and struggling to function as a result? Is the child over- or under-responding to the sensory input from the environment and this causes them to feel overwhelmed or confused about what is happening around them? The child's internal and external perception of the world must be understood so that their physical and sensory needs can be met consistently.

5.2.1.3 *Correction*

The goal of Correction Principals is to help a child match their behavior to the demands of the environment. However, changes in behavior are not facilitated through reward or punishment. Instead, correction starts with the deeply felt safety, positive regard, and value that the child feels within the caregiver-child relationship. Behavior is viewed as communication related to the child expressing specific needs. Then the caregiver can partner with the child to teach them to use their behavior more effectively.

TBRI[R] prioritizes understanding of the child's internal state and feelings of threat or safety to contextualize behavior (Lynch & Mahler, 2021). When a child is able to regulate and connect to others, successful participation in all of the activities of living is possible.

5.2.2 *Neurosequential Model of Therapeutics*

Neurosequential Model of Therapeutics (NMT$_{tm}$) was developed by psychologist Bruce Perry and is organized around the hierarchical way in which the brain develops (Perry, 2009). During sensitive periods of development, the brainstem forms the foundation for physiological homeostasis in the body and brain. At the next level, the limbic system develops to process emotions adaptively and facilitate emotional attachment within relationships. Finally, the cortex allows for inhibiting impulses, problem solving and using higher-level skills, like language. This model provides a conceptual framework for guiding treatment for people who have experienced trauma that matches the treatment to the level of the brain in which the individual is struggling.

NMT encourages an understanding of the impact of trauma on the brain so that treatment can be targeted to the area that is not fully developed. For example, patterned, rhythmic, repetitive somatosensory experiences are necessary to calm the fight or flight response and facilitate physiological regulation. Integration of frequent nurturing and connection experiences, at the child's just-right level of tolerance for social engagement, is necessary to build the capacity to relate to others and recognize people as safe, predictable and a source of comfort. Finally, when the child is regulated, teaching a child cognitive strategies for coping and problem solving and practicing these strategies in the context in which they need to be used, can allow the child to generalize these skills over time in order to function effectively in any setting.

5.2.3   Trauma Focused Cognitive Behavioral Treatment

Trauma Focused Cognitive Behavioral Treatment (TF-CBT) is an evidenced-based approach for treating individuals that have experienced maltreatment (Cohen et al., 2018). In general, a Cognitive Behavioral Frame focuses on modifying thoughts that might influence maladaptive behaviors. When applied with the addition of the trauma lens, considerations for the individual's history and the impact of maltreatment on the body and brain are woven into the treatment plan. This type of treatment requires special training and is considered a goal standard, particular for children and adults with the ability to communicate thoughts and feelings using verbal language (McGuire et al., 2021).

TF-CBT includes three multi-element phases (Cohen et al., 2018). Phase one focuses on Skill Building. Psychoeducation for the parent and child provides insight into the impact of trauma on the brain and how these changes influence behavior. Children and caregivers develop and practice calming strategies to address the physiological and emotional trauma response. For example, treatment might include incorporating mindfulness or breathing strategies. In this phase, coping skills are implemented into daily life to manage thoughts and feelings that arise when the child is triggered by something in their environment.

Phase two focuses on helping the child develop their trauma narrative. This is done when the child is stable and unfolds slowly, at a pace that the child can tolerate while simultaneously employing the coping strategies learned during Phase One. The child is able to process their experiences and gain understanding of context and impact with the support of the strong therapeutic alliance.

In Phase Three, the youth has the opportunity to share their trauma narrative with their caregiver, who is carefully prepared to support the child through this process. During this phase, the child and the caregiver work to enhance their connection and communication skills. They develop a safety plan to map out how the child-caregiver team will handle future triggering experiences and how the child will stay safe and feel safe as they move though daily life.

5.3   Conclusion

In summary, child maltreatment impacts the developmental structure and functioning of the brain. Best practice when working with this population includes gathering an understanding of the child's cognitive and developmental functioning through comprehensive evaluation. Then, an individualized treatment plan can provide the experiences necessary to support healing and rich, meaningful, and robust participation in everyday life. Through this process, individual experiences, strengths, and culture of the individual is honored and incorporated into holistic, trauma-informed care.

References

Ainamani, H. E., Rukundo, G. Z., Nduhukire, T., Ndyareba, E., & Hecker, T. (2021). Child maltreatment, cognitive functions and the mediating role of mental health problems among maltreated children and adolescents in Uganda. *Child and Adolescent Psychiatry and Mental Health, 15*(1). https://doi.org/10.1186/s13034-021-00373-7

Achenbach, T. M., & Rescorla, L. A. (2001). *Manual for the child behaviour checklist (CBCL)*. Burlington, VT: ACER.

American Academy of Child and Adolescent Psychiatry (2023, September). *Posttraumatic Stress Disorder (No. 70)*. Retrieved from https://www.aacap.org/AACAP/Families_and_Youth/Facts_for_Families/FFF-Guide/Posttraumatic-Stress-Disorder-PTSD-070.aspx

Armstrong, J., Carlson, E. B., & Putnam, F. (n.d.). *Adolescent Dissociative Experiences Scale- II (A-DES)*. Retrieved from https://www.emdrworks.org/Downloads/a-des.pdf

Atchison, B. J. (2007). Sensory modulation disorders among children with a history of trauma: A frame of reference for speech-language pathologists. *Language, Speech, and Hearing Services in Schools, 38*(2), 109–116. https://doi.org/10.1044/0161-1461(2007/011)

Atchison, B., & Morkut, B. (2017). Developmental trauma disorder. In B. J. Atchison, & D. K. Dirette (Eds.), *Conditions in occupational therapy: Effect of occupational performance* (pp. 323–355). Lippincott Williams & Wilkins.

Ayre, K., & Krishnamoorthy, G. (2020). *Trauma informed behaviour support: A practical guide to developing resilient learners.* University of Southern Queensland. Retrieved from https://open.umn.edu/opentextbooks/textbooks/936

Bayley, N. (2005). *Bayley scales of infant and toddler development,* Third Edition, https://doi.org/10.1037/t14978-000

Beery, K. E., & Beery, N. A. (2010). *Beery VMI. Administration, scoring and teaching manual: The Beery-Buktenica developmental test of visual-motor integration with supplemental developmental tests of visual perception and motor skills.* Bloomington, MN: PsychCorp.

Berntson, G. G., & Khalsa, S. S. (2021). Neural circuits of interoception. *Trends in Neurosciences, 44*(1), 17–28. https://doi.org/10.1016/j.tins.2020.09.011

Becker-Weidman, A. (2009). Effects of early maltreatment on development. *Child Welfare, 88*(2), 137–161. https://www.jstor.org/stable/48623259

Bledsoe, N., & Shepherd, J. (1982). A study of reliability and validity of a preschool play scale. *American Journal of Occupational Therapy, 36,* 783–788.

Bremness, A., & Polzin, W. (2014). Commentary: Developmental trauma disorder: A missed opportunity in DSMV. *Journal of the Canadian Academy of Child and Adolescent Psychiatry = Journal de l'Academie canadienne de psychiatrie de l'enfant et de l'adolescent, 23*(2), 142–145.

Briere, J. (1996). *Trauma symptom checklist for children (TSCC)* [Database record]. APA PsycTests. https://doi.org/10.1037/t06631-000

Briggs, E. C., Nooner, K., & Amaya-Jackson, L. M. (2021). Assessment of PTSD in children and adolescents. In M. J. Friedman, P. P. Schnurr, & T. M. Keane (Eds.), *Handbook of PTSD: Science and practice* (pp. 299–313). The Guilford Press.

Bridges, L. J., Grolnick, W. S., & Connell, J. P. (1997). Infant emotion regulation with mothers and fathers. *Infant Behavior & Development, 20*(1), 47–57. https://doi.org/10.1016/S0163-6383(97)90060-6

Brown, S. M., Rodrigues, K. E., Smith, A. D., Ricker, A., & Williamson, A. A. (2022). Associations between childhood maltreatment and behavioral sleep disturbances across the lifespan: A systematic review. *Sleep Medicine Reviews.* https://doi.org/10.1016/j.smrv.2022.101621

Buhler-Wassmann, A. C., & Hibel, L. C. (2021). Studying caregiver-infant co-regulation in dynamic, diverse cultural contexts: A call to action. *Infant Behavior & Development, 64,* Article 101586. https://doi.org/10.1016/j.infbeh.2021.101586

Bunting, L., Davidson, G., McCartan, C., Hanratty, J., Bywaters, P., Mason, W., & Steils, N. (2018). The association between child maltreatment and adult poverty- A systematic review of longitudinal research. *Child Abuse and Neglect, 77.* https://doi.org/10.1016/j.chiabu.2017.12.022

Children's Bureau: An Office of the Administration for Children and Families (2022). *Child Maltreatment, 2021.* Retrieved from https://www.acf.hhs.gov/cb/data-research/child-maltreatment

Ciolino, C., Hyter, Y., Suarez, M., & Bedrosian, J. (2021). Narrative and other pragmatic language abilities of children with a history of maltreatment. *Sig 1 Language Learning and Education.* https://doi.org/10.1044/2020_PERSP-20-00136

Cohen, M. (1997). *Children's memory scale.* San Antonio, TX: The Psychological Corporation.

Cohen, J. A., Deblinger, E., & Mannarino, A. P. (2018). Trauma focused cognitive behavioral therapy for children and families. *Psychotherapy Research, 28*(1), 47–57, https://doi.org/10.1080/10503307.2016.1208375

Cohen, E., Dr, Chazan, S., Lerner, M., & Maimon, E. (2010). Posttraumatic play in young children exposed to terrorism: An empirical study. *Infant Mental Health Journal, 31*(2), 159–181. https://doi.org/10.1002/imhj.20250

Colarusso, R. P., & Hammill, D. D. (2015). *Motor Free Visual Perception Test-4*. WPS. Retrieved from https://www.wpspublish.com/mvpt-4-motor-free-visual-perception-test-4

Conners, C. K., Sitarenios, G., Parker, J. D. A., & Epstein, J. N. (1998). Revision and restandardization of the conner teacher rating scale (CTRS-R): Factor structure, reliability, and criterion validity. *Journal of Abnormal Child Psychology, 26*, 279–291.

Davis, A. S., Moss, L. E., Nogin, M. M., & Webb, N. E. (2014). Neuropsychology of child maltreatment and implications for school psychologists. *Psychology in the Schools, 52*(1), 77–91. https://doi.org/10.1002/pits.21806

Dong, M., Anda, R. F., Felitti, V. J., Dube, S. R., Williamson, D. F., Thompson, T. J., Loo, C. M., & Giles, W. H. (2004). The interrelatedness of multiple forms of childhood abuse, neglect, and household dysfunction. *Child Abuse & Neglect, 28*(7), 771–784. https://doi.org/10.1016/j.chiabu.2004.01.008

Dunn, W. (2014). *Sensory profile 2*. Bloomington, MN: Psych Corp.

Brown, C., & Dunn, W. (2002). *Adolescent/adult sensory profile*. San Antonio, TX: Psychological Corporation.

DuPaul, G. J., Power, T. J., Anastopoulos, A. D., & Reid, R. (n.d.). *ADHD Rating Scale-IV (ADHD-RS-IV: Home Version)* [Database record]. APA PsycTests. https://doi.org/10.1037/t05638-000

Folio, R. M. (2000). *PDMS-2: Peabody developmental motor scales*. Austin, TX: Pro-Ed.

Ford, J. D., Spinazzola, J., van der Kolk, B., & Chan, G. (2022). Toward an empirically based developmental trauma disorder diagnosis and semi-structured interview for children: The DTD field trial replication. *Acta Psychiatrica Scandinavica, 145*(6), 628–639. https://doi.org/10.1111/acps.13424

Fortson, B. L., Klevens, J., Merrick, M. T., Gilbert, L. K., & Alexander, S. P. (2016). *Preventing child abuse and neglect: A technical package for policy, norm, and programmatic activities*. Atlanta, GA: National Center for Injury Prevention and Control, Centers for Disease Control and Prevention.

Friedrich, W. N., Grambsch, P., Damon, L., Hewitt, S. K., Koverola, C., Lang, R. A., Wolfe, V., & Broughton, D. (1992). *Child sexual behavior inventory (CSBI)*.

Gardner, M. J., Thomas, H. J., & Erskine, H. E. (2019). The association between five forms of children maltreatment and depressive and anxiety disorders: A systematic review and meta-analysis. *Child Abuse and Neglect*. https://doi.org/10.1016/j.chiabu.2019.104082

Gerge, A. (2020). What neuroscience and neurofeedback can teach psychotherapists in the field of complex trauma: Interoception, neuroception and the embodiment of unspeakable events in treatment of complex PTSD, dissociative disorders and childhood traumatization. *European Journal of Trauma &Amp; Dissociation, 4*(3), 100164. https://doi.org/10.1016/j.ejtd.2020.100164

Geva, R., & Feldman, R. (2008). A neurobiological model for the effects of early brainstem functioning on the development of behavior and emotion regulation in infants: Implications for prenatal and perinatal risk. *Journal of Child Psychology and Psychiatry, 49*(10), 1031–1041.

Gilbert, R., Widom, C. S., Browne, K., Fergusson, D., Webb, E., & Janson, S. (2009). Burden and consequences of child maltreatment in high-income countries. *The Lancet, 373*(9657), 68–81. https://doi.org/10.1016/s0140-6736(08)61706-7

Goldstein, S., & Naglieri, J. A. (2014). *Handbook of executive functioning.* Springer. https://doi.org/10.1007/978-1-4614-8106-5.pdf

Gioia, G. A., Isquith, P. K., Guy, S. C., & Kenworthy, L. (2015). *BRIEF2: Behavior rating inventory of executive function* (2nd ed.). Pyschological Assessment Resources.

Graf, N., Zanca, R. M., Song, W., Zeldin, E., Raj, R., & Sullivan, R. M. (2022). Neurobiology of parental regulation of the infant and its disruption by trauma within attachment. *Frontiers in Behavioral Neuroscience, 16.* https://doi.org/10.3389/fnbeh.2022.806323

Hall, B. J. (2020). Assessment of PTSD in non-western cultures. *The Oxford Handbook of Traumatic Stress disorders, Second Edition.* https://doi.org/10.1093/oxfordhb/9780190088224.013.22

Hart, H., & Rubia, K. (2012). Neuroimaging of child abuse: A critical review. *Frontiers in Human Neuroscience, 6,* 52. https://doi.org/10.3389/fnhum.2012.00052

Henry, J., Black-Pond, C., & Richardson, M. M. (2010). *CTAC Trauma Screening Checklist.* Retrieved from https://wmich.edu/sites/default/files/attachments/u248/2014/Trauma%20screening%20checklist%200-5%20rev%2011-13-1.pdf

Hodgdon, H. B., Blaustein, M., Kinniburgh, K., Peterson, M. L., & Spinazzola, J. (2016). Application of the ARC model with adopted children: Supporting resilience and family well-being. *Journal of Child Adolescent Trauma, 9,* 43–54.

Howe, D., Brandon, M., Hinings, D., & Schofield, G. (1999). *Attachment theory, child maltreatment and family support.* Macmillan Press LTD.

Humphreys, K. L., LeMoult, J., Wear, J. G., Piersiak, H. A., Lee, A., & Gotlib, I. H. (2020). Child maltreatment and depression: A meta-analysis of studies using the childhood trauma questionnaire. *Child Abuse and Neglect.* https://doi.org/10.1016/j.chiabu.2020.104361

Hyter, Y. D., & Jackson, J. J. (2010). *Pragmatic protocol-revised (ages 4–6; 6–9; and 9–15). [Unpublished document.]* Kalamazoo: Western Michigan University.

Hyter, Y. D. (2021). Childhood maltreatment consequences on social pragmatic communication: A systematic review of the literature. *Perspectives of the ASHA Special Interest Grou, 6,* 262–287. *https://doi.org/10.1044/2021_PERSP-20-00222*

Hyter, Y. D., & Applegate, E. B. (2012). *Assessment of Pragmatic Language and Social Communication (APLSC).* Unpublished Beta Research Version. Kalamazoo, MI.

Hyter, Y., Henry, J., Atchison, B., Sloane, M., Black-Pond, C., & Shangraw, K. (2003). Children affected by trauma and alcohol exposure. *ASHAWire.* https://doi.org/10.1044/leader.FTR2.08212003.6

Ionio, C., Ciuffo, G., & Landoni, M. (2021). Parent-infant skin-to-skin contact and stress regulation: A systematic review of the literature. *International*

Journal of Environmental Research and Public Health, 18(9), 4695. https://doi.org/10.3390/ijerph18094695

Jenness, J. L., Peverill, M., Miller, A. B., Heleniak, C., Robertson, M. M., Sambrook, K. A., Sheridan, M. A., & McLaughlin, K. A. (2021). Alterations in neural circuits underlying emotion regulation following child maltreatment: A mechanism underlying trauma-related psychopathology. *Psychological Medicine, 51*(11), 1880–1889. https://doi.org/10.1017/S0033291720000641

Jeon, M. S., & Bae, E. B. (2022). Emotions and sensory processing in adolescents: The effect of childhood traumatic experiences. *Journal of Psychiatric Research, 151*, 136–143. https://doi.org/10.1016/j.jpsychires.2022.03.054

Jonson-Reid, M., Kim, J., Porterfield, S., & Han, L. (2004). A prospective analysis of the relationship between reported child maltreatment and special education eligibility among poor children. *Child Maltreatment.* https://doi.org/10.1177/1077559504269192

Kaczmarczyk, M., Wingenfeld, K., Kuehl, L. K., Otte, C., & Kinkelmann, K. (2018). Childhood trauma and diagnosis of major depression: Association with memory and executive function. *Psychiatry Research.* https://doi.org/10.1016/j.psychres.2018.10.071

Kaufman, A. S., & Kaufman, N. L. (1998). *K-TEA: Kaufman test of educational achievement: Brief form.* Circle Pines, MN: American Guidance Service.

Kelly, A. M. C., Di Martino, A., Uddin, L. Q., Shehzad, Z., Gee, D. G., Reiss, P. T., Margulies, D. S., Castellanos, F. X., & Milham, M. P. (2009). Development of anterior cingulate functional connectivity from late childhood to early adulthood. *Cerebral Cortex, 19*(3), 640–657. https://doi.org/10.1093/cercor/bhn117

Kisely, S., Strathearn, L., & Najman, J. M. (2020). Child maltreatment and mental health problems in 30-year-old adults: A birth cohort study. *Journal of Psychiatric Research.* https://doi.org/10.1016/j.jpsychires.2020.06.009

Kisley, S., Abajobir, A. A., Mills, R., Strathearn, L., Clavarino, A., & Najman, J. M. (2018). Child maltreatment and mental health problems in adulthood: birth cohort study. *British Journal of Psychiatry.* https://doi.org/10.1192/bjp.2018.207

Kommers, D. R., Joshi, R., van Pul, C., Feijs, L., Bambang Oetomo, S., & Andriessen, P. (2018). Changes in autonomic regulation due to Kangaroo care remain unaffected by using a swaddling device. *Acta Paediatrica, 108*(2), 258–265. https://doi.org/10.1111/apa.14484

Kovacs, M. (2010). *Children's depression inventory.* Pearson. https://www.pearsonassessments.com/store/usassessments/en/Store/Professional-Assessments/Personality-%26-Biopsychosocial/Children%27s-Depression-Inventory-2/p/100000636.html

Lynch, A., & Mahler, K. (2021). Trauma effects on neurobiological, social, emotional, and motor function: Considerations for occupation. In A. Lynch, R. Ashcraft & L. Tekell (Eds.), *Trauma, occupation and participation: Foundations and population considerations in occupational therapy* (pp. 19–41). AOTA Press.

March, J. S., Parker, J. D. A., Sullivan, K., Stallings, P., & Conners, C. K. (1997). The multidimensional anxiety scale for children (MASC): Factor structure, reliability, and validity. *Journal of the American Academy of Child & Adolescent Psychiatry, 36*(4), 554–565. https://doi.org/10.1097/00004583-199704000-00019

Martinez, W., Polo, A. J., & Zelic, K. J. (2014). Symptom variation on the trauma symptom checklist for children: A within-scale meta-analytic review. *Journal of Traumatic Stress, 27*, 655–663. https://doi.org/10.1002/jts.21967

McCrory, E., De Brito, S. A., & Viding, E. (2010). Research review: The neurobiology and genetics of maltreatment and adversity. *Journal of Child Psychology and Psychiatry, 51*(10), 1079–1095. https://doi.org/10.1111/j.1469-7610.2010.02271.x

McGuire, A., Steele, R. G., & Singh, M. N. (2021). Systematic review on the application of trauma-focused cognitive behavioral therapy (TF-CBT) for preschool-aged children. *Clinical Child and Family Psychology Review, 24.* https://doi.org/10.1007/s10567-020-00334-0

Miller, L. J. (2014). *Sensational kids: Hope and help for children with sensory processing disorder.* New York, NY: Perigee.

Mutti, M., Martin, N. M., Sterling, H., & Spalding, N. (2018). *ATP Assessments.* Retrieved from https://www.academictherapy.com/detailATP.tpl?eqskudatarq=2073-2

Op den Kelder, R., Van den Akker, A. L., Geurts, H. M., Lindauer, R. J. L., & Overbeek, G. (2018). Executive functions in trauma-exposed youth: A meta-analysis. *European Journal of Psychotraumatology, 9*(1), 1450595. https://doi.org/10.1080/20008198.2018.1450595

Perry, B. D. (2009). Examining child maltreatment through a neurodevelopmental lens: Clinical applications of the neurosequential model of therapeutics. *Journal of Loss and Trauma, 14*(4), 240–255, https://doi.org/10.1080/15325020903004350

Prince-Embury, S. (2006). *Resiliency Scales for Children & Adolescents: A Profile of Personal Strength.* Retrieved from https://www.pearsonassessments.com/store/usassessments/en/Store/Professional-Assessments/Behavior/Resiliency-Scales-for-Children-%26-Adolescents%3A-A-Profile-of-Personal-Strengths/p/100000655.html

Purvis, K. B., Cross, D. R., Dansereau, D. F., & Parris, S. R. (2013). Trust-based relational intervention (TBRI): A systematic approach to complex developmental trauma. *Child & Youth Services, 34*(4), 360–386. https://doi.org/10.1080/0145935X.2013.859906

Putnam, F. W. (1990). *Child dissociative checklist.* PsyTESTS.

Ranjbar, N., Erb, M., Mohammad, O., & Moreno, F. A. (2020). Trauma-informed care and cultural humility in the mental health care of people from minoritized communities. *Focus (American Psychiatric Publishing), 18*(1), 8–15. https://doi.org/10.1176/appi.focus.20190027

Romano, E., Babchishin, L., Marquis, R., & Fréchette, S. (2015). Childhood maltreatment and educational outcomes. *Trauma, Violence & Abuse, 16*(4), 418–437. https://doi.org/10.1177/1524838014537908

Schonning, V., Sivertsen, B., Hysing, M., Dovran, A., & Askeland, K. (2022). Child maltreatment and sleep in children and adolescents: A systematic review and meta-analysis. *Sleep Medicine Reviews.* https://doi.org/10.1016/j.smrv.2022.101617

Serafini, G., Gonda, X., Pompili, M., Rihmer, Z., Amore, M., & Engel-Yeger, B. (2016). The relationship between sensory processing patterns, alexithymia, traumatic childhood experiences, and quality of life among patients with unipolar and bipolar disorders. *Child Abuse & Neglect, 62,* 39–50. https://doi.org/10.1016/j.chiabu.2016.09.013

Sparrow, S. S., Cicchetti, D. V., & Saulnier, C. A. (2016). *Vineland adaptive behavior scales third edition.* Pearson.

Struck, N., Krug, A., Yuksel, D., Stein, F., Schmitt, S., Meller, T., Brosch, K., Dannlowski, U., Nenadić, I., Kircher, T., & Brakemeier, E. L. (2020). Childhood maltreatment and adult mental disorders - the prevalence of different types of maltreatment and associations with age of onset and severity of symptoms. *Psychiatry Research, 293,* 113398. https://doi.org/10.1016/j.psychres.2020.113398

Su, Y., D'Arcy, C., Yuan, S., & Meng, X. (2019). How does childhood maltreatment influence ensuing cognitive functioning among people with the exposure of childhood maltreatment? A systematic review of prospective cohort studies. *Journal of Affective Disorders, 252,* 278–293. https://doi.org/10.1016/j.jad.2019.04.026

Suga, A., Uraguchi, M., Tange, A., Ishikawa, H., & Ohira, H. (2019). Cardiac interaction between mother and infant: enhancement of heart rate variability. *Scientific Reports, 9*(1). https://doi.org/10.1038/s41598-019-56204-5

Sylvestre, A., Bussieres, E., & Bourchard, C. (2016). Language problems among abused and neglected children: A meta-analytic review. *Child Maltreatment, 21*(1), 47–58. https://doi.org/10.1177/1077559515616703

Teicher, M. H., Samson, J. A., Anderson, C. M., & Ohashi, K. (2016). The effects of childhood maltreatment on brain structure, function and connectivity. *Nature Reviews Neuroscience, 17*(10), 652–666. https://doi.org/10.1038/nrn.2016.111

Thomason, M. E., & Marusak, H. A. (2017). Toward understanding the impact of trauma on the early developing human brain. *Neuroscience, 342,* 55–67. https://doi.org/10.1016/j.neuroscience.2016.02.022

Toth, S. L., & Manly, J. T. (2018). Developmental consequents of child abuse and neglect: Implications for intervention. *Child Developmental Perspectives.* https://doi.org/10.1111/cdep.12317

Tottenham, N., & Sheridan, M. (2009). A review of adversity, the amygdala and the hippocampus: A consideration of developmental timing. *Frontiers in Human Neuroscience.* https://doi.org/10.3389/neuro.09.068.2009

Valentino, K., Cicchetti, D., Toth, S., & Rogosch, F. (2006). Mother–child play and emerging social behaviors among infants from maltreating families. *Developmental Psychology, 42,* 474–485. https://doi.org/10.1037/0012–1649.42.3.474

van der Kolk, B. A., Pynoos, R. S., Cicchetti, D., Cloitre, M., D'Andrea, W., Ford, J. D., Lieberman, A. F., Putnam, F. W., Saxe, G., Spinazzola, J., Stolbach, B. C., & Teicher, M. (2009, February 1). *Proposal to include a developmental trauma disorder diagnosis for children and adolescents in DMS-V.* Retrieved June 29, 2022 from https://www.cttntraumatraining.org/uploads/4/6/2/3/46231093/dsm-v_proposal-dtd_taskforce.pdf

Wade, T. J., Bowden, J., & Sites, H. J. (2018). Child maltreatment and motor coordination deficits among preschool children. *Journal of Child and Adolescent Trauma, 11*(2), 159–162. https://doi.org/10.1007/s40653-017-0186-4

Way, I., Applegate, B., Cai, X., Kimball-Franck, L., Black-Pond, C., Yelsma, P., Roberts, E., Hyter, Y., & Muliett, M. (2010). Children's alexithymia measure (CAM): A new instrument for screening difficulties with emotional expression. *Journal of Child and Adolescent Trauma, 3*, 303–318.

Westby, C., Burda, A., & Mehta, Z. (2003). Asking the right questions in the right ways. *The ASHA Leader.* https://doi.org/10.1044/leader.FTR3.08082003.4

Wiig, E. H., Semel, E. M., & Second, W. (2013). *Celf-5: Clinical evaluation of language fundamentals.* Bloomington, MN: Pearson.

Wilson, K. R., Hansen, D. J., & Li, M. (2011). The traumatic stress response in child maltreatment and resultant neuropsychological effects. *Aggression and Violent Behavior, 16*, 87–97. https://doi.org/10.1016/j.avb.2010.12.007

Wechsler, D. (2014). *Manual for the wechsler intelligence scale for children fifth edition.* San Antonio, TX: The Psychological Corporation.

Yoshida, S., Kawahara, Y., Sasatani, T., Kiyono, K., Kobayashi, Y., & Funato, H. (2020). Infants show physiological responses specific to parental hugs. *IScience, 23*(4), 100996. https://doi.org/10.1016/j.isci.2020.100996

Zarse, E. M., Neff, M. R., Yoder, R., Hulvershorn, L., Chambers, J. E., & Chambers, R. A. (2019). The adverse childhood experiences questionnaire: Two decades of research on childhood trauma as a primary cause of adult mental illness, addiction, and medical diseases. *Cogent Medicine, 6*(1), 1581447. https://doi.org/10.1080/2331205x.2019.1581447

6 The Impact of Post-Traumatic Stress on Cognitive-Communication in Multilingual Children and Adults

Sulare Telford Rose and Jennifer Rae Myers

6.1 Case Study

Mariana is a 35-year-old migrant who speaks several dialects of Spanish and English. Several months ago, Mariana was diagnosed with a complicated mild traumatic brain injury because of a serious car accident. While most of her physical and sensory symptoms have resolved, she continues to experience significant language difficulties. Her partner suggested she sees a speech-language clinician for further evaluation.

*During the initial assessment, Mariana freely uses her full semiotic resources (e.g., Spanish, English, gestures) to communicate with the clinician – also known as **translanguaging**.[1] When the clinician asks Mariana if she had previously received speech-language services, she informs them that she had received services as a young child due to a significant language delay after several years of neglect from her aunt. She had moved in with her aunt at the age of seven shortly after her parents died in a car accident.*

Based on the case scenario above, consider the following questions:

1 How might the traumatic experience of her parent's death and subsequent neglect from her aunt have impacted Mariana's language skills as a multilingual child? What about the possible trauma from her recent car accident as a multilingual adult?
2 What are some possible explanations for why trauma may have impacted Mariana's language skills and overall use?
3 What is the role of the speech-language clinician in this context?
4 What culturally responsive and trauma-informed considerations should be made for Mariana as a multilingual who experienced trauma?

If you're struggling to answer any or even all the questions above, don't worry. The goal of this chapter is to discuss the potential impact of trauma on language skills among multilinguals through the following objectives

DOI: 10.4324/9781003225270-7

1 Describe the relationship between trauma and language.
2 Explore theories on the relationship between trauma and multilingualism.
3 Discuss important culturally responsive considerations concerning trauma-informed services for multilingual clients.

"Language starts as an affective experience – a cry in the dark." (Caruth, 1987)

6.2   Introduction

As humans, language is our primary means of communication. It influences how we experience and interpret the world around us. What starts as coos and cries to indicate happiness or pain later develops into words, phrases, and discourse to do the same. Given the connection between language and emotion in our human experience, we must explore the relationship between trauma and language.

6.2.1   *Trauma and Language*

What is the impact of trauma on language, particularly for multilingual individuals? To understand its impact, it is important to first examine the concept of trauma. Trauma, by its simplest definition, is the impact of a disturbing experience or disturbing experiences. Not only can a traumatic event be emotional, psychological, and/or physical in nature, an individual's response to trauma, **posttraumatic stress** (PTS)–can also manifest as emotional, psychological, and physical symptoms. **Adverse childhood experiences** (ACE's) are traumatic experiences that occur in childhood. Such experiences include neglect, abuse, economic hardship, household dysfunction and neighborhood crime. Exposure to ACEs can yield long-term consequences well into adulthood including disrupted neurodevelopment, mental health issues, increased health complications, social and cognitive disabilities, and early death (Herzog & Schmahl, 2018; Monnat & Chandler, 2015).

Research has found that the language skills of children who are abused and/or neglected are delayed compared to their peers (Sylvestre et al., 2016). Age also matters: the younger the child, the bigger the impact abuse and neglect have on language. Language impairments have been documented not just in children, but in adults with a history of trauma. In individuals with a diagnosis of **posttraumatic stress disorder** (PTSD), exposure to trauma-salient stimuli has been shown to have a negative effect on both language and memory retrieval, as shown through decreased activity in Broca's area – the area responsible for verbal production (Rauch et al., 1996; Shin et al., 1999).

PTSD is a mental health condition that may develop as a result of experiencing a traumatic event. Symptoms are persistent and severe, characterized by intrusive thoughts, recurrent distress, as well as flashbacks and avoidance of triggers related to the trauma experienced. Research has also shown that PTSD can directly or indirectly disrupt cognitive processes such as executive function, memory, and language (Hayes et al., 2012; Hoge et al., 2008; Myers et al., 2022; Qureshi et al., 2011). It is reported that lifetime exposure to trauma in adults may be as high as 90% (Forman-Hoffman et al., 2016; Kilpatrick et al., 2013). While only a small portion of individuals who experience trauma go on to develop PTSD, minoritized groups are disproportionately affected. It has been reported that in the United States, at least 8 in 100 women and 4 in 100 men will meet the criteria for a PTSD diagnosis in their lifetime (Gradus, 2007), with Blacks and African Americans[2] more likely to develop PTSD than whites (Roberts et al. 2010).

It is important to note that PTSD and posttraumatic stress (PTS) are not the same. Also known as posttraumatic stress syndrome (PTSS), PTS has similar symptoms to PTSD that are less intense and shorter in duration (Sparks, 2018). Equally important, studies have shown that PTSD may be underreported and underdiagnosed due to the limited accuracy of assessment techniques, differences in symptom presentation, unreliable memory, or avoidance of the trauma (Dyb et al., 2003; Miele & O'Brien, 2010; Schreier et al., 2005; Van Zyl et al., 2008). Regardless of the presence or absence of a formal PTSD diagnosis, the impact of trauma exposure on individuals and society remains extensive.

The relationship between trauma and language is both complex and dynamic in nature. Language can be weaponized, resulting in trauma (e.g., verbal abuse; hate speech), but can also be affected by a traumatic event (e.g., language delay due to neglect). An individual's response to trauma may result in difficulties learning, using, and retaining a language, abandoning a language, or taking refuge in silence (Busch, 2020). As highlighted in Table 6.1, all components of language may be impacted by trauma and vice versa. Even the absence of language, such as the denial of the right to speak or the silence in which an event is enclosed, can be associated with trauma.

6.2.2   *Trauma and Multilingualism*

Do you or someone you know use or understand more than one language? If your answer is yes, it's not surprising because multilingualism is a common phenomenon experienced by many people around the globe. It is estimated that more than half of the world's population is **multilingual**; that is,

Table 6.1 Examples of the Bidirectional Relationship between Trauma and Language based on Bloom and Lahey's 1978 Language Model

Language component	Definition	How language can be traumatizing	How language can be impacted by trauma
Content	Meaning of language (semantics)	Certain words or phrases may trigger intrusions and flashbacks of a traumatic event (e.g., verbal abuse)	Trauma-related stress can impact cognitive processes making it difficult for an individual to remember words, concepts required to understand the intended meaning behind certain words or phrases
Form	Language structure (phonology, morphology, syntax)	The sound of a language, accent, or dialect may be associated to a traumatic event resulting in an individual to avoid the language	Individuals experiencing trauma may struggle with structuring their thoughts in a logical and coherent manner which may be reflected in disorganized or fragmented discourse
Use	Social use of language (pragmatics)	Being ignored or marginalized in social settings due to language differences may cause an individual to refrain from using certain languages socially	The psychological impact of trauma may affect an individual's desire to participate in social situations due to trauma-related fear or anxiety

the ability to use or understand two or more languages (Romaine, 2017). The terms multilingual and bilingual are often used interchangeably to denote the use of more than one language system, which is reflected in this chapter. In the United States, 67.8 million people speak a language other than English. While Spanish is the second most spoken language followed by Chinese, Tagalog and Vietnamese, there are 380 different languages spoken in the nation (U.S. Census Bureau, 2021).

Trauma can have a significant impact on brain mechanisms for language learning in multilingual children (Kaplan et al., 2016; Myles et al., 2018) and adults (Gordon, 2011; Johnson, 2018; Kartal et al., 2019). Multilingual children who have been abused or neglected resulting in structural

brain changes may have a difficult time developing the necessary skills required for language acquisition (O'Neill et al., 2016). This maltreatment
may result in language delays or disorders in their first (L1) or second (L2)
language as the areas associated with language may not have been adequately stimulated during language development. For multilingual adults,
research has shown that trauma-related symptoms such as the inability
to concentrate, memory problems, anxiety, verbal recluse, and headaches
negatively impact on the ability to learn a second language (McDonald,
2000; Santoro, 1997; Söndergaard & Theorell, 2004; Ying, 2001). PTS
can make second or subsequent language acquisition challenging as language learning requires control, connection, and meaning – processes often
disrupted by trauma (Herman, 1992, p. 33; Isserlis, 2000). While most
of the literature on adults is based on English as an Additional Language
(EAL) refugees, these findings likely extend to other trauma-exposed multilingual adult populations. The remaining part of this section explores
several multilingual populations often impacted by unique trauma.

6.2.3   Immigrants and Refugees

Migration is the primary reason for the diverse linguistic landscape (multilingualism) in the United States. In 2019, the United States had approximately 44.9 million immigrants which is the highest in the history of the
nation (Jocelyn, 2022; U.S. Census Bureau, 2021). While immigrants may
leave their homelands to settle in the United States for greater economic
and or educational opportunities or to be reunited with family members (Drachman, 2014), refugees are "forcibly displaced" and may also
be fleeing their home country due to "persecution, conflict, violence, human rights violations or events seriously disturbing public order" (United
Nations High Commissioner for Refugees, 2021). The ongoing wars in
many countries such as Yemen, Sudan, and Ukraine may also lead to an increased number of refugees coming to the United States to flee war and war
conditions, further contributing to the linguistic complexity of the United
States (Jordan et al, 2022). (To read more about the impact of trauma on
refugees, refer to Chapter 3 by Westby.)

   In their efforts to assimilate and succeed in the new country, immigrants,
and refugees from a variety of English-speaking countries often attempt to
learn the receiving country's variation of English. For example, immigrants
and refugees from India may try to acquire the US. White American dialect. They, therefore, become multilingual with varying levels of linguistic
competency in each language. Children of first-generation immigrants are
often simultaneous and sequential multilingual speakers thus further contributing to this linguistic diversity. They learn their heritage language(s) at
home and in communities and learn the societal language (some variation

of English) in educational institutions, through media, and other social settings. The ability to successfully acquire the host language can help to cope with stress related to migration (Archuleta & Lakhwani, 2016). This is why translanguaging, which will be discussed in greater detail later in this chapter, can serve as a valuable practice in this context.

Regardless of the reason for their migration, many immigrants and refugees find themselves experiencing the negative consequences of trauma whether prior to or post-immigration. The Latino/a population, particularly Spanish language speakers from Mexico constitute the largest immigrant population in the United States and are at high risk for PTS due to their minoritized status and conflicts in their homelands. While the first generation of Latino/a immigrants may experience trauma themselves, their children may also be affected by secondary trauma, as its impact can be passed on intergenerationally (Cerdeña et al., 2021; Phipps & Degges-White, 2014). This is known as transgenerational or **intergenerational trauma,** which can result in mental and physical health issues due to unresolved trauma and the subsequent response that can be inherited from parents or other individuals from previous generations. In the case of children with migrant or refugee parents, intergenerational trauma is often a result of systemic oppression from their homeland or host country (or both) and includes such events as genocide and institutional exclusion, or exploitation. (To read more about intergenerational trauma, refer to Chapter 2 by Archibald & Archibald.)

6.2.4   Deaf and Hard-of-Hearing Communities

Individuals who are Deaf or hard-of-hearing are often multilingual, using visual and spoken and/or written languages to communicate. They are considered **bimodal bilinguals** as the languages they use exist in different modalities such as sign language and spoken language (Lillo-Martin, 2016). Deaf multilinguals are very linguistically diverse, depending on various factors including their degree of hearing loss, the onset of deafness, social networks they have developed, and various acquisition and use of their languages (Grosjean, 2008).

Studies have shown that children and adults who are Deaf or hard-of-hearing multilinguals may be more susceptible to trauma (Anderson et al., 2016; Black & Glitman, 2006; Øhre et al., 2015). Factors such as social isolation, increased family conflict, and deprivation of language development may contribute to why individuals from deaf communities are at greater risk for trauma (Anderson et al., 2016). Some individuals who are deaf or hard-of hearing often feel pressured to assimilate to the culture of their hearing peers, with some attempting to "pass" as hearing (Aldalur et al., 2021; Goffman, 1963). The stress associated with trying to identify with the hearing culture may lead to trauma and related psychological issues (Aldalur et al., 2021; Grushkin, 1996). Alternatively, Deaf or hard-of-hearing people may feel pressured to be fluent in their minoritized language (Aldalur et al., 2021). The burden of dual cultural pressures may impact fluency of the acquisition of languages due to the conflict. However, research has shown embracing a deaf, hearing, or multicultural identity has reported significantly higher levels of well-being than those with neither deaf nor hearing identity (Chapman & Dammeyer, 2017). Therefore, a strong cultural identity may be a protective factor regarding trauma.

6.2.5   *African American Language Speakers*

African American Language (AAL) is a centuries-old language with unique grammatical, vocabulary, phonological, pragmatic, and accent features. AAL, also known as African American English, originated from the various African languages and English dialects during the era of slavery and evolved into a distinct linguistic system of communication. While AAL has been extensively researched, the connection between PTS and the use of AAL has been significantly understudied. However, the historical and current prejudice, discrimination, and racism toward Blacks and African Americans who speak AAL make a strong case for why this connection warrants further study. Oppression of Blacks and African Americans can be traced using AAL as a marker of social and economic isolation (Smith, 2016; Rickford et al., 2015). The study of **raciolinguistics** examines how race and language are interrelated. Language plays a crucial role in constructing and perpetuating racial hierarchies in a society and can be used as a tool to marginalize and discriminate against certain racial and ethnic groups (Alim et al., 2016; Rosa & Flores, 2017). Additionally, language practices are not only influenced by race but also shape racial identities (Alim et al., 2016). **Linguistic profiling** – or the practice of using an individual's dialect or accent to make inferences about them–often results in discriminatory practices toward AAL speakers (Baugh, 2003). This is known as linguistic racism which perpetuates inequality and stigmatizes AAL (Baker-Ball, 2019; Baugh, 2003). For instance, studies have shown that linguistic profiling of AAL has resulted in workplace, housing, and income discrimination (Grogger, 2011; Purnell et al., 1999; Rickford, 1999).

The use of AAL can also be the subject of racial microaggressions, which studies have shown can result in trauma and other negative health outcomes (Bryant-Davis, 2007; Bryant-Davis & O'Campo, 2005; Lewis & Neville, 2015; Nadel et al., 2019; Sue, 2010; Sue et al., 2007). **Microaggressions** are subtle, everyday comments or behaviors that communicate bias toward historically marginalized groups (e.g., commenting on how well a non-White American speaks White American English).

Microaggressions often impact multilinguals across different populations and can have long-lasting detrimental effects given the close ties between language and identity. Research suggests trauma related to racial or ethnic identity may result in long-term behavioral and personality changes (Anderson & Stevenson, 2019; Carter & Sant-Barket, 2015). The stigma associated specifically with the use of AAL can facilitate cultural isolation and the pressure to adopt White American English ideologies to reduce socio-cultural challenges (Lyn, 2022). Therefore, there is a critical need to reduce the negative perception toward AAL and support the use of AAL as a valuable form of social and cultural capital.

There is significant diversity in language status and cultural identity among multilinguals, as they can acquire languages in many different ways. Consequently, multilingual language acquisition may look different for an individual depending on their unique personal and cultural characteristics. Moreover, the languages acquired can represent distinct ways of thinking, feeling, and interacting with the world (Grosjean, 2010; Castaño et al., 2007). Individuals may also represent themselves differently depending on their language (Ramírez-Esparza & García-Sierra, 2014; Grosjean, 2010; Santiago-Rivera et al., 2009). In the context of trauma, the multilingual identity of the individual (e.g., how, and when they learned additional languages) may determine how they use language to respond to trauma.

6.3 Theoretical Considerations for the Relationship Between Trauma and Multilingualism

To fully understand the relationship between trauma and multilingualism, we must consider each role language may play for multilingual clients in both processing and expressing their PTS. We must also remember the interaction between trauma and language in general and how that may be impacted by being multilingual–culturally, cognitively, and of course, linguistically. In this section, we briefly cover three theories that explore this complex relationship.

6.3.1 Multilingualism as a Mediating Effect

Acculturation stress are stressors associated with the unique experience of leaving one's native culture for another culture. One important part of acculturation, or the adaptation process, is communication. For immigrants and refugees, acquisition of the host country's language is a known protective factor. Research has shown it acts as a buffer against stress often associated with adapting to a new environment and helps individuals complete day-to-day activities (Beiser & Hou, 2001; Leong et al., 2013). However, if an individual has difficulty acquiring the host language, they may experience additional stress, which can negatively impact their mental health and predict general distress, anxiety, and PTSD (Kartal & Kiropoulos, 2016; Schweitzer et al., 2011). Functionally, it can have detrimental effects on social integration including participation in the employment market and other social environments (Birman et al., 2014; Doucerain et al., 2015).

From a theoretical perspective, Kartal et al.'s (2019) model of the mediating effect of second language acquisition on PTS proposes that trauma exposure has a direct impact on mental health and an indirect impact on mental health through its connection with secondary language acquisition. Therefore, the more acquired the secondary language is (host language), the less impact the trauma will likely have. Moreover, trauma indirectly increases vulnerability to stress-related conditions as it reduces an individual's ability to deal with additional stress (Lindencrona, 2008; Matheson et al., 2008). This theory supports evidence that refugees with severe PTSD symptoms acquire the host language at a significantly slower rate (Sondergaard & Theorell, 2004). PTSD symptoms have been associated with impairment in cognitive functions such as automatic mental processing and memory (Kanagaratnam & Asbjørnsen, 2007; Sondergaard & Theorell, 2004); it may partially explain difficulties in acquiring the host language. (See Westby (this volume) regarding the impact of trauma on autobiographical memory.)

Familiarity with a host language is a crucial part of the acculturation process (Kartel et al., 2019). During this time, refugees and migrants are attempting to participate in the new culture of the host country while still maintaining their culture of origin and their identity (Berry, 1997). As one might imagine, the stress that may arise from this negotiation associated with the acquisition of the host language can become a significant risk factor (Berry, 1997; Bogic et al., 2012). Based on the belief that multilingualism has a mediating effect, difficulty with second (third or fourth) language acquisition not only exacerbates preexisting PTS and other mental health conditions but also inhibits functional adaptation to a new cultural landscape.

6.3.2   Competition for Limited Cognitive Resources

Trauma can alter neural networks in the brain with potentially long-term negative consequences (see both Hyter & Suarez, this volume for a discussion of the impact that trauma has on the brain). Premises of the noticing hypothesis (Schmidt, 1990, 2010) are that (1) learners do not automatically encode an additional language, and (2) for language acquisition to occur, they must first attend to and process the additional language for it to be acquired. Therefore, language acquisition may be cognitively affected by PTS. PTS symptoms (e.g., ruminating on the traumatic event) can drain brain networks associated with attentional control resulting in limited cognitive resources for language learning (Yehuda, 2016).

Memory is another cognitive process needed for new language acquisition but can also be consumed by PTS. When multilinguals experience PTS it can negatively impact memory by disrupting the brain areas associated with recalling facts, events, procedures, and emotions which are also associated with language areas including the prefrontal cortex and hippocampus. This translates to difficulties in encoding, storing and retrieving new language information, including vocabulary, and syntax (Johnson, 2018).

Limited cognitive resources may also result in misinterpreted behaviors. For example, adults learning English (or another language) in formal classes may have difficulties paying attention during class or attending class regularly due to the pervasive nature of PTS, which may be perceived as lack of motivation (Kerka, 2002). Socially, intrusive thoughts and triggers related to the traumatic event(s) may cause multilinguals to avoid social interactions altogether, thereby reducing language exposure opportunities and use. The lack of language exposure is especially important concerning the role of language in the reduction or exacerbation of acculturation stress.

6.3.3   *Code-Switching as a Defensive Mechanism*

Language is intimately connected to an individual's identity and culture. As a result, language may serve as a coping mechanism for multilinguals who engage in code-switching (Javier, 1989; Mahootian, 2020). **Code-switching,** or the practice of alternating between two or more languages, adds complexity and depth to the role of language as multilinguals who engage in code-switching likely use each language for different purposes. This is different from translanguaging which emphasizes the use of linguistic resources rather than switching between separate language codes. Javier (1989) proposed the idea that multilinguals use code-switching under stress, consciously or subconsciously, as a defensive mechanism to avoid or minimize the emotional impact associated with one of the languages. This is supported by other studies that show an individual's first language (L1) is preferred for emotional expression (Ayçiçeği & Harris, 2004), while their second language (L2) is used for emotional detachment (Ayçiçeği & Harris, 2004; Javier & Alpert, 1986; Tausczik & Pennebaker, 2010).

According to Javier (1989), this is due to the phenomenon of language independence which is when an individual acquires and maintains two distinct representational processes for each language resulting in independent linguistic organization. It implies that different cognitive and emotional processes are associated with, organized, and activated by the two languages separately. This has been demonstrated in a number of studies as it relates to emotion and trauma. Kolers (1963) found that words associated with emotion (e.g., pain) elicited dissimilar associations in languages among bilinguals, whereas words associated with concrete objects (e.g., chair) elicited similar associations. Findings from Greenfield and Fisherman's 1975 study revealed that Spanish/English-speaking multilinguals were more likely to use Spanish in intimacy-related situations and English in occupation-related situations. More recently, Ladegaaud (2018) found that survivors of trauma who speak more than one language may prefer speaking about their traumatic event in their non-dominant language in an attempt to emotionally distance themselves from the trauma.

Although some literature suggests that L1 is the preferred language for emotional expression, other research indicates that it may not be the case. For instance, because L2+ is often acquired formally (e.g., school), researchers argue that it does not involve personal emotional identity as much as their L1 and therefore, the use of L1 for emotional expression may be more of a reflection of language dominance. (Dewaele, 2010; Thass-Thienemann, 1973). Additionally, multilinguals may utilize code-switching to select the expression that best represents their emotional state which may be due to perceived language emotionality, or the emotional repertoire of a given language (Dewaele, 2010; Pavlenko, 2004). While it may not be clear if code-switching truly serves as a defensive mechanism, the relationship between trauma and multilingualism is evident. It may be the case that it acts both as a defensive and coping mechanism depending on factors such as language fluency and trauma resilience.

As clinicians, it is imperative that we are culturally responsive, especially in the context of providing trauma-informed services for bilingual clients. In the next section we'll discuss important culturally responsive considerations concerning trauma-informed services for bilingual clients.

6.4   General Guidelines for Trauma-Informed Care for Speech-Language-Hearing Professionals

In speech-language-hearing sciences, conversations regarding trauma-informed care have dated back to as early as 1974 (O'Toole, 1974). Despite this, formal guidelines and research to practice were not in place. However, within the past decade, a few researchers have increased the dissemination of empirical research regarding trauma-informed care. Table 6.2 summarizes the recommendations and considerations for trauma-informed care that arose from the field of speech-language-hearing sciences.

Table 6.2 General Guidelines for Trauma-Informed Care for Speech-Language-Hearing Professionals

Population	Guideline	Reference
Adults	Speech-Language Professionals (SLPs) can identify intimate partner violence due to the nature of the work.	Ballan and Freyer (2019)
Children	Assess pragmatic language skills. Focus on narrative language when evaluating pragmatic language skills.	Hyter (2021), Di Sante et al. (2019)
	Assess verbal, visual, and working memory.	Hwa Froelich (2012)
	Differentiate whether non-mainstream cultural disciplinary practices are harmless or harmful. Only report harmful behavior even when insipid within a culture.	Westby (2007)
Children & Adults	Work with social workers, counselors, and psychologists.	Hyter (2021), Ballan and Freyer (2019), Rupert and Bartlett (2022)
	Incorporate culturally responsive assessment & intervention methods.	Hyter and Salas-Provance (2023), Hyter (2021)
	Help clients construct a trauma narrative in collaboration with a counselor (Ciolino et al., 2021; Hyter, 2021; Deblinger et al., 2011) – "a story about the history of their trauma and its effect on their life."	Ciolino et al (2021), Schauer et al. (2011), O'Brien and Sutherland (2007)
	Incorporate a relationship development framework.	Hwa Froelich (2022)
	Develop relationships of trust and safety.	Hyter (2016, 2021), Hyter and Ciolino (2017, 2018), Purvis et al (2013), O'Brien and Sutherland (2007), Yehuda (2016)
	Include trauma inquiry in the speech-language-hearing assessment process.	Rupert and Bartlett (2022)

(*Continued*)

Table 6.2 (Continued)

Population	Guideline	Reference
	Identify trauma response in individuals.	Hyter (2021)
	Report identified abuse.	O'Toole (1974), Hwa-Froliech (2012)
	Advocate for clients who've experienced trauma.	Hyter (2012)
	Educate self on the relationship between executive processes and emotional behavioral challenges in youth.	Moreno- Manso et al. (2021)
	Educate oneself on the relationship between language difficulties and neglect/abuse.	Dumont et al. (2019), Sylvestre et al. (2017), Sylvestre et al. (2012), Sylvestre and Mérette (2010)

6.4.1 General Recommendations for Culturally Responsive Care for Multilingual Clients in Speech-Language-Hearing Sciences

A trauma-informed speech-language clinician adheres to culturally responsive practice. To ignore one's cultural and linguistic status entirely is to ignore the client. Much of how we (humankind) perceive the world, operate, value, and problem-solve is shaped by our cultural perspectives (Hyter & Salas-Provance, 2023). Gillespie (2016) recounts that for many Indigenous Americans who entered mainstream classrooms, the cultural and linguistic experiences that accompanied them were not welcomed. This experience is true for many other American forced and voluntary immigrants and refugees who constitute marginalized cultures and speak/use dialects/languages of their communities. While some individuals were stripped of their cultural and linguistic identities, others suppressed and hid them to assimilate into society and to avoid the perpetuation of historical prejudice and racism that led to intergenerational historical trauma.

As speech-language clinicians, it is our ethical responsibility to understand multilingualism and tailor our practices to assess and treat multilingual clients effectively. We must do so in a fashion that does not perpetuate the egregious misdiagnosis of multilingual individuals that has plagued our profession from its inception. Culturally responsive practice for multilingual/multicultural clients requires an extended skill set beyond what is needed to evaluate speakers of the host language (which is English in the US context) and the majority dialect. The authors provide general recommendations for working with multilingual clients. While the information provided is not exhaustive, it provides foundational tools and strategies for practice.

It is important to note that multilingualism is an asset that should be fostered and nourished. As language specialists, we should encourage our clients to continue using their home language and dialect alongside the use of their second language(s) in all facets of society. In doing so, we counteract the societal and political narratives that have historically suppressed diversity. As vocal advocates for multilingualism, we bring awareness to the value of our client's cultural and linguistic diversity. In Tables 6.3 and 6.4, the authors provide general practical guidelines gleaned from the literature that provides a roadmap for working with multilingual clients.

6.5 Recommendations for Culturally Responsive, Trauma-Informed Care for Bilingual Clients

This section of the chapter presents the Multilingual UPLIFT approach as a recommendation developed by the authors Drs. Sulare Telford Rose and Jennifer Rae Myers for culturally responsive trauma-informed care for multilingual individuals with minoritized status. While not exhaustive, the Multilingual UPLIFT approach is a supplement to be used in conjunction with other culturally responsive trauma-informed practices that address the intersectionality of trauma and minoritized ethnic and linguistic status. The approach melds recommendations that emerged from the fields of anthropology, psychology, speech-language-hearing sciences, education, and linguistics on multilingualism and trauma and takes a broader non-traditional perspective of multilingualism. It also takes into account that individuals who speak more than one language or "dialect" are all multilinguals. It accounts for linguistic codes of communication that may not hold political power and therefore not be given the status of an official language within society. As renowned linguist Max Weinreich states, the difference between language and dialect is politics (Wolfram & Schilling-Estes, 2016). Therefore, this approach adheres to the linguistic definition of a language, which is a code communication that has its own semantics, pragmatics, morphology, syntax, and phonology, whether spoken, written or signed. The Multilingual UPLIFT approach aims to promote change in clinical practice and dismantle socio-political practices that promote Eurocentric monolingual ideals that lead to re-traumatization.

The approach includes (1) Upholding the cultural and linguistic values of the client, (2) Listening to the collective narratives of the client, (3) Implementing a transdisciplinary approach to trauma-informed care, (4) Facilitating access to essential resources, (5) Fostering use of the home language and sustained bilingualism, and (6) Terminating current ideologies

Table 6.3 General Guidelines for Assessment of Multilingual Clients

Population	Guideline	Reference
Children & Adults	Exercise cultural responsiveness and cultural humility.	Hyter and Salas-Provance (2023)
	Practice honest self-reflection. Reflect on your "beliefs, dispositions, and attitudes about culture, diversity, race, privilege, socioeconomic status, and globalized populations through resources in our field" Lindsay Nurse et al. (2021, p. 204)	Lindsay Nurse et al. (2021), Hyter and Salas-Provance (2023)
	Research the client's culture, language, and community prior to assessing their cognitive, linguistic, and literacy abilities.	Ladson-Billings (2011)
	Develop an expanded view of bilingualism and of who is bilingual (i.e., anyone who speaks or understands two or more languages which include creoles and dialects).	Karem and Washington (2021), Telford Rose et al. (2020)
	Understand that bilinguals are not two separate monolinguals. Children particularly, may have language abilities in one language that they do not have in the other.	Mahootian (2020), Shin (2018)
	Conduct assessments in all the languages the client speaks (Paradis et al., 2011; Soto et al., 2020). If the clinician does not have linguistic competencies in the client's language(s); use interpreters, translators and transliterators in the assessment process.	American Speech-Language-Hearing Association, (n.d.), Kayser (1995)
	Understand bilingual language development to include phenomena that differ from monolinguals such as translanguaging, code-switching, language transfer, language interference, fossilization, BICS, CALP, language independence etc.	Mahootian (2020), Shin (2018)
	Build long-term partnerships with cultural and linguistic brokers.	Hamilton and Ramos-Pizarro (2020)

(Continued)

Table 6.3 (Continued)

Population	Guideline	Reference
	Penn (2011) states that these brokers should be "individuals who act as a repository of world knowledge and serve the role of bridging, linking, or mediating between groups or persons of differing cultural backgrounds, not only for interpreting services but for providing insight into the life experience of the client."	Friedland and Penn (2003), Hseih (2007)
	Modified and adapted assessments should have linguistic, cultural, and metric equivalence.	Peña (2007)
	Ensure that selected standardized assessment tools have been normed on the population you wish to assess.	
	Identify if assessment protocols have situational, format, value or linguistic biases.	Taylor and Payne (1983)
	A convergence assessment approach where multiple assessment data is collected is the recommended approach for bilingual assessment. Castilla-Earls et al. (2020) suggest using four methods: language experience questionnaires; bilingual language, speech sample analysis; evaluation of learning potential; and standardized testing.	Castilla-Earls et al. (2020), Telford Rose et al. (2020)
	Do not assume that because a clinician or educator speaks more than one language that they are automatically experts in the field of bilingualism. Becoming a culturally competent practitioner requires training, particularly on typical bilingual development and disorders.	Hamilton and Ramos Pizzaro (2020)
	Develop an expanded view of bilingualism and of who is bilingual (i.e., anyone who speaks or understands two or more languages, which include creoles and dialects).	Karem and Washington (2021), Telford Rose et al. (2020)

(Continued)

Table 6.3 (Continued)

Population	Guideline	Reference
Children	Ladson-Billings (2001) recommends learning the student's "culture and community, use student culture as a context for learning, and promote flexible use of local and global culture."	Gillispie (2016)
	Learn about dual language development.	Paradis et al. (2011)
	Use teacher and parent reports as an essential process in culturally responsive assessment especially for bilingual assessment.	Kan et al. (2020)
	Note that bilingual children "who are at-risk for having a communication disorder may have poorer receptive vocabulary skills in their home language compared to typically developing children."	Kan et al. (2020)
	Note that bilingual children whose parents and teachers are concerned about their communication skills may also be at an increased risk for having a communication disorder.	Kan et al. (2020)
	Using dynamic assessment and response to intervention (RTI) models or any assessment model that requires monitoring a client's progress over time is a critical approach to clinical decision-making.	Hyter and Salas-Provance (2023), Castilla-Earls et al. (2020), Kan et al. (2020)

Table 6.4 General Guidelines for Intervention of Multilingual Clients

Population	Guideline	References
Children and adults	Exercise cultural humility.	Hyter and Salas Provance (2023)
	Address problems of racism within the clinical and educational community.	Winer (2009)
	Incorporate materials and resources that reflect the client's local and global culture and language.	Caesar and Nelson (2013)
	Incorporate literature, media and other resources that were written not only in the language of the client but reflect true cultural elements.	Winer (2009)
	Cultural modifications to mainstream intervention programs and tailoring intervention strategies and procedures to "clients and caregivers cultural background/interaction style/priorities" are foundational to foundational to ensure culturally responsive treatment implementation.	Guiberson and Ferris (2019)
	Use culturally appropriate materials.	Source not provided.
Children	Foster relationships with the parents/guardians, and communities that our bilingual clients live in.	Pham and Tipton (2018), Kohnert et al. (2005), Caesar and Nelson (2013)
	Clarify misconceptions to parents regarding bilingualism. Many parents of bilingual children hold the false premise that using the home language with children will hinder the development of their children's second language.	Pham and Tipton (2018), Kohnert et al. (2005)
	Encourage parents to foster home language or heritage and literacy development through "rich and frequent exposure" to the language. Pham & Tipton (2018) suggest that parents enroll children in weekend heritage language classes, schedule classes, schedule frequent trips to the parents' country of origin, and speak and read to their children in their home language.	Guiberson and Ferris (2019), Pham and Tipton (2018), Mendez et al. (2015), Caesar and Nelson (2013)

(Continued)

Table 6.4 (Continued)

Population	Guideline	References
	Support the development of the home/heritage language in the clinical and classroom environments through bilingual and cross-linguistic intervention. Monolingual SLPs should consider first working on speech or language skills that are common across both languages. Using cognates to begin vocabulary development has been cited in the literature. However, beware of false cognates.	Pham and Tipton (2018)
	Incorporate the home/heritage language into intervention planning, even when the educator does not speak the home language of the student/client.	Telford Rose (2023)
	Provide "purposeful, consistent and systematic" intervention in the client's home/heritage language, which allows for cross-linguistic transfer and better linguistic, educational, social-emotional, and psychological gains.	Mendez et al. (2015)
	Use technology to support development of the client's first language especially when the clinician does not speak that language. "Collaborations with BI ([bilingual) SLPs, paraprofessionals, professionals in related fields, interpreters, and families are essential in designing and implementing intervention programs that promote the development of a child's L1 alongside gains in English."	Telford Rose (2023), Adams et al. (2018), Pham et al. (2011) Pham et al. (2011), Kohnert (2007), Kohnert et al. (2005)
	Organize a buddy system with other children in the classroom or clinical settings who speak the language or are a part of the culture that the client is from, especially if he/she/they have followed a similar path.	Winer (2009)
	Keep reference sources such as dictionaries that are in the client's language, such as Caribbean English Creoles, Amharic, or Spanish dictionaries.	Winer (2009)

of linguistic imperialism. Figure 6.1 presents a summary of the Multilingual UPLIFT Approach to Trauma-Informed Care.

While many of the Multilingual UPLIFT Approach recommendations are cited across the literature and are already presented in the previous section, the approach emphasizes the aspects that are particularly pertinent for working with multilingual clients who experience trauma and PTS. The goal of this approach is to provide a meaningful and accessible guideline for improving practice in the field. The elements of the Multilingual UPLIFT Approach to Trauma-Informed Care will be presented in reverse order, as the lower levels are foundational.

6.5.1   T – Terminate Current Ideologies of Linguistic Imperialism

Foundational to the Multicultural UPLIFT approach to Trauma-Informed Care is the "termination of current ideologies of linguistic imperialism." Our ideology invariably shapes our practice. Therefore, the first step to reducing trauma in bilingual clients is to shift the ideologies that cause trauma and re-traumatization. The term linguistic imperialism was coined by Phillipson (1992). Philipson defines linguistic imperialism in part as interlocking

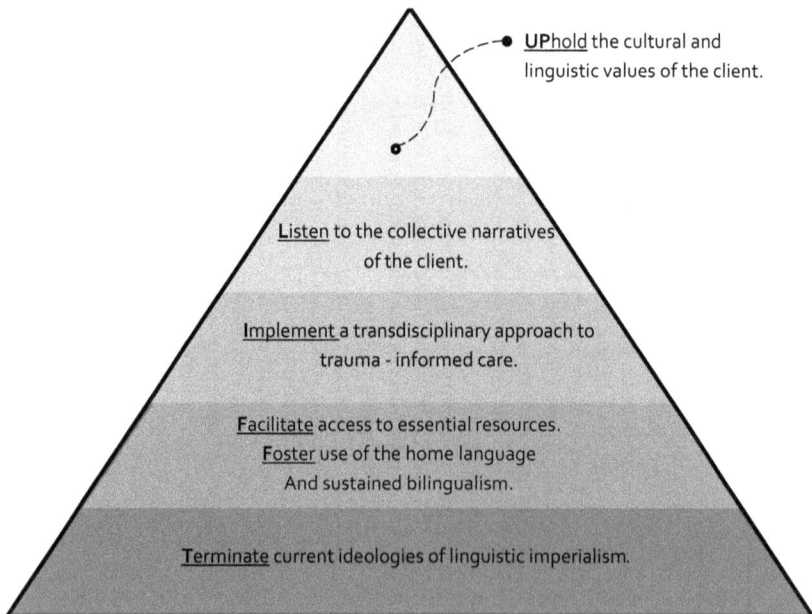

Figure 6.1 Multilingual UPLIFT Approach to Trauma-Informed Care.

with a structure of imperialism in culture, education, the media, communication, the economy, politics, and military activities. Linguistic Imperialism, a form of linguicism, a favoring of one language over others in ways that parallel societal structuring through racism, sexism, and class... Linguicism serves to privilege users of the standard forms of the dominant language, which represent convertible linguistic capital.

(Phillipson, 2012, p. 1)

Philipson (2012) provides an expansive and context-driven definition in his Encyclopedia of Applied Linguistics chapter.

If we reflect on our clinical practices, we can begin to identify ways in which we perpetuate ideologies that support linguistic imperialism. Linguistic imperialism is so finely embedded in our clinical and educational systems that we often fail to recognize them, especially when they do not directly affect us or our own families or community. However, once we begin to recognize them, we can begin to shift our own practices and provide more equitable services to our clients including those who are monolingual speakers of non-mainstream languages (in the US context, any language other than English) and multilingual individuals. While we cannot individually dismantle the systems and structures that shape our society, we can take a step in that direction by changing our own practices and advocating for the rights of others.

Take this example from one of the authors who experienced linguicism while working in the school system as a bilingual clinician. The author had recently completed a bilingual assessment for a bilingual Spanish (dominant) -English-speaking school-age child. The parents of the client were recent immigrants from a Spanish-dominant country. Furthermore, they had few linguistic skills in English. The child was diagnosed with a language delay. The author's supervisor at the educational site encouraged her to advise the child's parents to only speak with their child in English as speaking Spanish and English would confuse her. While the supervisor may have been well-meaning, this recommendation was problematic clinically and ethically. Everyone should have the right to speak and use the language(s) of their choice and to pass on their linguistic heritage to their children. Also, children who receive support in both their home language and societal language often demonstrate more significant gains over time linguistically, academically, socially, and emotionally than their peers who do not receive bilingual support.

Terminating these ideologies of linguistic imperialism will take more than just individual speech-language clinicians making changes, but rather concerted institutional and societal changes, which include changing policy, curriculum, etc. See Cushing (2023) and Ortega et al. (2022) for expanded ways to enforce these changes. In addition to the recommendations of Cushing (2023) and Ortega et al. (2022), the authors recommend that speech-language-hearing training programs and professional organizations designate specific and required courses on Sociolinguistics or Raciolinguistics for all students for pre-service and practicing clinicians. The second recommendation is to examine curricular training materials, client resource, professional, and discipline documentation with a team of people from diverse communities across age groups and expertise to identify ways that these materials may perpetuate linguistic imperialism. The final recommendation is to collectively work to change the systems within and beyond our field that systematically reinforce linguistic imperialism.

6.5.2   F – Facilitate Access to Essential Resources

Torres (2010) posits that when working with bilingual individuals particularly those who are newcomers to the host country, clinicians should consider external factors that may hinder their involvement such as access to resources. Torres (2010) recommends:

1 Connecting clients and their families to "information regarding local immigrant rights organizations and specific options such as the U Visa (Fontes, 2005)."
2 Providing assistance during holidays and back-to-school events such as giving out clothing, can goods, school supplies.
3 "Facilitating access to community after-school programs and participation in organizations in the neighborhood, such as Big Brother and Big Sister programs, or the Boys and Girls Club."
4 Informing clients about their rights.
5 Connecting families with victim rights advocates.
6 Facilitating access to transportation.

It should be noted that one should not automatically assume that every bilingual client does not have access to financial and other resources. Therefore, understanding the needs of clients is of importance.

6.5.3   F – Foster Use of the Home Language and Sustained Multilingualism

"Implicit in culture-informed care is the expectation that language access services are integrated into all aspects" (Im & Swan, 2021). When working with multilingual clients, especially adult clients, we may find that many of them are most comfortable using their first or native language. Torres (2010) recommends the use of culture/language matched dyads, where the clinician and client share the same culture and language as a culturally responsive trauma-informed approach with bilingual clients. While this is optimal, culture/language matched dyads may not always be possible with speech-language-hearing professionals and their clients as the majority of US-based speech-language clinician are monolingual speakers of English. In this case, as Im et al. (2021) suggest, having language access services where the client can speak their preferred language with an interpreter present, may be an alternative method to practice. However, the use of a third party in the client-clinician relationship may not be the optimal trauma-informed approach as the third party may not be one the client trusts or to whom they wish to disclose information about themselves. As such, the authors suggests use of technology such google translate or similar tools to facilitate culturally responsive trauma-informed communication in the clinician-client dyads, and also call for speech-language clinicians to engage in the development of technology to support multilingual clients in therapy (Telford Rose, 2023).

Clinicians however should be aware that "choosing to use one language versus another can have social consequences for a bilingual speaker" (Arizmendi, 2022). For example,

> If the speaker chooses to use Spanish, she may encounter social obstacles such as being perceived as unable to speak English, salespeople questioning her ability to afford the goods in the store, or simply enduring negative looks or glances from people who are not accepting of another language being spoken in the community. If the speaker chooses to use English, the majority language, she is less likely to encounter these same types of negative social ramifications. Choosing to use Spanish, in this context, can lead to increased stress.
>
> (Arizmendi, 2022)

As such we may find clients who would much prefer to speak in their more dominant native language but who may choose to speak with clinicians using English, even when other language options are presented. While some clients may prefer to speak their native language, others may not because of fear of being looked down upon or feeling the need to impress the clinician regarding their adeptness in the host language (which is English in the United States). It is therefore the work of a culturally responsive trauma-informed clinician to dismantle these societal trauma-inducing realities by counteracting the narrative, one clinician at a time, while simultaneously advocating against the racially charged linguistic imperialist policies and systems. One way that the authors recommend doing this is by demonstrating to the client that we as professionals value their non-mainstream language(s). This can be done by:

1 Posting signs in our clinical settings that have multiple languages.
2 Using pictures and decor that depict our clients' culture and language.
3 Learning the basics of the client's language, like greetings and idioms.
4 Clearly stating that our clients are welcome to use their native or preferred language with us.
5 Saying that we value their language and culture.
6 Demonstrating genuine interest in cultural norms and perspectives. (This genuineness can only come about when we learn and exercise cultural and linguistic humility).
7 Learning and asking the client and or caregivers to teach us new words without being patronizing.
8 Acknowledging that when one's first language development/rehabilitation is supported then we see greater gains in both languages.
9 Advocating for clients when others in the community discourage or dissuade clients from using their native language.
10 Providing paperwork, brochures and other written material in both the client's native language and the majority or host language.
11 Encouraging translanguaging.
12 Advocate to change policy and systems that perpetuate the use of certain types of English only in the classroom, clinical and other settings (See Cushing, 2023).

An important note for the culturally responsive, trauma-informed clinician working with multilingual clients, is to understand that it is not our role to force the client to do anything they are not comfortable with, which includes using their first language in the clinical setting; clients should always have the power to do with what they are most comfortable. As highlighted in Myers & Telford Rose (2022), multilingual clients may not use their native languages because they are trying to distance themselves from the language in which they experience the trauma. We do not want to stimulate re-traumatization; however, fostering an environment in which their native language is encouraged, welcomed and promoted, is the goal.

As aforementioned in this chapter, translanguaging and code-switching are normal phenomena among multilingual individuals. Building upon the approach of fostering use of the home language and sustained bilingualism, supports this notion. If our clients are unable to fully express themselves using one language or the other, encourage them to use both languages whenever necessary. Many multilingual clients may not even be aware that this is occurring, but encouraging them to bring their whole selves, is a key element in culturally responsive, trauma-informed care. This is important both for the diagnostic process in which both/all languages should be tested and seen as one whole of the linguistic abilities of our multilingual clients in the therapeutic sessions.

While representation is important in clinical practice, it is equally as important for speech-language clinicians, healthcare providers, and educators to work concertedly to dismantle existing structures that perpetuate linguistic trauma. A major part of this is to bring to light that "linguistic racism" is part of the larger societal issue linked to racism and discrimination. Cushing (2023) provides specific strategies in this area.

6.5.4   I – Implement a Transdisciplinary Approach to Trauma-Informed Care

A transdisciplinary approach to trauma-informed care has been cited across the literature (Hyter & Ciolino, 2018; Ciolino et al., 2021; Hyter, 2021; Myers & Telford Rose, 2022). Myers & Telford Rose (2022) promote collaborative transdisciplinary care among speech-language clinicians, educators, and scholars, psychologists, social workers, occupational therapists, and cultural/linguistic brokers as a possible key to providing holistic care and elevating our discipline-specific culturally responsive care for bilingual individuals suffering from posttraumatic stress. The authors expand on the Myers & Telford Rose (2022) recommendations by suggesting the inclusion of ELL teachers into the transdisciplinary approach when working with bilinguals. The literature highlights that immigrants who have experienced trauma report having difficulty acquiring a second language especially among adults, secondary to their trauma exposure. Additionally, including occupational therapists, families, and the clients themselves as part of the team can lead to effective outcomes. Figure 6.2 depicts the transdisciplinary approach to culturally responsive, trauma-informed care for bilingual individuals which builds on the Myers & Telford Rose recommendations (2022).

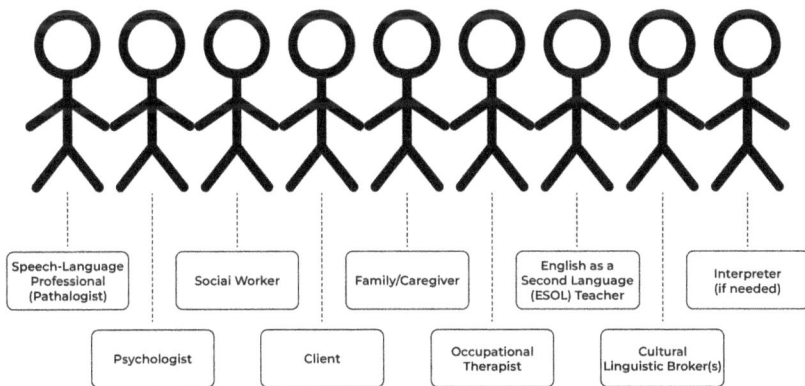

Figure 6.2 Transdisciplinary Model to Trauma-Informed Care for Bilinguals.

6.5.5   L – Listen to the Collective Narratives of the Client

Context matters – researching the historical, community, and personal narratives of the client broadens awareness of the client and the impacts of trauma on their lives. Many marginalized communities such as Native Americans, African Americans, and Jews experienced long-lasting historical traumas which have intergenerational effects that continue to perpetuate trauma today. Therefore, listening to documentaries and reading historical accounts and stories that depict the historical traumas of your client's community, is essential in fostering an environment of care and reducing re-traumatization (DeGruy-Leary, 2017). It is essential that you do this research with the understanding that you'll never fully understand the impact because you've never walked in the client's shoes. However, empathy is essential. "Empathy requires believing people. The quickest path to an empathic miss is to evaluate + judge what people are sharing through the lens of our lived experiences vs listening and believing" (Brown, 2020).

Additionally, staying abreast of current news, laws, or actions – especially those related to immigration, health, and race – that impact communities in which we serve is essential. One such law that was recently passed in Florida (SB 148) states that one cannot discuss topics that would make people feel uncomfortable about past heinous actions such as slavery. A part of the bill reads

> An individual, by virtue of his or her race or sex, does not bear responsibility for actions committed in the past by other members of the same race or sex. An individual should not be made to feel discomfort, guilt, anguish, or any other form of psychological distress on account of his or her race.

This law may cause re-traumatization, hurt, fear and continued distrust among the victims of slavery and genocide. This can cause re-traumatization because the law fails to acknowledge the history of systems that led to racial and linguistic imperialism and may cause a sense of hopelessness and fear among clients that they will continue to be ill-treated and their history and language does not matter.

The clinician should also listen to narratives from community members from the client's ethnic group to gain understanding of the perceived impact on their community. We often may not be aware of impact if we are not affected, thus it is our job to listen and inquire. Innovation and ideas for change do not start outside the community in which we aim to adjust our practices. Our clients and their caregivers are also essential parts of the team. They are the experts on themselves and their community. So in the case of working with bilingual clients and their caregivers, clinicians ought to employ an ethnographic approach to service delivery. It centers the clients as experts on themselves, their communities and their needs. Therefore, when conducting the case history, it is important to ask clients what their specific needs and wants are in terms of the work with the speech-language clinicians, and to collect extensive data on the client's language history, language preferences, and their migration history. However, it is also important to remember that due to historic prejudices, racism, and widespread anti-immigration sentiments in the current socio-political climate, our clients may be suffering from posttraumatic slave syndrome or other traumas (that are secondary to systemic racism) and racial inequities and therefore may be leery to share any information with clinicians that they believe may jeopardize their future and safety (DeGruy-Leary, 2005; Woods-Jaegar et al., 2022). Therefore, building mutual trust is an important element in working with our clients and may not happen overnight. Practicing patience and having a more long-term and ongoing approach to case history and data collection, are therefore pertinent. Trust should be earned and not simply given because of our roles. Demonstrating trustworthiness is critical and frankly, not all of us are. The holistic narrative collective narratives provide context which will help to improve assessment and intervention practices.

6.5.6   UP – Uphold the Cultural and Linguistic Values of the Client

At the top of the pyramid is the principle of upholding our clients' cultural and linguistic values. This cannot be achieved without adhering to the aforementioned practices. At its core, upholding clients' cultural and linguistic values requires communication and understanding of what they need and want from our services, even if these differ from our own practice. This allows us to entertain educational and clinical practices that may bring healing to the client, even if they juxtapose with western views. No cultural way of doing things is inferior. Psychology scholarship tells us that some cultures use different methods to bring healing, such as dance in the Ubuntu of Africa (Bryant Davis, 2019). While there is not much empirical evidence to support this thrust, people know and understand themselves and their culture better than we do. We ought to uphold their traditions and incorporate them into clinical practice to meet the needs of our clients and we should ascribe value to their cultural variations in educational and clinical practice (Bryant Davis, 2019).

6.6   Chapter Summary

This chapter explores trauma and language among multilingual children and adults. Posttraumatic stress can result in language delay or deficits in multilingual individuals. Certain multilingual populations such as immigrants and refugees, individuals from deaf or hard-of-hearing communities, and individuals who speak AAL often experience unique traumas related to their linguistic identity, adding an additional layer of challenges as language is the source of trauma.

There are several theoretical considerations when examining the relationship between trauma and multilingualism. Multilingualism has a mediating effect, particularly for immigrants and refugees where the fluency of the host language may interact with the presence or severity of PTS. The potential competition for limited cognitive resources between trauma and language may also offer insight into the intrusive effects of trauma on language as well as consequences of language as the trauma. Lastly, code-switching may serve as a defense mechanism for multilinguals. The use of code-switching to avoid or minimize the emotional impact associated with one of the languages has been established in the literature; however, some research suggests it may be more of a reflection of language dominance.

As clinicians serving multilinguals who have experienced trauma, the UP-LIFT model is a recommended approach for culturally responsive trauma-informed care. The UPLIFT model instructs clinicians to understand and treat multilingual clients without perpetuating the egregious misdiagnosis of multilinguals. This includes encouraging clients to utilize translanguage, building long-term partnerships with cultural and linguistic brokers, and dismantling institutional socio-political practices that promote Eurocentric monolingual ideals that lead to re-traumatization. Thus, our role and ethical responsibility to address the "whole" multilingual client in this context of trauma is paramount to their therapeutic success.

By now, we hope you have a clearer understanding of the complex relationship between PTS and language among multilinguals as well as the role of the speech-language professionals as a trauma-informed culturally responsive clinician. Stories like Mariana from the vignette at the beginning of the chapter are not uncommon; therefore, it is important to consider the cultural, cognitive, and linguistic needs of our multilingual clients who have experienced trauma. While research in this domain is still growing, ongoing efforts are bringing much needed attention to this dynamic and critical issue.

Notes

1 When defining translanguaging, Vogel and Garcia (2017) stress that *all* language users, not just bilingual and multilingual languagers, employ a range of codes, strategies, and modes for meaning making.
2 Blacks and African Americans refer to all people of African descent including those not born in the U.S.

References

Adams, A. M., Glenberg, A. M., & Restrepo, M. A. (2018). Moved by reading in a Spanish-speaking, dual language learner population. *Language, Speech, and Hearing Services in Schools, 49*(3), 582–594. https://doi.org/10.1044/2018_lshss-16-0032

Aldalur, A., Pick, L. H., & Schooler, D. (2021). Navigating deaf and hearing cultures: An exploration of deaf Acculturative stress. *The Journal of Deaf Studies and Deaf Education, 26*(3), 299–313. https://doi.org/10.1093/deafed/enab014

Alim, H. S., Rickford, J. R., & Ball, A. F. (2016). *Raciolinguistics: How language shapes our ideas about race*. Oxford University Press.

American Speech-Language-Hearing Association. (n.d.). *Collaborating with interpreters, transliterators, and translators*. American Speech-Language-Hearing Association. Retrieved from https://www.asha.org/practice-portal/professional-issues/collaborating-with-interpreters/

Anderson, M. L., Wolf Craig, K. S., Hall, W. C., & Ziedonis, D. M. (2016). A pilot study of deaf trauma survivors' experiences: Early traumas unique to being deaf in a hearing world. *Journal of Child & Adolescent Trauma, 9*(4), 353–358. https://doi.org/10.1007/s40653-016-0111-2

Anderson, R. E., & Stevenson, H. C. (2019). RECASTing racial stress and trauma: Theorizing the healing potential of racial socialization in families. *American Psychologist, 74*(1), 63–75. https://doi.org/10.1037/amp0000392

Archuleta, A. J., & Lakhwani, M. (2016). Posttraumatic stress disorder symptoms among first-generation Latino youths in an English as a second language school. *Children & Schools, 38*(2), 119–127. https://doi.org/10.1093/cs/cdw005

Arizmendi, G. (2022). Bilingual Therapies Symposium 2022. In *Executive Function and Learning During COVID-19: A Call for Trauma Informed Care [Oral Presentation]*. Bilingual Therapies, Virtual.

Ayçiçeği, A., & Harris, C. (2004). BRIEF REPORT bilinguals' recall and recognition of emotion words. *Cognition and Emotion, 18*(7), 977–987. https://doi.org/10.1080/02699930341000301

Baker-Bell, A. (2019). Dismantling anti-Black linguistic racism in English language arts classrooms: Toward an anti-racist Black language pedagogy. *Theory Into Practice, 59*(1), 8–21. https://doi.org/10.1080/00405841.2019.1665415

Baugh, J. (2003). Linguistic profiling. In A. Ball, S. Makoni, G. Smitherman, A. K. Spears, & F. B. Thiong'o (Eds.), *Black linguistics: Language, society and politics in Africa and the Americas* (pp. 155–168). Routledge.

Beiser, M., & Hou, F. (2001). Language acquisition, unemployment and depressive disorder among Southeast Asian refugees: A 10-year study. *Social Science & Medicine, 53*(10), 1321–1334. https://doi.org/10.1016/s0277-9536(00)00412-3

Berry, J. W. (1997). Immigration, acculturation, and adaptation. *Applied Psychology, 46*(1), 5–34. https://doi.org/10.1111/j.1464-0597.1997.tb01087.x

Ballan, M. S., & Freyer, M. (2019). Intimate partner violence and women with disabilities: The role of speech-language pathologists. *American Journal of Speech - Language Pathology (Online), 28*(4), 1692–1697. https://doi.org/10.1044/2019_AJSLP-18-0259

Birman, D., Simon, C. D., Chan, W. Y., & Tran, N. (2014). A life domains perspective on acculturation and psychological adjustment: A study of refugees from the former Soviet Union. *American Journal of Community Psychology, 53*(1–2), 60–72. https://doi.org/10.1007/s10464-013-9614-2

Black, P. A., & Glickman, N. S. (2006). Demographics, psychiatric diagnoses, and other characteristics of North American deaf and hard-of-Hearing inpatients. *Journal of Deaf Studies and Deaf Education, 11*(3), 303–321. https://doi.org/10.1093/deafed/enj042

Bloom, L., & Lahey, M. (1978). *Language development and language disorders.* John Wiley & Sons.

Bogic, M., Ajdukovic, D., Bremner, S., Franciskovic, T., Galeazzi, G. M., Kucukalic, A., Lecic-Tosevski, D., Morina, N., Popovski, M., Schützwohl, M., Wang, D., & Priebe, S. (2012). Factors associated with mental disorders in long-settled war refugees: Refugees from the former Yugoslavia in Germany, Italy and the UK. *British Journal of Psychiatry, 200*(3), 216–223. https://doi.org/10.1192/bjp.bp.110.084764

Brown, B. (2020, November 9). *Empathy requires believing people. the quickest path to an empathic miss is to evaluate+judge what people are sharing through the lens of our lived experiences vs listening and believing. convo with @aikobethea here: Https://t.co/onegn1urtb https://t.co/b6mv55rs5v pic.twitter.com/ajknkackcw.* Twitter. Retrieved from https://twitter.com/BreneBrown/status/1325865811496595456

Bryant-Davis, T. (2007). Healing requires recognition. *The Counseling Psychologist, 35*(1), 135–143. https://doi.org/10.1177/0011000006295152

Bryant-Davis, T. (2019). The cultural context of trauma recovery: Considering the posttraumatic stress disorder practice guideline and intersectionality. *Psychotherapy, 56*(3), 400–408. https://doi.org/10.1037/pst0000241

Bryant-Davis, T., & Ocampo, C. (2005). The trauma of racism. *The Counseling Psychologist, 33*(4), 574–578. https://doi.org/10.1177/0011000005276581

Busch, B., & McNamara, T. (2020). Language and trauma: An introduction. *Applied Linguistics, 41*(3), 323–333. https://doi.org/10.1093/applin/amaa002

Caesar, L., & Nelson, N. (2013). Picturing literacy success. *The ASHA Leader, 18*(2). https://doi.org/10.1044/leader.ftr4.18022013.np

Carter, R. T., & Sant-Barket, S. M. (2015). Assessment of the impact of racial discrimination and racism: How to use the race-based traumatic stress symptom scale in practice. *Traumatology, 21*(1), 32–39. https://doi.org/10.1037/trm0000018

Caruth, E. G. (1987). Language in intimacy and isolation: Transitional dilemma, transformational resolution. *Journal of the American Academy of Psychoanalysis, 15*(1), 39–49. https://doi.org/10.1521/jaap.1.1987.15.1.39

Castaño, M. T., Biever, J. L., González, C. G., & Anderson, K. B. (2007). Challenges of providing mental health services in Spanish. *Professional Psychology: Research and Practice, 38*(6), 667–673. https://doi.org/10.1037/0735-7028.38.6.667

Castilla-Earls, A., Bedore, L., Rojas, R., Fabiano-Smith, L., Pruitt-Lord, S., Restrepo, M. A., & Peña, E. (2020). Beyond scores: Using converging evidence to determine speech and language services eligibility for dual language learners.

American Journal of Speech-Language Pathology, 29(3), 1116–1132. https://doi.org/10.1044/2020_ajslp-19-00179

Cerdeña, J. P., Rivera, L. M., & Spak, J. M. (2021). Intergenerational trauma in Latinxs: A scoping review. *Social Science & Medicine, 270*, 113662. https://doi.org/10.1016/j.socscimed.2020.113662

Chapman, M., & Dammeyer, J. (2017). The significance of deaf identity for psychological well-being. *The Journal of Deaf Studies and Deaf Education, 26*(4), 567–567. https://doi.org/10.1093/deafed/enw078

Cushing, I. (2023). Challenging anti-Black linguistic racism in schools amidst the 'what works' agenda. *Race Ethnicity and Education, 26*(3), 257–276. https://doi.org/10.1080/13613324.2023.2170435

Degruy-Leary, J. A. (2005). *Post traumatic slave syndrome: America's legacy of enduring injury and healing.* Milwaukie, Oregon: Uptone Press.

Degruy-Leary, J. A. (2017). *Post traumatic slave syndrome: America's legacy of enduring injury and healing.* Joy DeGruy Publications.

Dewaele, J. (2010). *Emotions in multiple languages.* Palgrave Macmillan.

Di Sante, M., Sylvestre, A., Bouchard, C., & Leblond, J. (2019). The pragmatic language skills of severely neglected 42-month-old children: Results of the ELLAN study. *Child Maltreatment, 24*(3), 244–253. https://doi.org/10.1177/1077559519828838

Doucerain, M. M., Varnaamkhaasti, R. S., Segalowitz, N., & Ryder, A. G. (2015). Second language social networks and communication-related acculturative stress: The role of interconnectedness. *Frontiers in Psychology, 6.* https://doi.org/10.3389/fpsyg.2015.01111

Drachman, D. (2014). Immigrant and refugees. In A. Gitterman (Ed.), *Handbook of social work practice with vulnerable and resilient populations* (pp. 366–391). Columbia University Press.

Dumont, F., Tarabulsy, G. M., Sylvestre, A., & Voisin, J. (2019). Children's emotional self-regulation in the context of adversity and the association with academic functioning. *Child Psychiatry & Human Development, 50*(5), 856–867. https://doi.org/10.1007/s10578-019-00888-3

Dyb, G., Holen, A., Brænne, K., Indredavik, M. S., & Aarseth, J. (2003). Parent-child discrepancy in reporting children's post-traumatic stress reactions after a traffic accident. *Nordic Journal of Psychiatry, 57*(5), 339–344. https://doi.org/10.1080/08039480310002660

Fontes, L. A. (2005). *Child Abuse and Culture.* New York: Guilford Press.

Forman-Hoffman, V. L., Bose, J., Batts, K. R., Glasheen, C., Hirsch, E., Karg, R. S., Huang, L. N., & Hedden, S. L. (2016). Correlates of lifetime exposure to one or more potentially traumatic events and subsequent posttraumatic stress among adults in the United States: Results from the mental health surveillance study, 2008--2012. In CBHSQ data review. (p. 1–49). Substance Abuse and Mental Health Services Administration (US).

Friedland, D., & Penn, C. (2003). Conversation analysis as a technique for exploring the dynamics of a mediated interview. *International Journal of Language & Communication Disorders, 38*(1), 95–111. https://doi.org/10.1080/13682820304811

Gillispie, M. (2016). Need for culturally responsive literacy instruction in Native American communities. *Perspectives of the ASHA Special Interest Groups, 1*(14), 56–68. https://doi.org/10.1044/persp1.sig14.56

Goffman, E. (1963). *Stigma: Notes on the management of spoiled identity.* Prentice Hall.

Gordon, D. (2011). Trauma and second language learning among Laotian refugees. *Journal of Southeast Asian American Education and Advancement, 6*(1). https://doi.org/10.7771/2153-8999.1029

Gradus, J. L. (2007). *Epidemiology of PTSD.* National Center for PTSD.

Greenfield, L., & Fishman, J. A. (1975). Situational measures of normative language views of person, place and topic among Puerto Rican bilinguals. In J. A. Fishman, R. L. Cooper, & R. Ma (Eds.), *Bilingualism in the barrio* (pp. 233–252). Bloomington: Indiana University Press.

Grogger, J. (2011). Speech patterns and racial wage inequality. *Journal of Human Resources, 46*(1), 1–25. https://doi.org/10.1353/jhr.2011.0017

Grosjean, F. (2008). The bilingualism and biculturalism of the Deaf. *Studying bilinguals.* Oxford University Press.

Grosjean, F. (2010). Personality, thinking and dreaming, and emotions in bilinguals. *Bilingual: Life and reality.* Harvard University Press.

Grushkin, D. A. (1996). *Academic, linguistic, social and identity development in hard of hearing adolescents educated within an ASL/English bilingual/bicultural educational setting for deaf and hard of hearing students* [Doctoral dissertation]. ProQuest Dissertations and Theses Global.

Guiberson, M., & Ferris, K. P. (2019). Early language interventions for young dual language learners: A scoping review. *American Journal of Speech-Language Pathology, 28*(3), 945–963. https://doi.org/10.1044/2019_ajslp-idll-18-0251

Hamiliton, A. F., & Ramos-Pizarro, C. A. (2020). Assimilation and language assumptions - why english isn't "better". In A. F. Hamilton, C. A. Ramos-Pizarro, J. F. Rivera Pérez, W. González, & K. L. Beverly-Ducker (Eds.), *Exploring cultural responsiveness: Guided scenarios for communication sciences and disorders (CSD) professionals.* ASHA Press.

Hayes, J. P., VanElzakker, M. B., & Shin, L. M. (2012). Emotion and cognition interactions in PTSD: A review of neurocognitive and neuroimaging studies. *Frontiers in Integrative Neuroscience, 6.* https://doi.org/10.3389/fnint.2012.00089

Herman, J. L. (1992). *Trauma and recovery.* New York: Basic Books.

Herzog, J. I., & Schmahl, C. (2018). Adverse childhood experiences and the consequences on neurobiological, psychosocial, and somatic conditions across the lifespan. *Frontiers in Psychiatry, 9.* https://doi.org/10.3389/fpsyt.2018.00420

Hoge, C. W., McGurk, D., Thomas, J. L., Cox, A. L., Engel, C. C., & Castro, C. A. (2008). Mild traumatic brain injury in U.S. soldiers returning from Iraq. *New England Journal of Medicine, 358*(5), 453–463. https://doi.org/10.1056/nejmoa072972

Hwa-Froelich, D. (2012). Childhood maltreatment and communication development. *Perspectives on School-Based Issues, 13*(2), 43–53. https://doi.org/10.1044/sbi13.2.43

Hwa-Froelich, D. A. (Ed.). (2022). *Social communication development and disorders.* Taylor & Francis.

Hsieh, E. (2007). Interpreters as co-diagnosticians: Overlapping roles and services between providers and interpreters. *Social Science & Medicine, 64*(4), 924–937.

Hyter, Y. D. (2012). Complex trauma and prenatal alcohol exposure: Clinical implications. *Perspectives on School-Based Issues, 13*(2), 32–42. https://doi.org/10.1044/sbi13.2.32

Hyter, Y. D. (2021). Childhood maltreatment consequences on social pragmatic communication: A systematic review of the literature. *Perspectives of the ASHA Special Interest Groups, 6*(2), 262–287. https://doi.org/10.1044/2021_persp-20-00222

Hyter, Y. D., & Ciolino, C. (2017). Providing SLP services through a trauma informed lens. In *Seminar presented at the annual convention of the American Speech-Language-Hearing Association, Los Angeles, CA*.

Hyter, Y. D., & Ciolino, C. (2018, March). *Trauma and pragmatic language, social communication and trauma informed SLP practice. Seminar presented at the Annual Convention of the Michigan Speech-Language-Hearing Association, Kalamazoo, MI, United States*.

Hyter, Y. D., & Salas-Provance, M. B. (2023). *Culturally responsive practices in speech, language and hearing sciences* (2nd ed.). Plural Publishing.

Im, H., & Swan, L. E. (2021). Working towards culturally responsive trauma-informed care in the refugee resettlement process: Qualitative inquiry with refugee-serving professionals in the United States. *Behavioral Sciences, 11*(11), 155. https://doi.org/10.3390/bs11110155

Isserlis, J. (2000). *Trauma and the adult English language learner.* Center for Applied Linguistics & National Clearinghouse for Bilingual Education.

Javier, R. A. (1989). Linguistic considerations in the treatment of bilinguals. *Psychoanalytic Psychology, 6*(1), 87–96. https://doi.org/10.1037/0736-9735.6.1.87

Javier, R. A., & Alpert, M. (1986). The effect of stress on the linguistic generalization of bilingual individuals. *Journal of Psycholinguistic Research, 15*(5), 419–435. https://doi.org/10.1007/bf01067723

Jocelyn, J. (2022). *The Perspective of Haitian Parents on Heritage Language Maintenance In Children with Speech-Language Disorders* [Doctoral dissertation]. ProQuest Dissertations and Theses Global.

Johnson, R. (2018). Trauma and learning: Impacts and strategies for adult classroom success. *MinneTESOL Journal, 34* (1–9). https://minnetesoljournal.org/wp-content/uploads/2018/11/Johnson-2018-Trauma-and-Learning_Impacts-and-Strategies-for-Adult-Classroom-Success.pdf

Jordan, M., Kanno-Youngs, Z., & Shear, M. D. (2022, March 24). United States Will Welcome Up to 100,000 Ukrainian Refugees. *NY Times.* Retrieved from https://www.nytimes.com/2022/03/24/us/ukrainian-refugees-biden.html

Kan, P. F., Huang, S., Winicour, E., & Yang, J. (2020). Vocabulary growth: Dual language learners at risk for language impairment. *American Journal of Speech-Language Pathology, 29*(3), 1178–1195. https://doi.org/10.1044/2020_ajslp-19-00160

Kanagaratnam, P., & Asbjørnsen, A. E. (2007). Executive deficits in chronic PTSD related to political violence. *Journal of Anxiety Disorders, 21*(4), 510–525. https://doi.org/10.1016/j.janxdis.2006.06.008

Kaplan, I., Stolk, Y., Valibhoy, M., Tucker, A., & Baker, J. (2016). Cognitive assessment of refugee children: Effects of trauma and new language acquisition. *Transcultural Psychiatry, 53*(1), 81–109. https://doi.org/10.1177/1363461515612933

Karem, R. W., & Washington, K. N. (2021). The cultural and diagnostic appropriateness of standardized assessments for dual language learners: A focus on Jamaican preschoolers. *Language, Speech, and Hearing Services in Schools, 52*(3), 807–826. https://doi.org/10.1044/2021_lshss-20-00106

Kartal, D., Alkemade, N., & Kiropoulos, L. (2019). Trauma and mental health in resettled refugees: Mediating effect of host language acquisition on posttraumatic stress disorder, depressive and anxiety symptoms. *Transcultural Psychiatry, 56*(1), 3–23. https://doi.org/10.1177/1363461518789538

Kartal, D., & Kiropoulos, L. (2016). Effects of acculturative stress on PTSD, depressive, and anxiety symptoms among refugees resettled in Australia and Austria. *European Journal of Psychotraumatology, 7*(1). https://doi.org/10.3402/ejpt.v7.28711

Kayser, H. G. (1995). *Bilingual speech-language pathology: An Hispanic focus.* Singular Pub. Group.

Kerka, S. (2002). *Journal writing as an adult learning tool* (ERIC Document Reproduction Service No. ED470782). ERIC Clearinghouse on Adult Career and Vocational Education.

Kilpatrick, D. G., Resnick, H. S., Milanak, M. E., Miller, M. W., Keyes, K. M., & Friedman, M. J. (2013). National estimates of exposure to traumatic events and PTSD prevalence using *dsm-iv* and *dsm-5* criteria. *Journal of Traumatic Stress, 26*(5), 537–547. https://doi.org/10.1002/jts.21848

Kohnert, K., Yim, D., Nett, K., Kan, P. F., & Duran, L. (2005). Intervention with linguistically diverse preschool children. *Language, Speech, and Hearing Services in Schools, 36*(3), 251–263. https://doi.org/10.1044/0161-1461(2005/025)

Kolers, P. A. (1963). Interlingual word associations. *Journal of Verbal Learning and Verbal Behavior, 2*(4), 291–300. https://doi.org/10.1016/s0022-5371(63)80097-3

Ladegaard, H. J. (2018). Codeswitching and emotional alignment: Talking about abuse in domestic migrant-worker returnee narratives. *Language in Society, 47*(5), 693–714. https://doi.org/10.1017/s0047404518000933

Ladson-Billings, G. (2011). Is meeting the diverse needs of all students possible? *Kappa Delta Pi Record, 47*(sup1), 13–15. https://doi.org/10.1080/00228958.2011.10516716

Leong, F., Park, Y. S., & Kalibatseva, Z. (2013). Disentangling immigrant status in mental health: Psychological protective and risk factors among Latino and Asian American immigrants. *American Journal of Orthopsychiatry, 83*(2–3), 361–371. https://doi.org/10.1111/ajop.12020

Lewis, J. A., & Neville, H. A. (2015). Construction and initial validation of the gendered racial microaggressions scale for Black women. *Journal of Counseling Psychology, 62*(2), 289–302. https://doi.org/10.1037/cou0000062

Lillo-Martin, D., Quadros, R. M., & Chen Pichler, D. (2016). The development of bimodal bilingualism. *Epistemological issue with keynote article "The development of bimodal bilingualism: Implications for linguistic theory" by Diane Lillo-Martin, Ronice Müller de Quadros and Deborah Chen Pichler, 6*(6), 719–755. https://doi.org/10.1075/lab.6.6.01lil

Lindencrona, F. (2008). *Strategies for a health promoting introduction for newly-arrived refugees and other immigrants.* Institutionen för klinisk neurovetenskap/ Department of Clinical Neuroscience.

Lindsay Nurse, K. T., Gardner, K., & Brea, M. R. (2021). Operationalizing culturally responsive research practices: Documenting the communication skills of children with confirmed or possible exposure to the Zika virus in Saint Lucia, West Indies. *Perspectives of the ASHA Special Interest Groups, 6*(1), 191–206. https://doi.org/10.1044/2020_persp-19-00140

Lyn, K. O. (2022). Negotiating African American language, identity, and culture in the urban classroom. *Journal of Black Studies, 53*(8), 780–795. https://doi.org/10.1177/00219347221115035

Mahootian, S. (2020). *Bilingualism.* Routledge.

Matheson, K., Jorden, S., & Anisman, H. (2007). Relations between trauma experiences and psychological, physical and neuroendocrine functioning among Somali refugees: Mediating role of coping with acculturation stressors. *Journal of Immigrant and Minority Health, 10*(4), 291–304. https://doi.org/10.1007/s10903-007-9086-2

McDonald, S. (2000). Trauma and second language learning. *The Canadian Modern Language Review, 56*(4), 690–696. https://doi.org/10.3138/cmlr.56.4.690

Miele, D., & O'Brien, E. J. (2010). Underdiagnosis of posttraumatic stress disorder in at risk youth. *Journal of Traumatic Stress, 23*(5), 591–598. https://doi.org/10.1002/jts.20572

Monnat, S. M., & Chandler, R. F. (2015). Long-term physical health consequences of adverse childhood experiences. *The Sociological Quarterly, 56*(4), 723–752. https://doi.org/10.1111/tsq.12107

Myers, J. R., Solomon, N. P., Lange, R. T., French, L. M., Lippa, S. M., Brickell, T. A., Staines, S., Nelson, J., Brungart, D. S., & Coelho, C. A. (2022). Analysis of discourse production to assess cognitive communication deficits following mild traumatic brain injury with and without posttraumatic stress. *American Journal of Speech-Language Pathology, 31*(1), 84–98. https://doi.org/10.1044/2021_ajslp-20-00281

Myers, J. R., & Telford, S. R. (2022). A preliminary report of trauma impact on language skills in bilingual adults: A case for trauma-informed services. *HPHR, 62.* Retrieved from https://hphr.org/62-article-rose/

Myles, P., Swenshon, S., Haase, K., Szeles, T., Jung, C., Jacobi, F., & Rath, B. (2018). A comparative analysis of psychological trauma experienced by children and young adults in two scenarios: Evacuation after a natural disaster vs forced migration to escape armed conflict. *Public Health, 158*, 163–175. https://doi.org/10.1016/j.puhe.2018.03.012

Méndez, L. I., Crais, E. R., Castro, D. C., & Kainz, K. (2015). A culturally and linguistically responsive vocabulary approach for young Latino dual language learners. *Journal of Speech, Language, and Hearing Research, 58*(1), 93–106. https://doi.org/10.1044/2014_jslhr-l-12-0221

Nadal, K. L., Erazo, T., & King, R. (2019). Challenging definitions of psychological trauma: Connecting racial microaggressions and traumatic stress. *Journal for Social Action in Counseling & Psychology, 11*(2), 2–16. https://doi.org/10.33043/jsacp.11.2.2-16

O'Brien, J., & Sutherland, R. J. (2007). Evidence for episodic memory in a Pavlovian conditioning procedure in rats. *Hippocampus, 17*(12), 1149–1152. https://doi.org/10.1002/hipo.20346

Øhre, B., Uthus, M. P., Von Tetzchner, S., & Falkum, E. (2015). Traumatization in deaf and hard-of-Hearing adult psychiatric outpatients. *Journal of Deaf Studies and Deaf Education, 20*(3), 296–308. https://doi.org/10.1093/deafed/env013

Ortega, P., Martinez, G., Aleman, M. A., Zapien-Hidalgo, A., & Shin, T. M. (2022). Recognizing and dismantling Raciolinguistic hierarchies in Latinx health. *AMA Journal of Ethics, 24*(4), E296–304. https://doi.org/10.1001/amajethics.2022.296

O'Neill, L., Fraser, T., Kitchenham, A., & McDonald, V. (2016). Hidden burdens: A review of intergenerational, historical and complex trauma, implications for Indigenous families. *Journal of Child & Adolescent Trauma, 11*(2), 173–186. https://doi.org/10.1007/s40653-016-0117-9

O'Toole, T. J. (1974). The speech clinician and child abuse. *Language, Speech, and Hearing Services in Schools, 5*(2), 103–106. https://doi.org/10.1044/0161-1461.0502.103

Paradis, J., Genesee, F., & Crago, M. B. (2011). *Dual language development and disorders: A handbook on bilingualism and second language learning* (2nd ed.). Brookes Publishing.

Pavlenko, A. (2004). L2 influence and L1 attrition in adult bilingualism. *Studies in Bilingualism*, 47. https://doi.org/10.1075/sibil.28.04pav

Peña, E. D. (2007). Lost in translation: Methodological considerations in cross-cultural research. *Child Development, 78*(4), 1255–1264. https://doi.org/10.1111/j.1467-8624.2007.01064.x

Pham, G., Kohnert, K., & Mann, D. (2011). Addressing clinician–client mismatch: A preliminary intervention study with a bilingual Vietnamese–English preschooler. *Language, Speech, and Hearing Services in Schools, 42*(4), 408–422. https://doi.org/10.1044/0161-1461(2011/10-0073)

Pham, G., & Tipton, T. (2018). Internal and external factors that support children's minority first language and English. *Language, Speech, and Hearing Services in Schools, 49*(3), 595–606. https://doi.org/10.1044/2018_lshss-17-0086

Phillipson, R. (1992). *Linguistic imperialism*. Oxford University Press.

Phillipson, R. (2012). Linguistic imperialism. *The Encyclopedia of Applied Linguistics*. https://doi.org/10.1002/9781405198431.wbeal0718

Phipps, R. M., & Degges-White, S. (2014). A new look at Transgenerational trauma transmission: Second-generation Latino immigrant youth. *Journal of Multicultural Counseling and Development, 42*(3), 174–187. https://doi.org/10.1002/j.2161-1912.2014.00053.x

Purnell, T., Idsardi, W., & Baugh, J. (1999). Perceptual and phonetic experiments on American English dialect identification. *Journal of Language and Social Psychology, 18*(1), 10–30. https://doi.org/10.1177/0261927x99018001002

Purvis, K. B., Cross, D. R., Dansereau, D. F., & Parris, S. R. (2013). Trust-based relational intervention (TBRI): A systemic approach to complex developmental trauma. *Child & Youth Services, 34*(4), 360–386. https://doi.org/10.1080/0145935x.2013.859906

Qureshi, S. U., Long, M. E., Bradshaw, M. R., Pyne, J. M., Magruder, K. M., Kimbrell, T., Hudson, T. J., Jawaid, A., Schulz, P. E., & Kunik, M. E. (2011). Does PTSD impair cognition beyond the effect of trauma? *Journal of Neuropsychiatry, 23*(1), 16–28. https://doi.org/10.1176/appi.neuropsych.23.1.16

Ramírez-Esparza, N., & García-Sierra, A. (2014). The bilingual brain: Language, culture & identity. In V. Benet-Martinez & Y. Hong (Eds.), *The Oxford handbook of multicultural identity* (pp. 35–56). Oxford University Press.

Rauch, S. L. (1996). A symptom provocation study of posttraumatic stress disorder using positron emission tomography and script-driven imagery. *Archives of General Psychiatry, 53*(5), 380. https://doi.org/10.1001/archpsyc.1996.01830050014003

Rickford, J. R., Duncan, G. J., Gennetian, L. A., Gou, R. Y., Greene, R., Katz, L. F., Kessler, R. C., Kling, J. R., Sanbonmatsu, L., Sanchez-Ordoñez, A. E., Sciandra, M., Thomas, E., & Ludwig, J. (2015). Neighborhood effects on use of African-American Vernacular English. *PNAS Proceedings of the National Academy of Sciences of the United States of America, 112*(38), 11817–11822. https://doi.org/10.1073/pnas.1500176112

Rickford, J. R. (1999). *African American Vernacular English: Features, evolution, educational implications*. Wiley-Blackwell.

Roberts, A. L., Gilman, S. E., Breslau, J., Breslau, N., & Koenen, K. C. (2010). Race/ethnic differences in exposure to traumatic events, development of post-traumatic stress disorder, and treatment-seeking for post-traumatic stress disorder in the United States. *Psychological Medicine, 41*(1), 71–83. https://doi.org/10.1017/s0033291710000401

Romaine, S. (2017). Multilingualism. In M. Aronoff & J. Rees-Miller (Eds.), *The handbook of linguistics* (2nd ed., pp. 541–556). Wiley-Blackwell.

Rosa, J., & Flores, N. (2017). Unsettling race and language: Toward a raciolinguistic perspective. *Language in Society, 46*(5), 621–647. https://doi.org/10.1017/s0047404517000562

Rupert, A. C., & Bartlett, D. E. (2022). The childhood trauma and attachment gap in speech-language pathology: Practitioners' knowledge, practice, and needs. *American Journal of Speech-Language Pathology, 31*(1), 287–302. https://doi.org/10.1044/2021_ajslp-21-00110

Santiago-Rivera, A. L., Altarriba, J., Poll, N., Gonzalez-Miller, N., & Cragun, C. (2009). Therapists' views on working with bilingual Spanish–English speaking clients: A qualitative investigation. *Professional Psychology: Research and Practice, 40*(5), 436–443. https://doi.org/10.1037/a0015933

Santoro, N. (1997). Why won't they talk: The difficulties of engaging victims of trauma in classroom interaction. *TESOL in Context, 7*(2), 14–18.

Schauer, M., Neuner, F., & Elbert, T. (2011). *Narrative exposure therapy: A short-term treatment for traumatic stress disorders* (2nd ed.). Hogrefe Publishing.

Schmidt, R. W. (1990). The role of consciousness in second language learning. *Applied Linguistics, 11*(2), 129–158. https://doi.org/10.1093/applin/11.2.129

Schmidt, R. (2010). Attention, awareness, and individual differences in language learning. In W. M. Chan, S. Chi, K. N. Cin, J. Istanto, M. Nagami, J. W. Sew, T. Suthiwan, & I. Walker (Eds.), *Proceedings of CLaSIC 2010*, Singapore,

December 2–4 (pp. 721–737). Singapore: National University of Singapore, Centre for Language Studies.

Schreier, H., Ladakakos, C., Morabito, D., Chapman, L., & Knudson, M. M. (2005). Posttraumatic stress symptoms in children after mild to moderate pediatric trauma: A longitudinal examination of symptom prevalence, correlates, and parent-child symptom reporting. *The Journal of Trauma: Injury, Infection, and Critical Care, 58*(2), 353–363. https://doi.org/10.1097/01.ta.0000152537.15672.b7

Schweitzer, R. D., Brough, M., Vromans, L., & Asic-Kobe, M. (2011). Mental health of newly arrived Burmese refugees in Australia: Contributions of pre-migration and post-migration experience. *Australian & New Zealand Journal of Psychiatry, 45*(4), 299–307. https://doi.org/10.3109/00048674.2010.543412

Shin, D. S. (2018). Multimodal mediation and argumentative writing: A case study of a multilingual learner's metalanguage awareness development. In R. Harman (Ed.), *Bilingual learners and social equity: Critical approaches to systemic functional linguistics* (pp. 225–242). Springer.

Shin, L. M., McNally, R. J., Kosslyn, S. M., Thompson, W. L., Rauch, S. L., Alpert, N. M., Metzger, L. J., Lasko, N. B., Orr, S. P., & Pitman, R. K. (1999). Regional cerebral blood flow during script-driven imagery in childhood sexual abuse-related PTSD: A pet investigation. *American Journal of Psychiatry, 156*(4), 575–584. https://doi.org/10.1176/ajp.156.4.575

Smith, S. (2016). African American ebonics: Discourse & discursive practice—a Chicago case study of historical oppression. *Howard Journal of Communications, 27*(4), 311–326. https://doi.org/10.1080/10646175.2016.1197867

Sparks, S. W. (2018). Posttraumatic stress syndrome: What is it? *Journal of Trauma Nursing, 25*(1), 60–65. https://doi.org/10.1097/jtn.0000000000000343

Sue, D. W. (2010). *Microaggressions in everyday life: Race, gender, and sexual orientation.* John Wiley & Sons.

Sue, D. W., Capodilupo, C. M., Torino, G. C., Bucceri, J. M., Holder, A. M., Nadal, K. L., & Esquilin, M. (2007). Racial microaggressions in everyday life: Implications for clinical practice. *American Psychologist, 62*(4), 271–286. https://doi.org/10.1037/0003-066x.62.4.271

Sylvestre, A., Bussières, È., & Bouchard, C. (2016). Language problems among abused and neglected children. *Child Maltreatment, 21*(1), 47–58. https://doi.org/10.1177/1077559515616703

Sylvestre, A., Desmarais, C., Meyer, F., Bairati, I., & Leblond, J. (2017). Prediction of the outcome of children who had a language delay at age 2 when they are aged 4: Still a challenge. *International Journal of Speech-Language Pathology, 20*(7), 731–744. https://doi.org/10.1080/17549507.2017.1355411

Sylvestre, A., Desmarais, C., Meyer, F., Bairati, I., Rouleau, N., & Mérette, C. (2012). Factors associated with expressive and receptive language in French-speaking toddlers clinically diagnosed with language delay. *Infants & Young Children, 25*(2), 158–171. https://doi.org/10.1097/iyc.0b013e31823dca22

Sylvestre, A., & Mérette, C. (2010). Language delay in severely neglected children: A cumulative or specific effect of risk factors? *Child Abuse & Neglect, 34*(6), 414–428. https://doi.org/10.1016/j.chiabu.2009.10.003

Söndergaard, H. P., & Theorell, T. (2004). Language acquisition in relation to cumulative posttraumatic stress disorder symptom load over time in a sample of resettled refugees. *Psychotherapy and Psychosomatics, 73*(5), 320–323. https://doi.org/10.1159/000078849

Tausczik, Y. R., & Pennebaker, J. W. (2010). The psychological meaning of words: LIWC and computerized text analysis methods. *Journal of Language and Social Psychology, 29*(1), 24–54. https://doi.org/10.1177/0261927x09351676

Taylor, O. L., & Payne, K. T. (1983). Culturally valid testing. *Topics in Language Disorders, 3*(3), 8–20. https://doi.org/10.1097/00011363-198306000-00005

Telford Rose, S. (2023, January). Reaching multilingual children in their home language - @ASHA. Retrieved from https://leader.pubs.asha.org/do/10.1044/leader.FTR2.28012023.ai-treatment-slp.50/full/

Telford Rose, S. L., Payne, K. T., De Lisser, T. N., Harris, O. L., & Elie, M. (2020). A comparative phonological analysis of guyanese Creole and standard American English: A guide for speech-language pathologists. *Perspectives of the ASHA Special Interest Groups, 5*(6), 1813–1819. https://doi.org/10.1044/2020_persp-20-00173

Thass-Thienemann, T. (1973). The interpretation of language. *Volume 1. Understanding the symbolic meaning of language.* Jason Aronson, Incorporated.

Torres, A. (2010). *The Bilingual Integrative Trauma Treatment Program: A Guide for working with Latino Victims of Childhood Sexual Abuse and their Families.* Unpublished.

United Nations High Commissioner for Refugees. (2021). *Global Trends Report 2021.* Retrieved from https://www.unhcr.org/en-us/publications/brochures/62a9d1494/global-trends-report-2021.html?query=Global Trends Report 2021

US Census Bureau (2021, December 16). *Detailed languages spoken at home and ability to speak English for the population 5 years and over: 2009–2013.* Census.gov. Retrieved from https://www.census.gov/data/tables/2013/demo/2009-2013-lang-tables.html

Van Zyl, M., Oosthuizen, P., & Seedat, S. (2008). Post traumatic stress disorder: Undiagnosed cases in a tertiary inpatient setting. *African Journal of Psychiatry, 11*(2). https://doi.org/10.4314/ajpsy.v11i2.30263

Vogel, S., & Garcia, O. (2017). *Translanguaging.* Online publication. Retrieved from https://academicworks.cuny.edu/cgi/viewcontent.cgi?article=1448&context=gc_pubs

Wolfram, W., & Schilling-Estes, N. (2016). *American English: Dialects and variation.* Wiley-Blackwell.

Woods-Jaeger, B., Kleven, L., Sexton, C., O'Malley, D., Cho, B., Bronston, S., McGowan, K., & Starr, D. (2023). Two generations thrive: Bidirectional collaboration among researchers, practitioners, and parents to promote culturally responsive trauma research, practice, and policy. *Psychological Trauma: Theory, Research, Practice, and Policy, 15*(2), 181–188. https://doi.org/10.1037/tra0001209

Westby, C. E. (2007). Child maltreatment: A global issue. *Language, Speech, and Hearing Services in Schools, 38*(2), 140–148. https://doi.org/10.1044/0161-1461(2007/014)

Winer, L. (2009). Teaching English to Caribbean English creole-speaking students in the Caribbean and North America. In S. J. Nero (Ed.), *Dialects, Englishes, creoles, and education* (pp. 105–118). Routledge.

Woods-Jaeger, B., Kleven, L., Sexton, C., O'Malley, D., Cho, B., Bronston, S., McGowan, K., & Starr, D. (2023). Two generations thrive: Bidirectional collaboration among researchers, practitioners, and parents to promote culturally responsive trauma research, practice, and policy. *Psychological Trauma: Theory, Research, Practice, and Policy, 15*(2), 181–188. https://doi.org/10.1037/tra0001209

Yehuda, N. (2016). *Communicating trauma: Clinical presentations and interventions with traumatized children*. Routledge, Taylor & Francis Group.

Yehuda, R., Hoge, C. W., McFarlane, A. C., Vermetten, E., Lanius, R. A., Nievergelt, C. M., Hobfoll, S. E., Koenen, K. C., Neylan, T. C., & Hyman, S. E. (2015). Post-traumatic stress disorder. *Nature Reviews Disease Primers, 1*(1). https://doi.org/10.1038/nrdp.2015.57

Ying, Y. (2001). Psychotherapy with traumatized Southeast Asian refugees. *Clinical Social Work, 29*(1), 65–78.

Part II

Post-Traumatic Stress

Considerations Across the
Lifespan for Language Development
and Functioning

7 Post-Traumatic Stress

Child Language Development and Functioning

Na'ama Yehuda

7.1 Introduction

Communication defines our human experience. It is the process through which we convey information, express needs, share ideas, and understand others. All languages include content (semantics), form (morphology and syntax), and use (pragmatics) (Berman, 2004; Gleason & Ratner, 2009). Verbal communication includes speech sounds, the words we use and how we put them into sentences, as well as intonation, voice, and intention. Non-verbal communication conveys information through posture, facial expression, gestures, body-language, physical reaction, action, or inaction. Proficiency and familiarity with context and social customs, along with an understanding of idioms, puns, and expressions, all play a role in communication. Successful interaction fosters satisfaction, closeness, and ease. Failure, on the other hand, can lead to embarrassment, awkwardness, confusion, distance, and anger (Gleason & Ratner, 2009; Ninio & Snow, 1996; Schieflbusch, 1986).

Children's linguistic and cognitive abilities are still developing. They rely on caregivers who understand the child's preferences, needs, vocalizations, and behaviors, to help lessen communication failure, reward connection, and calm dysregulation. Such mediation may be less available to children who have been maltreated. Furthermore, it can be harder to accomplish for children who are themselves less available to interaction due to anxiety, illness, or developmental and communication difficulties (Cole et al., 2005; Kuttner, 2010; Schieflbusch, 1986; Yehuda, 2016).

The impact of posttraumatic stress on social pragmatic language and narrative has been covered in detail by Hyter in Chapter 4 of this volume. This chapter will examine the additional aspects of language development (semantics, morphology, syntax, and phonology) through the lens of their exquisite vulnerability to trauma, and the mechanisms by which meaning, context, content, form, and communication are affected by such stress. The added risks in children with developmental and communication disorders,

DOI: 10.4324/9781003225270-9

as well as possible assessment and intervention guidelines, needs, and recommendations will be noted, as well.

Two-and-a-half-year-old Bella spoke very little and did so mostly in single word utterances. She followed routines "with her eyes," and while she seemed mildly interested in daycare activities, she did not initiate contact nor indicate when she wanted an interaction continued. "She's passive till she cries," the daycare professional said, "and then good luck calming her." Bella threw long tantrums where nothing consoled her. "She doesn't even want to be held. Cries till she wears herself out to sleep. Makes me feel useless." Bella's mother escaped prolonged domestic violence several months after Bella was born. The last straw being when she had been thrown to the ground with the baby in her arms. Depressed, concussed, and in fear for both their lives, Bella's mother kept moving even after her abuser was behind bars. "What if he gets out?" she fretted. "Bella is already traumatized."

Five-year-old Cole rarely sat still. Teachers complained he "did not listen," required repeated prompting to follow directions (which he often failed to complete), was aggressive at the slightest provocation, and caused constant disruptions in class. "His sonar is on 24/7," his teacher sighed. "Information bounces off him. He's a smart kid, but wherever his brain is, it isn't on academics. Or on language, for that matter. Constant chatter but no straight answers from him." A year earlier, Cole had survived a housefire that burned the home to the ground, put the whole family in the hospital, and left his father and sister with burns and lingering disability. The ordeal also led to crushing debt for his family.

7.1.1   Language-Learning

There is no learning without engagement. This is especially true when it comes to language acquisition in children, whose cognitive, relational, and developmental abilities are still maturing. Language acquisition is a complex undertaking, yet when provided with good-enough exposure and opportunity, and if children have adequate perception, cognition, and attention, most do develop language, and many, more than one (Gleason & Ratner, 2009). How others interact with the child and how the child's perceptions, actions, and feelings are interpreted are paramount to how communication, relating, and meaning are formed (Cozolino, 2014; Gaensbauer, 2011; Hyter, 2021; Snow, 2019; Yehuda, 2016).

7.1.2   Experiences, Reaction, and Meaning

Infants and young children experience the world, their body, and the actions of others through their senses. Input from their environment forms the basis for the child's reactions to stimuli (Cross et al., 2017; Rizzolatti et al., 2004; van der Kolk, 2014), and it is through adults' responses and what those elicit in the baby, that meaning is established and patterns become hard-wired (see Suarez's Chapter 5 for more discussion about this hard-wiring). As children's brains develop, connections form between feelings, words, tone, sensations, movement, and more. Intricate associations weave semantics and pitch, intonation and meaning, faces and voices, feelings, movements, and sensory information. The brain is literally built and shaped by experiences, both good and bad (Albers et al., 2005; Cozolino, 2014; Cross et al., 2017; Fogassi & Ferrarri, 2007; Gaensbauer, 2011; Schore, 2012; Siegel, 2012; van der Kolk, 2014; Yehuda, 2016).

A baby for whom hands meant comfort may stop crying when someone reaches out to them. They may smile back at a grin. A child for whom hands meant pain might lash out or shut down even if reached to in kindness. They might look way in wariness when smiled at (Gaensbauer, 2011; Miller, 2005). How a child's brain 'interprets meaning' depends on that child's previous experiences, and posttraumatic responses can become the 'default path' when neurological connections formed during times of overwhelming stress are reinforced by activation from trauma reminders (Gaensbauer, 2011; Osofsky et al., 2017; Siegel, 2012; Schore, 2012).

7.1.3   Trauma and Language

Stress disrupts cognitive processes, language, and memory. It affects information processing, formulating, problem solving, and communication (also see Westby, Hyter, Suarez, and Collins et al.in Chapters 3–5 and 8, respectively). Overwhelming stress leads to traumatic events being encoded, retrieved, and communicated differently than everyday events (Cozolino, 2006; Herman, 1997; Silberg, 2013; van der Kolk, 2014). Dissociation, though an effective survival mechanism, can fragment traumatic events, thus further impacting encoding and processing (Attias & Goodwin, 1999; Levine & Mate, 2010; Putnam, 1997, 2006). Trauma evokes strong emotions while simultaneously disrupting the very integration that allows us to recognize, differentiate, name, and understand affect. In that sense, trauma defies words. Posttraumatic narrative can be incoherent and inconsistent and can seem overly dramatic or detached from feeling (Herman, 1997; van der Kolk, 2014).

Verbalizing trauma can be difficult even for those with mature language skills and world understanding. Even more so for children, whose language and conceptualization are still developing (Cozolino, 2006; Schore, 2001; Yehuda, 2016; Hyter, 2021, 2022; Sylvestre & Mérette, 2010; Sylvestre, 2021; Snow, 2021). What caregivers say or not say, do or not do, is interwoven into the child's knowledge and beliefs about the world. It becomes the child's reality. Children's experience of trauma can influence how they apply meaning, not only for trauma-related material, but in other interactions as well (Hyter, 2021; Romano et al., 2015; Yehuda, 2016).

7.2   Language Development – What Is Needed, What Goes Wrong

Language allows us to share thoughts, feelings, and ideas through verbal, gestural, and written modes. It incorporates expressive language, receptive language, and the use of language in context (pragmatics). Proficiency is often reflected in lexical diversity, sentence complexity, narrative sophistication, and the ideas one can convey and understand (Gleason & Ratner, 2009). To achieve proficiency, language development depends on the quality and context of exposure, as well as on opportunity, experience, availability, and ability (Eigsti & Cicchetti, 2004; Hyter, 2021; Putnam, 2006; Snow, 2021; Sylvestre, 2021; Yehuda, 2016).

7.2.1   *Vocabulary and Acquisition of Meaning*

Vocabulary represents the 'cache' of semantic items in one's language. It includes labels for persons, places, things, and actions, as well as descriptors such as adjectives, adverbs, prepositions, and temporal, spatial, sequential, and numerical words. Our lexicon (aka vocabulary) contains the words we use in sentences to express varied meanings (Gleason & Ratner, 2009).

Young children acquire vocabulary from their caregivers. The context in which words are used is what helps children derive meaning (Baron, 1992; Berman, 2004; de Boysson-Bardies, 1999; Ninio & Snow, 1996). Language acquisition is helped by responsive and sensitive caregiving, where both quantity and quality matter (Golinkoff et al., 2019). Words that are presented frequently enough, and in contexts that are relevant and timely to the child, are more likely to be acquired than words that are used rarely or are irrelevant to the child (Romeo et al., 2018). Caregivers shape semantics: the meaning they give something, verbally or through action, intonation, and consequence, is the meaning the child will learn.

Responsive caregivers who are sensitive to what and how the child is communicating, and who respond to the child's interests, facilitate language development. Such caregivers offer timely and relevant responses that encourage continued communication and support turn-taking where both child and adult are participants (Hudson et al., 2015; Yehuda, 2016; Sylvestre, 2021). They may comment on a child's actions and behavior, repeat vocalizations, interpret the child's needs, and offer answers to a child's direct or indirect questions and requests. They reciprocate. They give space for the child to respond, and respect cues from the child as to whether they want to continue an action or interaction or have had enough.

These experiences allow the child to listen, observe, make connections, attempt, and learn to use language both receptively and expressively (Hyter, 2021; Yehuda, 2016).

7.2.2   *Trauma and Language Development – What Goes Wrong*

Language acquisition depends on the quality, quantity, and context of exposure. Poor exposure, such as in neglect, can lead to limited cognitive and language capabilities (Albers et al., 2005; Beverly et al., 2008; Bowlby, 1997; Cohen, 2001; Cross, 2004; De Bellis, 2005, 2013; Hildyard & Wolfe, 2002; Hough & Kaczmarek, 2011; Miller, 2005; Milot et al., 2010; and many more). Research has shown that by age three, about one out of two children who experience neglect show serious delays in language development (Sylvestre & Mérette, 2010). Compared to peers, children who experienced neglect have smaller receptive vocabularies with less varieties of words, delayed lexical abilities, less advanced morphological and syntactic abilities, and weaker pragmatic skills (Romano et al., 2015; Sylvestre, 2021; Sylvestre et al., 2016; Hyter, 2021; Yehuda, 2016).

Children's early years are crucial for development, as genes, experiences, and environment interact to shape brain architecture and function (Bernard et al., 2017; Cross et al., 2017; Gaensbauer, 2011; Garner, 2013; Siegel, 2012). Children who experience maltreatment often miss out on the sensitive, reciprocal, and responsive interactions that are necessary for an optimal development. Children who experienced trauma have less opportunities to form connections for positive experiences, more exposure to negative experiences, and less support for managing and processing these negative experiences. Language acquisition also requires the child to be available to communicate. Overwhelming stress affects brain growth, regulation, and cognitive processes; and maltreatment in early years can impact how children's brains form and function, with ramifications for development and learning (Gaensbauer, 2011; Garner, 2013; Romano et al., 2015; van der Kolk, 2014). Indeed, children who experienced trauma have been found to have lexical and semantics difficulties in both receptive and expressive language, along with difficulties with language knowledge and use (Cozolino, 2014; Hyter, 2021; Putnam, 2006; Siegel, 2012; Snow, 2021; van der Kolk, 2014; Yehuda, 2004, 2005, 2011, 2016).

7.2.3   *Language Exposure in Maltreatment*

Language acquisition relies on exposure in varied contexts (Berman, 2004; Gleason & Ratner, 2009; Romeo et al., 2018). Rich exposure to language through narrative, inquiry, and literacy plays an important role in language expansion. For example, children whose caregivers read to them tend to have larger receptive vocabularies and better listening and processing skills than those whose caregivers do not (Gleason & Ratner, 2009; Heymann, 2010; Landry et al., 2006). Stories enrich connection, language structure, and semantic growth (Romeo et al., 2018; Yehuda, 2016). Both quality and quantity of exposure matter, as does the opportunity to interact and practice the use of language.

Communication is reciprocal. Learning it requires practice. It is common for children to make errors in using newly acquired language forms (e.g., "I see five mouses," "He taked it."). Sensitive caregivers respond with affectionate correction or re-phrasing. They applaud correct use with praise and delight. Such reactions reinforce the child's motivation to explore meaning and words. In contrast, children who experience maltreatment may not receive encouragement to experiment and have fewer opportunities to do so. Previous mockery or an expectation of failure might lead children to refrain from asking about or testing new words or expressions. This may further limit their opportunities to practice various aspects of language (Garner, 2013; Levendosky, 2003; Putnam, 2006; Yehuda, 2016).

Maltreatment poses a risk for language development. Children who experience maltreatment have less receptive vocabulary, use fewer lexical items, and have less effective expressive language than well-cared-for peers (De Bellis, 2005; Kurtz et al., 1993; Lum et al., 2015; Putnam, 1997, 2006; Sylvestre et al., 2016). A smaller store of words means fewer to draw on for comprehension and expression. Indeed, children with histories of maltreatment performed more poorly than peers who have not experienced maltreatment on receptive language measures (auditory comprehension, following directions), expressive language measures (mean length of utterance, speed of naming), and pragmatics measures (social discourse) (Ciolino et al., 2021; Hyter, 2021). Younger children were particularly vulnerable to the impact of maltreatment and were more negatively affected than children whose maltreatment occurred at an older age (Lum et al., 2015; Romano et al., 2015; Sylvestre & Mérette, 2010; Sylvestre et al., 2016).

The vocabulary of children who experience neglect tends to be the most affected (Albers et al., 2005; Miller, 2005; Putnam, 2006; Sylvestre & Mérette, 2010). It is not surprising that vocabularies suffer in children who have had little experience with interaction (e.g., orphanages), and whose interactions with caregivers were mostly limited to directive and repetitive utterances (e.g., "stop it!," "sit down," "give it to me!") (Miller, 2005; Yehuda, 2011, 2016). Children whose caregivers are overwhelmed (e.g., overstressed, disabled, unhoused), and unavailable to the child, are also at risk for having smaller vocabularies (Bartlett & Smith, 2017; Levendosky et al., 2003; Milot et al., 2010; Nabors et al., 2004).

7.2.4 Ability, Disability, and Availability

Exposure is not the only factor in vocabulary growth. The child's ability and availability matter, too. To make use of communication opportunities, children must be available to listen and able to process. Trauma can disrupt that. Even children who experienced trauma who have plenty of opportunities for interaction can be affected by how stress shuts down listening and learning (Cole et al., 2005; Romano et al., 2015; van der Kolk, 2014; Yehuda, 2004, 2016). Trauma and posttraumatic stress can make it difficult for children to attend during interactions, and be less able to process, store, and recall words, concepts, and names for things. Trauma itself can create scary associations and confusion about meaning, which can inhibit inquiry and exploration (Kuttner, 2010; Levendovsky et al., 2003; Schore, 2001; van der Kolk, 2014; Yehuda, 2016).

Born into violence, two-and-a-half-year-old Bella had learned to not draw attention to herself. She did not trust others to help her regulate. She feared loud voices and was terrified of being dropped. Even after escaping abuse, Bella's mother was often too depressed and overwhelmed to respond sensitively. Bella coped by withdrawing. Nowhere felt safe. The speech-language clinician collaborated with daycare personnel to offer deliberate, sensitive, responsive dyadic interaction and narrative. Trauma-informed, flexible ways to comfort and reassure Bella at the first sign of dysregulation were incorporated. Caregivers modulated their voices and pitch to support soothing. Story booklets and photos helped reinforce language, engagement, and vocalizations. Bella's mother accepted support for herself and carried over modeled interactions at home. Slowly but surely, Bella began reciprocating, approaching, requesting, and responding. She became curious. She relaxed. Her language expanded and soon included varied word combinations and sentences. She learned to protest and deny, seek comfort when upset, welcome, question, and correct. She took turns and showed interest in her peers. She reached developmental milestones and closed developmental gaps.

Trauma disruption can happen without maltreatment, too. Children who experience medical trauma may feel like their experiences have no words (Drew, 2007). They might lack the energy or resources to try. They may find interactions scary. Pain, malaise, and medications' side-effects can make listening difficult (Fuemmeler et al., 2002; Kazak et al., 2006; Kuttner, 2010). A child experiencing overwhelm is less available to process new information or retrieve vocabulary they already have.

A foundation of supportive experiences and a healthy baseline of prosocial and communication skills can help children regulate distress. They can build resilience and aid in moderating the impact of traumatic events (Bartlett & Smith, 2017; Racine et al., 2020). However, such a foundation can be harder to build for individuals whose communication skills are already compromised by any manner of developmental difficulties. Atypical development places children at a disadvantage for comprehending and processing everyday interactions, let alone traumatic ones. Developmental challenges can increase confusion and stress, which may further compromise availability for language-learning and communicating (Snow, 2021; Yehuda, 2006, 2011, 2016). To further complicate matters, disabilities themselves increase a child's risk for maltreatment, victimization, and trauma (Benedict et al., 1990; Crosse et al., 1993; Goldson, 1998; Hershkowitz et al., 2007; Sullivan et al., 1987, 1991; Sullivan & Knutson, 1998, 2000).

7.3   Language Aspects that are Vulnerable to Trauma

The ramifications of trauma on language in children, be it from insufficient exposure to sensitive and relevant communication, reduced opportunity, inability, preoccupation, fear, or combination thereof, can be serious. Language requires ongoing, flexible, and creative use to develop. Disruption during early childhood can have lasting effects (Hyter, 2022; Lum et al., 2018; Romano et al., 2015; Snow, 2019; Yehuda, 2016). While all language domains can be affected by trauma, some aspects appear especially vulnerable to chronic stress.

7.3.1   'Body State' and Emotive Vocabulary

Children who experienced trauma tend to use less body-state words such as: hungry, tired, thirsty, satisfied; have a smaller emotive vocabulary (i.e., words that describe feelings); and are likely to use primarily negative emotional states when they do use them (Pearce & Pezzot-Pearce, 2006; Putnam, 2006). Their 'feeling words' tend to be nonspecific (catchall "good," "bad," "sad", "mad") rather than emotions like excited, surprised, delighted, proud, hurt, worried, bored, etc. (Yehuda, 2005, 2016).

The paucity of body-state and emotive vocabulary can be partially explained by un-worded, ignored, and mislabeled experiences. If hunger is not named or attended to, if discomfort is left unexplained or is denied, if fatigue is not acknowledged; how would a child know what to call gurgles in their tummy, burn of a rash, droopiness of exhaustion, or pain of abuse? Another reason for a small emotive lexicon can be dissociation. When caregivers do not alleviate distress (let alone when they cause it!), young children may cope by shutting out their sensations, emotions, and discomfort. This can become their way of coping with the world (Gaensbauer, 2011; Levine & Mate, 2010; van der Kolk, 2014). While effective for survival, such detachment can make it harder for the child to associate words with an internal experience (Carter, 2002; Kuttner, 2010), Like Bella, children who experience trauma may not know how to utilize offered care or how to ask for it. When others then struggle to respond effectively to the child's needs, they may inadvertently reinforce the child's disconnection from body-states and emotive language (Yehuda, 2016).

Even when they know the words, children who experience trauma may find personal experiences confusing and scary to describe. If needs brought on suffering and care came with strings attached, children might find the very having of feelings and needs, triggering. It could feel safer to hide, deny, or disconnect from sadness, pain, hunger, anger, or fatigue (Silberg, 2013; van der Kolk, 2014; Yehuda, 2005).

Similar disconnection can take place in children who endure over-whelming medical situations (Kuttner, 2010). Children can become confused about the meaning and realness of their experiences (e.g., told "everything's okay" when things are not). They may believe that showing pain or expressing distress will lead to more hurt (e.g., if medical interventions felt like punishment). They might feel enraged that their caregivers 'let' others hurt them, yet also feel guilty for how expressions of pain upset or frighten their caregivers. Body sensations can be confusing, too (e.g., hunger when eating is forbidden). Words like "no" and "stop" may lose power as body boundaries become violable. In response, children who experience medical trauma can panic at any medical reminder or might dissociate and become numb (Carter, 2002; Kuttner, 2010; Yehuda, 2016). Being disconnected from one's own sensations and feelings can make it difficult to process and express one's experiences. It may also make it harder to recognize and label emotions in others (Gaensbauer, 2011; Fogassi & Ferrarri, 2007; Mitchel at al., 2020; van der Kolk, 2014). Indeed, children who experienced trauma can seem to lack empathy or have inconsistent interpretations for social situations (Hyter, 2021; Snow, 2019; Yehuda, 2011, 2016).

Children rely on caregivers to label and differentiate comfort from dis-comfort, pleasure from pain, worry from calm. To a child, if the adult is happy, it 'must' mean something good has happened; if the adult is sad, angry, frightened, it 'must' mean the child did something bad. Sensitive adults validate children's feelings even when these differ from their own. This helps children recognize and trust their own perceptions and that there can be more than one feeling—and view—of a situation. However, if the child's distress is ignored, dismissed, or shamed, they may remain confused (e.g., does being "happy" mean someone else has to be sad?) (Mitchel et al., 2020; Yehuda, 2016).

7.3.2   Cause and Effect

Cause and effect are learned. Babies who are well-cared-for learn to anticipate relief when their caregivers' approach. They may stop crying at the
sound of footsteps or a voice. As infants grow, they learn that calling out
brings people; smiling makes others smile back; throwing food on the floor
brings the dog. They learn that by moving a certain way, they can reach a
toy; that touching some things will bring on a firm "no!" (Cozolino, 2006;
Shore, 2012; Sigel, 2012; Yehuda, 2016). Repeated testing of actions and
reactions helps babies understand causation, supports a sense of agency,
and teaches the baby the effect of their actions, vocalizations, smiles, and
cries (Baron, 1992; de Boysson-Bardies, 1999; Cozolino, 2006; Ninio &
Snow, 1996; Schore, 2012; Siegel, 2012).

Acquiring cause and effect requires the opportunity to experiment. Children with insufficient opportunities for exploring and too few relational
exchanges, might not understand what could happen, how and why. Examples of such deprivation have been found in children who have been
institutionalized and suffered severe neglect (Albers et al., 2005; De Bellis,
2005; Miller, 2005; Yehuda, 2016), and where children spent hours con-
fined to cribs or strollers with limited access to activity and interaction.
Association may form (e.g., light turning on and caregivers' movement in
the room), but crying may not bring soothing, vocalizing may not bring
interaction. Babies who experience neglect show limited interest in initiat-
ing play, and even when provided with toys, may not know what to do
with them (Albers et al., 2005; Miller, 2005; Silberg, 2013; Yehuda, 2016).
They may not realize they can cause an effect, that voice can be used, that
people can bring relief.

Even if a child who experienced trauma has opportunities to experiment with their environment, their curiosity might be curtailed by stress
or frightening responses, and they may not connect interaction with a rewarding reciprocation (Gaensbauer, 2011; Mitchel et al., 2020; Yehuda,
2016). Children who are ill or injured may fear exploration, too. If movement was restricted or brought on pain, they might be afraid to try things
(Kuttner, 2010). Uncertainty can lead children who experience trauma to
limit vocalizations, social gestures, and exploratory play (Doesburg et al.,
2013; Ford & Courtois, 2013; Gaensbauer, 2011; Heller & Lapierre,
2012; Pearce & Pezzot-Pearce, 2006).

The development of cause and effect might also be affected by children's
belief that they are to blame (especially if reinforced by: "Look what you've
done! See what happens when you make noise/mess your diaper/spill").
Trapped between the need to affect change (get help, be fed, be held), and
fearing the consequences, children can become too overwhelmed to explore (Gomez-Perales, 2015; Silberg, 2013; Yehuda, 2016).

Cole was four when his home burned down. The fire started in the children's bedroom, possibly from a blanket tossed midsleep onto the heater. Cole's blanket. To him, this meant he was at fault. The burns, the pain, the "being locked" (hyperbaric chamber) felt like punishment. His father' and sister's suffering, his mother's stress; his fault. Bad things happen when you don't pay mind. He would not let down his guard. Sirens made him scared. Cole's body showed no scars, but he was still in survival mode. A language assessment showed spotty delays in both expressive and receptive language, with erratic attention span, disjointed narrative, and difficulty with reading and responding to social cues.

A trauma-informed approach helped Cole's teachers understand his reactions and behavior. Cole was offered in-class accommodations and tools for emotional and physiological regulation, along with narrative scaffolding for interaction. His signs of distress were monitored so support and reassurance could be provided before he became overwhelmed. Predictable routines and clear expectations helped, as did preparation when possible, and support during and after unexpected transitions. That, along with speech-language therapy to close language-learning gaps, assisted his understanding of what had happened and what current experiences meant. It enabled Cole to let in learning and let adults keep him safe. He discovered a love (and talent!) for art and drums. Life at home remained complicated, but his parents did their best to support him.

7.3.3 Sequence

Babies learn sequence through routines and the narrative and explanation that reinforce these routines: you are uncomfortable→ you cry→someone comes and attends to you→discomfort is removed→you feel better. The baby becomes familiar with the steps, so when the caregiver comes in holding a bottle or clean diaper, she knows she'll be tended to, and her discomfort resolved. Without exposure to basic predictability, babies may find it difficult to learn what to expect: food may or may not appear; a caregiver may pick the baby up or walk right past. The same sequence of events may lead to comfort or distress (Miller, 2005; Mitchel et al., 2020; Yehuda, 2016).

Children who experience maltreatment often struggle with sequence and temporal order (what happens first, second, etc.) (Nadeau & Nolin, 2013; Pearce & Pezzot-Pearce, 2006; Putnam, 1997, 2006; Yehuda, 2005, 2011, 2016). The reality of a child who experienced trauma can be incomprehensible: you play quietly and suddenly get hit; you leave for school not knowing where you'll sleep or if you will get to eat. When the child copes with stress by dissociating, they can miss parts of events, which can further reinforce feelings of unpredictability (Silberg, 2013; Waters, 2016). Children who experience trauma can struggle to understand how events unfold, not know how to explain why things happened, and treat a story as isolated events (Hyter, 2021, 2022; Yehuda, 2011, 2016).

For some children who experience trauma, the very reality of a sequence can be scary. "What happens next?" might trigger memories of painful sequences of events (you put pajamas on→go to sleep→dad comes into the room→does bad things). It could feel safer to not connect the dots, to not have to have it be a story with a beginning, middle, and end (Silberg, 2013; Waters, 2016; Yehuda, 2016).

7.3.4   *Literal, Ambiguous, and Symbolic Meaning*

Ambiguity, metaphor, and symbolism are part of language. Words can have more than one meaning (e.g., "Duck!"), as can the same sentence (e.g., "Is the window open?" by someone who is cold or sweaty). The meaning of expressions and metaphors may be far from that of the words themselves (e.g., "She's all ears") (Gleason & Ratner, 2009). When words do not match what children believe they heard, it can throw them off: they may look for what mommy had "in the back of her head all day"; may wonder if someone who "eats like a bird" is fed worms. Rich culture, literacy, legends, stories, and conversation, expose children to puns and idioms in narrated context (Eigsti & Cicchetti, 2004; Golinkoff et al., 2019). Over time, through responsive caregivers' clarification, and by observation and deduction, children learn to infer additional meanings (Berman, 2004; Gleason & Ratner, 2009; Heymann, 2010; Hudson et al., 2015; Ninio & Snow, 1996).

For that, children need to be available to process the context and meaning. Children who are overwhelmed, hypervigilant, or shut down, might struggle to do so (Siegel, 2012; van der Kolk, 2014). Children who experience trauma often miss nuances in stories and narrative. They can find symbolic language confusing, and the stress of confusion can further compromise processing (Ciolino et al., 2021; Hyter, 2021, 2022; Sylvestre, 2021). A 'tricky-sounding' language might remind a child who has a history of trauma of times when people said things she could not understand. The child might think she is being tricked on purpose or lied to. Children may get anxious, angry, and aggressive yet struggle to explain why (Yehuda, 2011, 2016).

7.4   Language Structure: Phonology, Morphology, and Syntax

7.4.1   *Phonology and Phonological Awareness*

Children with maltreatment histories are at risk for language, emotional, and behavioral difficulties, and impairment in academic performance (Romano et al., 2015). They often struggle with social cognition and executive functions and especially with mental flexibility, inhibition, and working memory, all of which are required for effective learning (Hyter, 2021). Phonological awareness and literacy skills rely on oral language skills, executive functions, and listening (Heymann, 2010; Landry et al., 2006). Children who do not listen well may find it difficult to decode subtle differences in sounds, to develop phonemic awareness and be interested in sound-to-symbol, phonetic information, rhymes, spelling, and other reading skills. Both hypervigilance and dissociation affect listening, auditory processing, and memory (Yehuda, 2016). Children who feel hypervigilant may focus on environmental and ambient noise to scan for signs of danger (van der Kolk, 2014), instead of on the subtle differences between speech sounds. Children who are feeling shut down may not listen well, either. They can have difficulty connecting new information with what they already know (Silberg, 2013; Waters, 2016).

Without adequate mastery of language, listening, and basic academic skills, children with histories of maltreatment are at increased risk for special-education placements, repeated grades, short-and long-term academic failure, school dropout, legal and employment issues, housing insecurity, and more (Pears et al., 2018; Putnam, 2006; Romano et al., 2015; Snow, 2019). In a study of school-aged children who had been adopted from orphanages into the U.S., a full third demonstrated reading disabilities even years after adoption, including delays in letter identification, which relies on phonological skills and auditory processing (Hough & Kaczmarek, 2011). The study's authors note that actual language-learning issues among such adoptees may be higher, as their criteria excluded children with sensory or cognitive disabilities. They describe a study by McGuinness and McKay where over half of parents of children adopted from institutions reported reading issues in their 9–13 years old children. Studies have shown that higher-order language and academic skills are negatively impacted by out of home residency (Pears et al., 2018; Romano et al., 2015), and indeed low reading scores were significantly correlated with higher age at adoption and longer time spent institutionalized (Hough & Kaczmarek, 2011). Exposure, opportunity, and availability form the base for learning. Clinical and research findings increasingly underscore the importance of early intervention for improving language competence, executive functions, listening skills, and academic achievement for children who have experienced maltreatment (Cole et al., 2005; Hough & Kaczmarek, 2011; Hyter, 2022; Kurtz et al., 1993; Landry et al., 2006; Snow, 2020, 2021).

7.4.2 *Morphology and Syntax*

Morphology and syntax are acquired through exposure to varied language forms. Both the quality and quantity of language forms that children are exposed to matter, as does the child's availability and ability to process and comprehend that information. Children who are exposed to only certain kinds of utterances (e.g., mostly directive and few descriptive, complex utterances), have few opportunities to learn the meaning and usage of more complex morphological and syntactic forms (Eigsti & Cicchetti, 2004; Golinkoff et al., 2019; Romano et al., 2015; Romeo et al., 2018). In addition, children who are too shutdown or too hypervigilant to listen, may miss opportunities to process complex sentences even when such syntactic structures are modeled, and therefore be less likely to comprehend and use them (Yehuda, 2016).

Eigsti and Cicchetti (2004) found that both vocabulary and expressive syntax were delayed in a group of five-year-old maltreated children compared to non-maltreated peers. Qualitative differences were noted in maternal utterances, as well. Mothers who maltreated directed fewer utterances toward their children and produced fewer of the kind that correlate with child language abilities. In their study of children adopted from Eastern-European orphanages, Hough & Kaczmarek (2011) found that over a third continued to score below average on morphology and syntax measures even several years post-adoption.

Children who had histories of trauma used simplified sentence structures, shorter utterances, and were more likely receive poor English/reading grades than non-maltreated peers (Eigsti & Cicchetti, 2004; Romano et al., 2015; Yehuda, 2016). The findings highlight how quantity, variety, and quality of caregiver language input matter in syntactic acquisition; and underscore the added vulnerability in high-risk populations. Language delays can exacerbate any existing difficulties that children are facing and lead to later cognitive, emotional, and social delays (Hyter, 2021; Pears et al., 2018; Snow, 2019, 2020; Trickett & McBride-Chang, 1995).

7.5   Practical Applications in Assessment and Intervention

7.5.1   *Trauma-Informed, Culturally Responsive Care*

Trauma disrupts communication and can impact many aspects of development (Cozolino, 2014; Gaensbauer, 2011; Schore, 2012; van der Kolk, 2014). It is paramount, therefore, that interaction with children who experienced trauma is done in a trauma-informed way. A trauma-informed approach requires that clinicians, caregivers, and educators realize the impact of trauma on children's development, behavior, communication, reactions, perceptions, language, and learning, as well as the possibility of and paths to recovery (Hyter, 2021; Yehuda, 2016). It also requires that professionals recognize the symptoms of maltreatment and posttraumatic activation, and that they integrate their knowledge about trauma into their practice and procedures. Not only should professionals work to minimize the impact of trauma, but they ought to ensure they avoid retraumatizing the child (Cole et al., 2005; Dombo & Anlauf Sabatino, 2019; Hyter, 2021; SAMHSA, 2014).

Trauma-informed environments best include careful policies, supportive infrastructure and staff-training that incorporates clinical and educational strategies, as well as cultural considerations. It is important to identify and correct barriers to care (e.g., misconceptions about trauma, burnout), and to develop environments that are sensitive to the needs of children who experienced trauma. Child professionals should be trained to recognize and address trauma-related manifestations by helping children with emotional regulation, creating a fair, and safe environment, offering supportive narrative and positive modeling, managing disruptive behavior, and reinforcing acceptable behavior. Emphasis should be placed on building children's sense of agency, and avoiding biases related to trauma (Cole et al., 2005; Dombo & Anlauf Sabatino, 2019; Hyter, 2021; Yehuda, 2016).

Community and culture are an integral part of communication, social interaction, and belonging. As such, culturally responsive approaches take the child's community, history, and culture into account, and engage in practices that can support building relationships of trust and safety. This includes participation in development and implementation of evidence-based assessments and interventions that consider cultural and social factors. It also requires advocacy for policies that identify and address risk-factors, and that reinforce individual and community resilience (Hough & Kaczmarek, 2011; Hyter & Salas-Provance, 2019; Hyter, 2022; Telford Rose & Myers, Chapter 6).

7.5.2   Recommendations for Assessment and Intervention

The risks of language delays across semantic, syntactic, and pragmatic skills in children who experienced trauma, indicate the need for speech-language evaluations and intervention for children with maltreatment and other trauma histories (Eigsti & Cicchetti, 2004; Snow, 2020, 2021; Sylvestre, 2021; Yehuda, 2016). At the same time, the increased trauma risks in children who manage disabilities and communication disorders (Benedict at al., 1990; Crosse et al., 1993; Goldson, 1998; Hershkowitz et al., 2007; Sullivan & Knutson, 2000), indicate the need for trauma-informed assessments and interventions with any child who is referred for clinical and educational support. Such assessments and interventions should account for cultural differences, dialects, and aspects specific to those learning a new language (e.g., migrants, refugees, adoptees); and strive to ensure that assessments and interventions are culturally sensitive and culturally appropriate (Hyter, 2022; Hyter & Salas-Provance, 2019).

Language assessments should examine all trauma-vulnerable aspects of language: vocabulary, emotion and body-state language, cause and effect, sequence, narrative production (in retelling as well as in generating), pragmatics, social cognition skills, and conversational skills (Hyter, 2021; Yehuda, 2011, 2016). Numeric, phonology, and morpho-syntactic forms should also be assessed (Pears et al., 2018; Romano et al., 2015; Snow, 2020). Care needs to be taken to not assume what children's association with context and concepts are (e.g., family visit as a happy event or grocery shopping as neutral). Children should be monitored for signs of posttraumatic activation, and their distress minimized (e.g., in standardized tests, explaining that some items are meant to be difficult, and the child isn't expected to know all the answers) (Yehuda, 2016).

Trauma impacts language, which can make it difficult for children who have experienced trauma to comprehend, process, and recount events. This has implications for forensic interactions (Hyter, 2021; Snow, 2020), but also for seemingly neutral everyday ones. It is important to support caregivers of children who experienced trauma, and to provide modeling for sensitive, rich, and relevant vocabulary, that is presented in varied morphological and syntactic contexts (Eigsti & Cicchetti, 2004). Every interaction is an opportunity to offer focused, positive presence that supports regulation and is responsive in ways relevant to the child (Bartlett & Smith, 2019; Hudson et al., 2015; Mitchel et al., 2020; Pears et al., 2018; Sylvestre, 2021; Yehuda, 2016).

Children with histories of maltreatment may have difficulty making connections between events. They may need assistance with identifying and understanding causation, responsibility, culpability, and consequence (Yehuda, 2016). Modeling connections in varied contexts can help children develop these abilities (Bartlett & Smith, 2019; Hyter, 2022). Everyday activities and routines can be turned into a story, with repetition and scaffolding to assist children with organizing ideas, identifying causes and effects, sequencing events, and determining the relationships and perspectives of story characters and people in their lives. Caregivers, educators, and clinicians can talk about events before, during, and after they take place. They can describe variations of the 'volume' of feelings in different contexts, create story books, utilize drawings or photos of activities, and retell the stories to reinforce familiarity (Yehuda, 2016).

Children who experienced trauma often miss instruction due to posttraumatic activation. Help for improving regulation and closing academic gaps is important for reducing stress, building connections, and supporting self-agency and resilience (Cole et al., 2005; Dombo & Anlauf Sabatino, 2019; Romano et al., 2015; Snow, 2020). Phonological, numerical, spatial, and temporal skills can be augmented through play, poems, rhymes, role play, listening, and literacy (Bartlett & Smith, 2019; Pears et al., 2019; Yehuda, 2016).

7.6   Look Ahead – Issues and Potential

There is a strong possibility that child professionals will have some children on their caseload whose maltreatment or trauma history is unknown (Hyter, 2021). In addition, trauma often co-occurs, and is in fact an added risk, with any developmental, emotional, behavioral, and educational difficulties. The impact of both trauma and disability can complicate etiology, differential diagnosis, and intervention (Yehuda, 2005, 2016). Clinical reality is further complicated by how current developmental, language, social, and academic measures often do not take maltreatment-related neurodevelopment into account (Hyter, 2021; Yehuda, 2016). The evidence for the impact of trauma on language development is there but is yet to be translated effectively into protocols that support early identification and interventions for children with impaired language skills through a trauma lens (Snow, 2020). It is important that speech-language clinicians be involved whenever children exhibit developmental strain, and even more so when trauma or maltreatment are a possibility.

The understanding of childhood trauma and its impact on language and communication has grown significantly in recent decades, as has the body of knowledge about protective factors, resilience, and potential for healing. This is heartening news for prevention, assessment, and intervention. Expanding transdisciplinary trauma-informed training, multidisciplinary interest, and collaboration can help both research and clinical applications. These can then be used to improve early detection and offer evidence-based assessment and intervention measures that will help ameliorate the impact of posttraumatic stress on children's language, communication, and development.

References

Albers, L., Barnett, E. D., Jenista, J. A., & Johnson, D. E. (Eds.) (2005). International adoption: Medical and developmental issues. *Pediatric Clinics of North America, 53*(5), 1221–1532. https://doi.org/10.1016/j.pcl.2005.08.001

Attias, R., & Goodwin, J. (1999). *Splintered reflections: Images of the body in trauma*. New York: Basic Books.

Baron, N. S. (1992). *Growing up with language: How children learn to talk*. Reading, MA: Addison-Wesley.

Bartlett, J. D., & Smith, S. (2019). The role of early care and education in addressing early childhood trauma. *American Journal of Community Psychology, 64* (3–4), 359–372. https://doi.org/10.1002/ajcp.12380

Benedict, M. I., White, R. B., Wulff, L. M., & Hall, B. J. (1990). Reported maltreatment of children with multiple disabilities. *Child Abuse & Neglect, 14*, 207–217. https://doi.org/10.1016/0145-2134(90)90031-N

Berman, R. (Ed.) (2004). *Language development across childhood and adolescence*. Philadelphia: John Benjamins.

Bernard, K., Lee, A. H., & Dozier, M. (2017). Effects of the ABC intervention on foster children's receptive vocabulary: Follow-up results from a randomized clinical trial. *Child Maltreatment, 22*(2), 174–179. https://doi.org/10.1177/1077559517691126

Beverly, B., McGuinness, T., & Blanton, D. (2008). Communication challenges for children adopted from the former Soviet Union. *Language, Speech, and Hearing Services in Schools, 39*, 1–11. https://doi.org/10.1044/0161-1461(2008/029)

Bowlby, J. (1997). *Attachment and loss. Vol. 1*. London: Random House.

Carter, B. (2002). Chronic pain in childhood and the medical encounter: Professional ventriloquism and hidden voices. *Qualitative Health Research, 12*(1), 28–41. https://doi.org/10.1177/104973230201200103

Ciolino, C., Hyter, Y. D., Suarez, M., & Bedrosian, J. (2021). Narrative and other pragmatic language abilities of children with a history of maltreatment. *Perspectives of the ASHA Special Interest Groups, 6*, 230–241. https://doi.org/10.1044/2020_PERSP-20-00136

Cohen, N. J. (2001). *Language impairment and psychopathology in infants, children, and adolescents*. Developmental Clinical Psychology and Psychiatry series, Vol. 45, Thousand Oaks, CA: Sage Publications.

Cole, S. F., O'Brien, J. G., Gadd, G., Ristuccia, J., Wallace, L., & Gregory, M. (2005). *Helping traumatized children learn: supportive school environments for children traumatized by family violence*. Boston: Massachusetts Advocates for Children.

Cozolino, L. (2006). *The neuroscience of human relationships: Attachment and the developing brain*. New York: Norton.

Cozolino, L. (2014). *The neuroscience of human relationships: Attachment and the developing social brain*. Second Edition, Norton Series on Interpersonal Neurobiology, USA: W. W. Norton & Company.

Cross, M. (2004). *Children with emotional and behavioural difficulties and communication problems: There is always a reason*. London: Jessica Kingsley Publishers.

Cross, D., Fani, N., Powers, A., & Bradley, B. (2017). Neurobiological development in the context of childhood trauma. *Clinical Psychology, 24*(2), 111–124. https://doi.org/10.1111/cpsp.12198

Crosse, S., Elyse, K., & Ratnofsky, A. (1993). *A report on the maltreatment of children with disabilities*. Washington, DC: National Center on Child Abuse and Neglect, U.S. Department of Health and Human Services.

De Bellis, M. D. (2005). The psychobiology of neglect. *Child Maltreatment, 10*(2), 150–172. https://doi.org/10.1177/1077559505275116

DeBellis, M. D., Woolley, D. P., & Hooper, S. R. (2013). Neuropsychological findings in pediatric maltreatment: Relationship of PTSD, dissociative symptoms, and abuse/neglect indices to neurocognitive outcomes. *Child Maltreatment, 18*(3), 171–183. https://doi.org/10.1177/1077559513497420

de Boysson-Bardies, B. (1999). *How language comes to children: From birth to two years*. Boston: Massachusetts Institute of Technology.

Doesburg, S. M., Chau, C. M., Cheung, T. P. L., Moiseev, A., Ribary, U., Herdman, A. T., Miller, S. P., Cepeda, I. L., Synnes, A., & Grunau, R. E. (2013). Neonatal pain-related stress, functional cortical activity and visual-perceptual abilities in school-age children born at extremely low gestational age. *Pain, 154*(10), 1946–1952. https://doi.org/10.1016/j.pain.2013.04.009

Dombo, E. A., & Anlauf Sabatino, C. (2019). *Creating trauma-informed schools: A guide for school social workers and educators*. New York: Oxford University Press.

Drew, S. (2007). 'Having cancer changed my life, and changed my life forever': Survival, illness legacy and service provision following cancer in childhood. *Chronic Illness, 3*, 278–295. https://doi.org/10.1177/1742395307085236

Eigsti, I., & Cicchetti, D. (2004). The impact of child maltreatment on expressive syntax at 60 months. *Developmental Science, 7*(1), 88–102. https://doi.org/10.1111/j.1467–7687.2004.00325.x

Fogassi, L., & Ferrarri, P. E. (2007). Mirror neurons and the evolution of embodied language. *Current Direction in Psychological Science, 16*(3), 136–141. https://doi.org/10.1111/j.1467-8721.2007.00491.x

Ford, J. D., & Courtois, C. A. (2013). *Treating traumatic stress disorders in children and adolescents: Scientific foundations and therapeutic models*. New York: Guilford Press.

Fuemmeler, B. F., Elkin, D. T., & Mullins, L. L. (2002). Survivors of childhood brain tumors: Behavioral, emotional, and social adjustment. *Clinical Psychology Review, 22*, 547–585. https://doi.org/10.1016/s0272–7358(01)00120-9

Gaensbauer, T. J. (2011). Embodied simulation, mirror neurons, and the reenactment of trauma in early childhood, *Neuropsychoanalysis: An Interdisciplinary Journal for Psychoanalysis and the Neurosciences, 13*(1), 91–107. https://doi.org/10.1080/15294145.2011.10773665

Garner, A. S. (2013). Home visiting and the biology of toxic stress: Opportunities to address early childhood adversity. *Pediatrics, 132*(Suppl. 2), S65–S73. https://doi.org/10.1542/peds.2013-1021D

Gleason, J. B., & Ratner, N. B. (2009). *The development of language*. 7th Edition, USA: Pearson Education, Inc.

Goldson, E. (1998). Children with disabilities and child maltreatment. *Child Abuse & Neglect, 22*, 663–667. https://doi.org/10.1016/S0145-2134(98)00046-5

Golinkoff, R. M., Hoff, E., Rowe, M. L., Tamis-LeMonda, C. S., & Hirsh-Pasek, K. (2019). Language matters: Denying the existence of the 30-million-word gap has serious consequences. *Child Development, 90*, 985–992. https://doi.org/10.1111/cdev.13128

Gomez-Perales, N. (2015). *Attachment-focused trauma treatment for children and adolescents: Phase-oriented strategies for addressing complex trauma disorders*. New York: Routledge Publishers.

Heller, L., & Lapierre, A. (2012). *Healing developmental trauma: How early trauma affects self-regulation, self-image, and the capacity for relationship*, 1st edition. Berkeley, CA: North Atlantic Books.

Herman, J. (1997). *Trauma and recovery: The aftermath of violence—from domestic abuse to political terror*. New York: Basic Books.

Heymann, K. L. (2010). *The sound of hope: Recognizing, coping with, and treating your child's auditory processing disorder*. New York: Ballantine Books.

Hershkowitz, I., Lamb, M. E., & Horowitz, D. (2007). Victimization of children with disabilities. *American Journal of Orthopsychiatry, 77*(4), 629–635. https://doi.org/10.1037/0002–9432.77.4.629

Hildyard, K. L., & Wolfe, A. W. (2002). Child neglect: Developmental issues and outcomes. *Child Abuse and Neglect, 26,* 679–695. https://doi.org/10.1016/s0145–2134(02)00341-1

Hough, S. D., & Kaczmarek, L. (2011). Language and reading outcomes in young children adopted from Eastern European orphanages. *Journal of Early Intervention, 33*(1), 51–74. https://doi.org/10.1177/1053815111401377

Hudson, S., Levickis, P., Down, K., Nicholls, R., & Wake, M. (2015). Maternal responsiveness predicts child language at ages 3 and 4 in a community-based sample of slow-to-talk toddlers. *International Journal of Language and Communication Disorders, 50*(1), 136–142. https://doi.org/10.1111/1460–6984.12129

Hyter, Y. D. (2021). Childhood maltreatment consequences on social pragmatic communication: A systematic review of the literature. *Perspectives of the ASHA Special Interest Groups, 6,* 262–287. https://doi.org/10.1044/2021_PERSP-20-00222

Hyter, Y. D. (2022). Language, social pragmatic communication, and childhood trauma. In I. Management Association (Ed.), *Research anthology on child and domestic abuse and its prevention* (pp. 874–908). IGI Global. https://doi.org/10.4018/978-1-7998-2261-5.ch004

Hyter, Y. D. (2023). Post-traumatic stress and social pragmatic communication. In Y. D. Hyter (Ed.), *Language research in post-traumatic stress* (pp. xx–xx). Routledge Publishers.

Hyter, Y. D., & Salas-Provance, M. B. (2019). *Culturally responsive practices in speech, language and hearing sciences*. San Diego, CA: Plural Publishing.

Kazak, A. E., Kassam-Adams, N., Schneider, S., Zelikovsky, N. Alderfer, M. A., & Rourke, M. (2006). An integrative model of pediatric medical traumatic stress. *Journal of Pediatric Psychology, 31*(4), 343–355. https://doi.org/10.1093/jpepsy/jsj054

Kuttner, L. (2010). *A child in pain: What health professionals can do to help*, 1st edition. Wales, UK: Crown House Publishing.

Kurtz, P. D., Gaudin, J. M., Wodarski, J. S., & Howing, P. T. (1993). Maltreatment and the school aged child: School performance consequences. *Child Abuse & Neglect, 17,* 581–589. https://doi.org/10.1016/0145–2134(93)90080-o

Landry, S. H., Swank, P. R., Smith, K. E., Assel, M. A., & Gunnewig, S. B. (2006b). Enhancing early literacy skills for preschool children: Bringing a professional development model to scale. *Journal of Learning Disabilities, 39,* 306–324. https://doi.org/10.1177/00222194060390040501

Levendosky, A. A., Huth-Bocks, A. C., Shapiro, D. L., & Semel, M. A. (2003). The impact of domestic violence on the maternal–child relationship and preschool-age children's functioning. *Journal of Family Psychology, 17*(3), 275–287. https://doi.org/10.1037/0893–3200.17.3.275

Levine, P. A., & Mate, G. (2010). *In an unspoken voice: How the body releases trauma and restores goodness*, 1st edition. Berkely, CA: North Atlantic Books.

Lum, J. A. G., Powell, M., Timms, L., & Snow, P. (2015). A meta-analysis of cross-sectional studies investigating language in maltreated children. *Journal of Speech, Language, and Hearing Research, 58*(3), 961–976. https://doi.org/10.1044/2015_JSLHR-L-14–0056

Lum, J. A. G., Powell, M., & Snow, P. C. (2018). The influence of maltreatment history and out-of-home care on children's language and social skills. *Child Abuse & Neglect, 76*, 65–74. https://doi.org/10.1016/j.chiabu.2017.10.008

Miller, L. C. (2005). *The handbook of international adoption medicine: A guide for physicians, parents, and providers*. New York: Oxford University Press.

Milot, T., St-Laurent, D., Éthier, L. S., & Provost, M. A. (2010). Trauma-related symptoms in neglected preschoolers and affective quality of mother-child communication. *Child Maltreatment, 15*, 293. https://doi.org/10.1177/1077559510379153

Mitchel, J., Tucci, J., & Tronick, E. (2020). *The handbook of therapeutic care for children: Evidence-informed approaches to working with traumatized children and adolescents in foster, kinship and adoptive care*. London and Philadelphia: Jessica Kingsley Publishers.

Nabors, L. A., Weist, M. D., Shugarman, R., Woeste, M. J., Mullet, E., & Rosner, L. (2004). Assessment, prevention, and intervention activities in a school-based program for children experiencing homelessness. *Behavior Modification, 28*, 565. https://doi.org/10.1177/0145445503259517

Nadeau, M. E., & Nolin, P. (2013). Attentional and executive functions in neglected children. *Journal of Child & Adolescent Trauma, 6*(1), 1–10. https://doi.org/10.1080/19361521.2013.733794

Ninio, A., & Snow, C. (1996). *Pragmatic development*. Boulder, CO: Westview Press.

Osofsky, J. D., Stepka, P. T., & King, L. S. (2017). *Treating infants and young children impacted by trauma: Interventions that promote healthy development (concise guides on trauma care series)*. American Psychological Association.

Pearce, J. W., & Pezzot-Pearce, T. D. (2006). *Psychotherapy of abused and neglected children*, 2nd Edition. New York: Guilford Press.

Pears, K. C., Kim, H. K., & Brown, K. L. (2018). Factors affecting the educational trajectories and outcomes of youth in foster care. In E. Trejos-Castillo & N. Trevino-Schafer (Eds.), *Handbook of foster youth* (pp. 208–222). New York: Routledge.

Putnam, F. W. (1997). *Dissociation in children and adolescents: A developmental perspective*. New York: Guilford Press.

Putnam, F. W. (2006). The impact of trauma on child development. *Juvenile and Family Court Journal, 57*(1), 1–11. https://doi.org/10.1111/j.1755-6988.2006.tb00110.x

Racine, N., Eirich, R., Dimitropoulos, G., Hartwick, C., & Madigan, S. (2020). Development of trauma symptoms following adversity in childhood: The moderating role of protective factors. *Child Abuse and Neglect, 101*, 104375. https://doi.org/10.1016/j.chiabu.2020.104375

Rizzolatti, G., & Craighero, L. (2004). The mirror-neuron system. *Annual Review of Neuroscience, 27*, 169–192. https://doi.org/10.1146/annurev.neuro. 27.070203.144230

Romano, E., Babchishin, L., Marquis, R., & Fréchette, S. (2015). Childhood maltreatment and educational outcomes. *Trauma, Violence, & Abuse, 16*(4), 418–437. https://doi.org/10.1177/1524838014537908

Romeo, R. R., Leonard, J. A., Robinson, S. T., West, M. R., Mackey, A. P., Rowe, M. L., & Gabrieli, J. D. (2018). Beyond the 30-million-word gap: Children's conversational exposure is associated with language-related brain function. *Psychological Science, 29*(5), 700–710. https://doi.org/10.1177/0956797617742725

SAMHSA (2014). *Substance abuse and mental health services administration. Samhsa's concept of trauma and guidance for a trauma-informed approach.* HHS Publication No. (SMA) 14–4884. Rockville, MD. https://store.samhsa.gov/ sites/default/files/d7/priv/sma14-4884.pdf

Schiefelbusch, R. L. (Ed.) (1986). *Language competence: Assessment and intervention.* London: College-Hill Press.

Schore, A. N. (2001). The early effects of trauma on right brain development, affect regulation, and infant health. *Infant Mental Health Journal, 22*, 201–269. https://doi.org/10.1002/1097-0355(200101/04)22:1<201::AID-IMHJ8>3.0. CO;2-9

Schore, A. N. (2012). *The science of the art of psychotherapy.* Norton Series on Interpersonal Neurobiology, USA: W. W. Norton & Company.

Siegel, D. A. (2012). *The developing mind: How relationships and the brain interact to shape who we are,* 2nd Edition. New York: The Guilford Press.

Silberg, J. L. (2013). *The child survivor: Helping developmental trauma and dissociation.* New York: Routledge Publishers.

Snow, P. C. (2019). Speech-language pathology and the youth offender: Epidemiological overview and roadmap for future speech-language pathology research and scope of practice. *Language, Speech, and Hearing Services in Schools, 50*(2), 324–339. https://doi.org/10.1044/2018_LSHSS-CCJS-18–0027

Snow, P. C. (2020). SOLAR: The science of language and reading. *Child Language Teaching and Therapy, 37*(3), 215–218. https://doi.org/10.1177/ 0265659020947817

Snow, P. C. (2021). Psychosocial adversity in early childhood and language and literacy skills in adolescence: The role of speech language pathology in prevention, policy, and practice. *Perspectives of the ASHA Special Interest Groups, 6,* 253–261 https://doi.org/10.1044/2020_PERSP-20-00120

Suarez, M. A., & Masselink, C. (2023). Neurodevelopmental impact of post-traumatic stress. In Y. D. Hyter (Ed.), *Language research in post-traumatic stress* (pp. xx–xx). Routledge.

Sullivan, P. M., Vernon, M., & Scanlan, J. M. (1987). Sexual abuse of deaf youth. *American Annals of the Deaf, 32*(4), 256–262. Retrieved from https://www.jstor. org/stable/44390241

Sullivan, P. M., Brookhouser, P. E., Scanlan, J. M., Knutson, J. F., & Schulte, L. E. (1991). Patterns of physical and sexual abuse of communicatively handicapped children. *Annals of Otology, Rhinology & Laryngology, 100*, 188–194. https:// doi.org/10.1177/000348949110000304

Sullivan, P. M., & Knutson, J. F. (1998). The association between child maltreat-ment and disabilities in a hospital-based epidemiological study, *Child Abuse & Neglect, 22*, 271–288. https://doi.org/10.1016/s0145-2134(97)00175-0

Sullivan, P. M., & Knutson, J. F. (2000). Maltreatment and disabilities: A population-based epidemiological study. *Child Abuse & Neglect, 24*, 1257–1274. https://doi.org/10.1016/s0145-2134(00)00190-3

Sylvestre, A., & Mérette, C. (2010). Language delay in severely neglected children: A cumulative or specific effect of risk factors? *Child Abuse & Neglect, 34*(6), 414–428. https://doi.org/10.1016/j.chiabu.2009.10.003

Sylvestre, A., Bussières, È.-L., & Bouchard, C. (2016). Language problems among abused and neglected children: A meta-analytic review. *Child Maltreatment, 21*(1), 47–58. https://doi.org/10.1177/1077559515616703

Sylvestre, A. (2021). Language difficulties among children experiencing neglect: A public health approach aimed at narrowing the gap. *Perspectives of the ASHA Special Interest Groups, 6*, 242–252 https://doi.org/10.1044/2020_PERSP-20-00116

Trickett, P., & McBride-Chang, C. (1995). The developmental impact of different types of abuse and neglect. *Developmental Review, 15*, 311–337. https://doi.org/10.1006/drev.1995.1012

van der Kolk, B. A. (2014). *The body keeps the score: Brain, mind and body in the healing of trauma*. New York: Viking.

Waters, F. S. (2016). *Healing the fractured child: Diagnosis and treatment of youth with dissociation*. New York: Springer Publishing Company, LLC.

Westby, C. E. (2023). Post-traumatic stress, autobiographical memory, and cultural neuroscience. In Y. D. Hyter (Ed.), *Language research in post-traumatic stress* (pp. xx–xx). Routledge.

Yehuda, N. (2004). Critical issues: Dissociation in schoolchildren: An epidemic of failing in disguise. *International Society for the Study of Dissociation NEWS, 22*, 8–9. Retrieved from https://www.academia.edu/11486175/Dissociation_in_school_children_an_epidemic_of_failing_in_disguise

Yehuda, N. (2005). The language of dissociation. *Journal of Trauma and Dissociation, 6*, 9–29. https://doi.org/10.1300/J229v06n01_02

Yehuda, N. (2011). Leroy (7 years old)—"It is almost like he is two children": Working with a dissociative child in a school setting. In Wieland's (Ed.), *Dissociation in Traumatized Children and Adolescents: Theory and clinical interventions* (pp. 285–341). New York: Routledge, Psychological Trauma Series.

Yehuda, N. (2016). *Communicating trauma: Clinical presentations and interventions with traumatized children*. New York: Routledge.

8 Addressing the Impact of Post-Traumatic Stress on Adolescent Language and Identity

An Interdisciplinary Approach

Ginger G. Collins, Jayna Mumbauer-Pisano, and Tobias Kroll

8.1 Introduction

The DSM-V-TR defines a traumatic event as one that involves death or threatened death, actual or threatened serious injury, or actual or threatened sexual violence. Trauma exposure could be through a direct experience or an indirect experience, such as witnessing a trauma happen to someone close or having repeated exposure to distressing details of a traumatic event (American Psychiatric Association, 2022). Relatedly, adverse childhood experiences (ACEs) are potentially traumatic events that occur before age 18. Researchers have identified ten ACEs including childhood abuse, neglect, and household challenges such as domestic violence, substance abuse, and having a family member incarcerated (Felitti et al., 1998). While ACEs span many traumatic situations children face, the list is not exhaustive. Scholars have argued to include exposure to systemic racism and interpersonal discrimination to the list of ACEs (Lanier, 2020), as well as classism, homophobia, xenophobia, transphobia, and ableism (Karatekin & Hill, 2019).

Exposure to trauma is an unfortunate reality for most youth. Two-thirds of individuals have experienced a traumatic event by age 16 (Copeland et al., 2007), and one in seven children have experienced child abuse and/or neglect (Center for Disease Control and Prevention, 2022). ACEs frequently co-occur in children. One in six adults reports experiencing four or more types of ACEs (Center for Disease Control and Prevention, 2022). While ACEs are common across socio-demographic strata, the frequency of ACEs is higher for females than males, individuals from low socioeconomic backgrounds, sexual minorities, and Black and Hispanic individuals compared to White individuals (Giano et al., 2020). Individuals with disabilities are also more likely to report higher ACE exposure compared

DOI: 10.4324/9781003225270-10

to individuals without a disability, with sexual abuse being the strongest association with disability status (Felitti et al., 1998).

ACEs are associated with numerous negative mental health outcomes. Exposure to childhood trauma or adversity accounts for 50% of the risk for the development of affective disorders, such as anxiety and depression (Hoppen & Chalder, 2018). There is also a strong association between trauma and suicide, with 41% of children with a trauma history reporting experiencing suicidal thoughts compared to 24% without a trauma history (Miller et al., 2013). While social support can act as an important protective factor for children who experience trauma, ACEs negatively impact young people's ability to form and sustain healthy relationships and are linked to negative interpersonal behaviors including social withdrawal, defiance, and aggression (Berkowitz, 2012; Clark et al., 2015).

8.2   Cognitive Development in Adolescence

Adolescence is a period of active neural development when the brain is particularly malleable, reorganizing itself in response to the pattern, intensity, and type of sensory, perceptual, and affective experiences to which it is exposed (Romeo, 2013). The rapid growth of neural connections paired with selective synaptic pruning leads to advances in memory, problem-solving, and increased capacity to process complex information (Arain et al., 2013). Adolescence is marked by changes in the brainstem and the limbic system. The brainstem is responsible for the "fight, flight, or freeze" reaction in response to perceived threats, and the limbic system is involved in the processing of memory and emotion (Casey et al., 2008; Romeo, 2013). Together, they play an integral role in the generation of emotions, attachment, motivation, and judgment.

During adolescence, there is greater activity (and reactivity) in the limbic system which often results in extreme emotional reactions to seemingly innocuous stimuli. Similar to how young children develop attachments to caregivers during early childhood, adolescents enter into another stage of attachment in which they seek the company of same-aged peers with similar interests with whom they can form interpersonal relationships (Herd & Kim-Spoon, 2021). Just as young children with secure attachment to caregivers experience a sense of safety that promotes exploration, adolescents experience validation and belonging through peer attachments that also promotes exploration. Typically developing adolescents usually develop meaningful friendships that help promote identity development through acceptance and opportunities to practice social skills. Adolescents' self-identity directly impacts their perceptions of belonging, and those that struggle with their own self-identity will likely struggle in relationships with others. Another hallmark of adolescence is an apparent decrease in motivation, which can be attributed to the lowered levels of dopamine experienced during this stage of development. Although dopamine is not released as easily, greater pleasure is experienced during adolescence when it is released. The intense feelings that result from a dopamine rush often lead to risk-taking and novelty-seeking behaviors at this age (Arain et al., 2013). These behaviors are further reinforced by the hyper-rational thought processes characteristic of this age. Adolescents are more likely to exaggerate the positive aspects of an experience while minimizing the potential dangers and risks.

Development of the prefrontal cortex plays a critical role in cognitive functioning in adolescence, in particular for abstract thinking, empathizing, and executive functioning (Blakemore & Choudhury, 2006). Abstract thinking can be thought of as the manipulation of self-generated thoughts (i.e., thoughts that are not directly connected to the environment). One must resist environmental distractions to think abstractly, and the ability to flexibly control whether one attends to self-generated thoughts or environmental distractions is supported by the prefrontal cortex (Dumontheil & Blakemore, 2012). Typically developing adolescents also experience an increase in empathy and gradually begin to reflect more on how their actions impact others. Empathy involves the ability to identify the mental states of others, which helps one understand and predict their intentions. Executive functioning refers to the ability to control and coordinate one's thoughts and behaviors and involves self-regulation, working memory, and cognitive flexibility. Numerous skills are dependent on executive functioning, including attention, organization, emotional regulation, and self-monitoring.

This period of adaptive neural growth is susceptible to interruption, and adolescents who have been exposed to trauma may experience a very different developmental trajectory. The malleable brains of those exposed to abuse and neglect are more likely to produce neurochemicals that result in neuro-inflammation, resulting in reduced executive functioning skills (Franke, 2014). Early trauma exposure has also been linked to a reduction in cognitive flexibility in adolescence, which frequently results in rigid thinking, perseveration, and poor ability to take another's perspective (Spann et al., 2012). Reduced cognitive flexibility can also negatively impact their ability to inhibit their responses to distracting stimuli in favor of goal-directed behavior. This often presents as difficulty with organizing and sequencing tasks to complete them in a timely fashion. In addition, early trauma exposure can negatively impact the development of empathetic awareness in adolescence, both of self and others (Levy et al., 2019). Behaviors associated with low empathetic awareness include limited or absent identification of and responsiveness to others' distress, as well as their own. This reduced awareness frequently results in difficulty inferring the emotions and interpreting the actions of others, leaving such adolescents feeling that others' actions are unpredictable and confusing. Cognitive inflexibility can also impact adolescents' ability to think abstractly; they may experience difficulty making generalizations and transferring knowledge from one context to another (Spann et al., 2012).

8.3   Language Development in Adolescence

Rapid growth in language development is apparent in early childhood, but children continue to hone their language skills throughout adolescence. Though language develops more gradually in adolescence, changes in syntax, semantics, and social-pragmatic skills are observable during these years. These developments are interdependent with the cognitive developments during the same time period (i.e., executive functioning, abstract thinking, capacity to empathize). Advances in language and cognition not only help adolescents succeed in academic contexts, but they also permit the speaker to communicate with greater clarity and efficiency across social and vocational situations. One of the hallmarks of adolescence is the increased importance placed on peer relationships and peer acceptance (Herd & Kim-Spoon, 2021), and successful peer relationships are often dependent on interpersonal communication skills (Spann et al., 2012). One's ability to think abstractly and flexibly becomes more refined during these years, as does the ability to interpret and integrate information and consider points of view that differ from one's own (Schickedanz et al., 2001). These cognitively sophisticated skills contribute to the development of complex language even as they are facilitated by it in mutually reinforcing feedback loops. What follows is a brief overview of these language developments and the role they play across communication contexts.

Typically developing adolescents demonstrate growth in their syntactic development through increased sentence length, greater syntactic complexity, and sophisticated use of cohesive devices (see Nippold, 1993 for detailed description). Sentences increase in length due to a variety of linguistic devices, including the elaboration of noun and verb phrases (Nippold et al., 1992), increased use of prepositional phrases, and use of low-frequency grammatical structures (e.g., cleft sentences, appositives). Increases in subordination are also common in adolescence. Students in the secondary grades produce more sentences containing subordinate clauses, such as nominal, adverbial, relative, and gerundive clauses, and more sentences containing multiple subordinate clauses (Nippold et al., 1992). Another hallmark of syntactic development at this age involves the use of inter-clausal and inter-sentential cohesive devices. For example, Nippold et al. (1992) found that the use and comprehension of adverbial conjuncts (e.g., *consequently, on the other hand, therefore*) gradually increase, starting in adolescence and continuing into early adulthood.

Nippold (1993) noted two particularly significant advances in semantic skills during adolescence— development of the literate lexicon and comprehension of figurative expressions. Both depend on highly developed metalinguistic skills that allow one to infer and interpret information from context. According to Nippold (2018), the literate lexicon refers to words that occur in academic contexts and are commonly morphologically complex, such as derived nominals (e.g., *recover* [verb] + *-y* = *recovery* [noun]) and derived adjectives (e.g., *meteor* [noun] + *-ic* = *meteoric* [adjective]). Abstract nouns and metacognitive verbs are also included in the literate lexicon. Abstract nouns refer to words that represent intangible entities (e.g., *justice, paradox*), inner states (e.g., *contentment, motivation*), and emotions (e.g., *serenity, apprehension*) (Nippold et al., 1999), whereas metacognitive verbs refer to "mental actions" (e.g., *decide, contemplate*) (Sun & Nippold, 2012). Figurative expressions (e.g., proverbs, idioms, metaphors), play an ever-increasing role in academic language in the secondary grades, and students' interpretations of these expressions gradually increases over the adolescent years.

Social-pragmatic language skills refer to the ability to use language in social contexts. The ability to infer the mental states of others (i.e., Theory of Mind) and read nonverbal cues that signal a communication partner's emotions is positively associated with more frequent socially competent behaviors and less frequent aggressive and withdrawn behaviors, better interpersonal negotiation skills, and greater peer approval (Slaughter et al., 2002). Interpersonal negotiation skills steadily improve throughout adolescence and require one to possess an awareness of others' wants, needs, and perspectives, the ability to reject short-term desires in favor of long-term outcomes, and the ability to focus on problem-solving that benefits all parties involved in a conflict (Nippold, 1993). Strong verbal ability is also associated with greater social competence and less frequent aggression, which positively impacts peer acceptance (Slaughter et al., 2002). Nippold (1993) noted that the use of popular slang terms is a verbal ability that holds much social capital among adolescents. Youth often prefer to use slang terms over more conventional vocabulary words because their usage signals in-group solidarity (De Klerk, 2005). For example, should an adolescent state, "Ignore Derrick—he's just flexing" instead of "Ignore Derrick—he's just showing off" to a peer, he is not only communicating what he thinks of Derrick, but also that he is privy to the particular language patterns preferred by that peer group.

Stunted cognitive development significantly impacts one's ability to develop complex language skills. In the secondary grades, much of students' semantic and syntactic growth occurs as a result of reading (Nippold, 2017,

2018), and successful reading comprehension involves executive functioning skills. Reading requires students to decode text while simultaneously allocating and managing their cognitive and attentional resources so that they can also focus on comprehending the text. Several studies have linked reading comprehension to working memory, planning and organization, and inhibition (e.g., Chiarenza, 1990; Sesma et al., 2009; Swanson, 2003). Students with reduced executive functioning often struggle with reading fluency due to difficulties in flexibly shifting from retrieving and interpreting background knowledge to attending to and interpreting print and new content. Flexible thinking is needed to draw inferences and conclusions, process redundant information, and interpret words or language that may be ambiguous. Impairments in these cognitive skills impede students' ability to comprehend the texts they read, which interferes with their learning of complex vocabulary and syntax.

Adolescents impacted by trauma often struggle to develop social-pragmatic skills. Negative past experiences contribute to their inherent distrust of others and make them disinclined to invest in intimate relationships. When underdeveloped cognitive skills result in difficulty taking another's perspective or integrating new information with previously learned information, social communication is often fragmented. At a time in development when the desire for peer acceptance is especially salient, adolescents with trauma histories often experience social rejection by their peers because they are viewed as socially inept. They often lack the interpersonal skills needed to navigate the increasingly complex social interactions of adolescence. Furthermore, alienation from their peers also increases the risk of being bullied.

8.4   Trauma and Adolescent Development

The transition from childhood to adulthood is challenging under optimal circumstances. Adolescents must learn to develop greater independence to prepare for their roles as autonomous adults. They are expected to continue to perform well academically and maintain peer relationships while gaining the knowledge and skills needed to obtain and maintain employment and engage with their communities after graduation (Davis, 2003). Erik Erikson believed these critical years of development constituted an "identity crisis" where adolescents are expected to come to terms with who they are and what they stand for and develop a sense of self, or "ego identity" (Erikson, 1980). Unfortunately, more than any other developmental stage, adolescence is associated with increased risk of trauma exposure, which often disrupts identity development (Darnell et al., 2019). In addition to the traumatic stressors experienced by adults, adolescents are more likely to encounter bullying, violence in the home and school and engage in high-risk behaviors such as drug experimentation (Hoppen & Chalder, 2018).

In addition, adolescence is the developmental period in which individuals are most vulnerable to the impact of trauma exposure because of the rapid physical, emotional, and social changes taking place (Darnell et al., 2019). These brain changes adversely impact the neurobiological systems responsible for emotional regulation, problem-solving, and behavior. As a result, adolescents struggling with traumatic stress are more likely to engage in risky behavior and more likely to underperform in school, which creates a cyclic effect when combined with the increased risk of exposure to traumatic events. In fact, ACEs exposure predicted disengaging school behaviors such as truancy, grade changes, and suspension in a sample of students at high risk for high school dropout (Iachini et al., 2016). During this tumultuous time of identity development and behavior change, traumatic stress in adolescents often goes unnoticed or rationalized as normal adolescent behavior rather than an impetus for mental health support. The intensity of adolescent emotional responses often leads to skepticism about their distress level by their adult caregivers, which can result in teens feeling invalidated or avoided while desperately seeking support.

Aside from being vulnerable to newly occurring trauma, adolescents may also carry within themselves the effects of earlier traumatic experiences. Adverse experiences in childhood have the potential to contribute to secondary stressors in adolescence, such as decreases in academic functioning, functioning in work settings, and establishing and maintaining social relationships (Darnell et al., 2019). How the impacts of developmental trauma are expressed varies, but there are four commonly agreed-upon domains of influence (Blaustein & Kinniburgh, 2015). The first domain involves *regulation*. Adolescents impacted by trauma often demonstrate a reduced ability to understand, tolerate, and manage their emotions and physiological states. When these skills are underdeveloped, these adolescents often turn to harmful coping strategies, such as substance use/abuse, self-destructive behaviors, or withdrawal. The second domain is centered around the development and maintenance of *safe, trusting relationships*. Adolescents with a history of trauma often experience intense vulnerability and distrust of others. While some respond to these feelings of mistrust with isolation and withdrawal, others engage in unhealthy relationships that often lead to further victimization. *Identity*, the third domain, is significantly influenced by an individual's experiences and relationships, including cultural beliefs and values. Because trauma-impacted adolescents' early experiences were often unpredictable, chaotic, and negative, many feel neither whole nor capable. They often doubt their own abilities to accomplish new tasks and struggle to envision succeeding in future endeavors. While this is true across socio-demographic strata, identity development is particularly disrupted for adolescents who identify as biracial, often facing heightened obstacles to identity development (Udry et al., 2003). The last domain involves *information processing*. An individual's capacity to absorb, process, and appropriately act upon internal and external information in a resourceful manner is negatively impacted by trauma. In addition to reduced executive functioning skills, these adolescents may also struggle to seek support to assist with problem-solving.

Despite the numerous difficulties that many adolescents who have experienced trauma may face, there are opportunities to promote resilience and help individuals recover, grow, and develop life goals. These opportunities include but are not limited to, the following: intentional inclusion of the adolescent in an adult community that fosters their growth and belonging; increased focus on shifting responsibility for any goals, intermediate or long-term, from interventionists to the adolescent themselves; and interprofessional collaboration to facilitate this shift in each area of functioning with which the individual may be struggling. We will detail some relevant factors and policies in the following section before introducing a case study.

8.5   Trauma-Informed Approaches to Treatment

The Substance Abuse and Mental Health Services Administration (SAMHSA, 2015) defines trauma-informed approaches as those that realize the impact of trauma, recognize the symptoms of trauma, respond by integrating knowledge about trauma policies and practices, and seek to reduce retraumatization. The six key concepts to be addressed include safety, trust, peer support, collaboration, empowerment, and consideration of cultural, historical, and gender issues (CDC, 2020). Because individuals experience trauma differently, intervention should be individualized to meet their specific needs. Collaborating with school-based mental health professionals is key in ensuring that practices are trauma-informed. Additionally, it should be noted that although school-based outcomes have traditionally focused heavily on academic domains, there has been increasing recognition and acceptance of the role social, emotional, behavioral, and mental health outcomes play in facilitating or impeding overall success in school (SAMHSA, 2015), factors that are also important to consider when helping students transition successfully to adulthood.

Fortunately, federal policies and services are designed to interrupt the potentially harmful outcomes often associated with early exposure to trauma and bolster proactive factors. Formal transition planning occurs in the schools as well as through the foster care system. Transition planning involves preparing adolescents for adulthood; school-based transition planning is focused on preparing students for life after they exit school, and transition planning through the foster care system is focused on pre-paring adolescents for life after emancipation.

Since the reauthorization of the Individuals with Disabilities Education Act (IDEA, 2004), students with an Individualized Education Plan (IEP) must have an individualized transition plan (ITP) included by the time they reach their 16th birthday. Postsecondary transition plans are designed to support overall student success, must be closely aligned with federal mandates, and should be carefully developed to integrate goals of (1) post-school employment, (2) education, (3) vocational training, (4) com-munity participation, and (5) healthy, independent living. As such, IEPs that include an ITP should include not only a focus on classroom success but also include focused preparation for successful postsecondary achieve-ments, including employment, independent living, and further training and/or education (Johnson, 2005). Transition planning begins with estab-lishing a transition team of school professionals whose expertise is aligned with the student's goals and needs. For students who have been exposed to abuse and/or neglect, this includes school professionals with expertise in trauma-informed practices.

Federal child welfare laws have undergone several changes in response to research revealing the negative impacts of trauma on developing brains. The development and maturation of the prefrontal cortex is not typically accomplished until around age 25 (e.g., Arain et al., 2013), and many studies suggest that this developmental period is further extended for indi-viduals who have been exposed to trauma (e.g., Delima & Vimpani, 2011; Nemeroff, 2016). It is estimated that approximately 90% of children in foster care have been exposed to trauma, with nearly half reporting expo-sure to four or more types of traumatic events (Stein et al., 2001). Given the high incidence of trauma exposure to children in foster care, laws to support the successful transition to adulthood through extended foster care were developed. The John H. Chafee Foster Care Program for Suc-cessful Transition to Adulthood (i.e., the *Chafee Program*) was created from the Foster Care Independence Act of 1999 (P.L. 106–169). This pro-gram enables states to provide support services (e.g., financial, housing, employment, education, counseling) that prepare adolescents for adult-hood. For example, the Chafee Program offers educational and training vouchers that can provide support for education and employment prepa-ration for individuals aged 14–26 years for up to five years. The Foster-ing Connections to Success and Increasing Adoptions Act of 2008 (P.L. 110–351) permits states to extend the age limit for foster care beyond 18 years. States have the option to permit individuals who have left foster care to return to foster care and receive the same services and supports as those who remained in care continuously. Additionally, because case management is a requirement of extended foster care, case managers will work with these young adults to help them get the services they need (e.g., counseling, speech-language intervention), even when they do not readily recognize the need for these services themselves.

8.6   Case Example

What follows is a case example of a hypothetical client who is approaching adulthood after a childhood characterized by trauma, instability, and issues of cultural identity including experiences of racism. After introducing the client's case history, it will be detailed how communicative and socioemotional issues intersect in the client, and how an speech-language professional (SLP) and a counselor jointly address them to facilitate the client's transition into adulthood.

8.6.1   *Trauma History*

Kayla is a 15-year-old female living on a reservation in the Mountain West region with a substantial history of trauma exposure. Until the age of seven, Kayla lived with her biological parents, who struggled with substance abuse. As a result, Kayla was often left in unsafe environments without supervision. During the times her parents were physically present, Kayla's emotional needs were rarely met. She witnessed her father enacting verbal and physical abuse on her mother numerous times. Kayla's father identifies as White and her mother as Indigenous, and much of the verbal abuse directed at her mother included racial slurs. Additionally, Kayla's parents routinely lacked the financial resources to meet basic family needs, such as heating, nutrient-rich foods, and running water. At age seven, Kayla's father was convicted of felony theft and incarcerated, at which time Kayla and her mother moved into her mother's maternal grandparents' home. Kayla indicated that she enjoyed living with her great-grandparents because their house was "calm." Although Kayla's mother made several attempts to overcome her drug addiction, she continued using and began dealing to support her habit. When Kayla was nine years old, her mother was convicted of possession with intent to distribute and was also incarcerated, after which Kayla was placed in her great-grandparents' custody. This home environment was advantageous in that the great-grandparents provided Kayla with the stability and emotional support she desperately needed, but they were very elderly and suffered from multiple medical conditions that often left them unable to meet some of Kayla's basic needs. She frequently ate highly processed snack foods (e.g., chips, candy) in place of meals, missed school, and did not receive adequate dental care because there was often no adult well enough to drive to the grocery store, school, or the dentist. Kayla was placed in foster care when she reached age 11 shortly after both of her great-grandparents died in a car accident. She has lived with the same foster parents since that time with plans to stay until she is emancipated.

8.6.2   *Language Development and Academic History*

Kayla was identified as having a language disorder at the end of third grade. Teachers from her earlier grades expressed concerns about her language skills, but because of her frequent absenteeism and the limited number of days the itinerant SLP provided services at the school each month, Kayla did not begin receiving language intervention until she was ten years old. Her language skills were characterized by underdeveloped vocabulary, reading, spelling, and writing skills. Kayla consistently produced short, simplistic sentences in both spoken and written modalities. Kayla also experiences some difficulty interpreting and producing social-pragmatic language. Kayla's teachers indicated that she struggles to follow classroom instructions, rarely completes homework assignments, and is generally minimally communicative and withdrawn. They also noted that Kayla has never really established any close peer relationships.

Kayla is beginning her freshman year of high school and just completed her triennial reevaluation to determine her eligibility for continued special education services. Because her 16th birthday will occur during this three-year cycle, Kayla's IEP must include a transition plan to prepare her for life after graduation in addition to her language intervention goals. The interdisciplinary team responsible for this plan included the school's SLP and counselor, who also involved teachers as needed.

8.6.2.1   *Interdisciplinary Intervention Planning*

After the school-based SLP and counselor re-evaluated Kayla's language skills and mental health functioning in the school setting, they met to discuss her relative strengths and growth areas, goals to be prioritized, and areas in which service provision overlapped. The counselor noted that although Kayla still struggles in school, she had fewer absences than in previous years and even found a class she enjoyed, Photography and Media Arts. She also noted that Kayla seems to struggle to regulate her emotions, especially when conflicts arose between teachers and students. Kayla found emotional regulation difficult and struggled to understand and use vocabulary words to describe and identify her emotions. In fact, the counselor noted that Kayla's underdeveloped vocabulary and limited responses to questions made evaluating her mental health needs challenging. For example, after a student (referring to her biracial identity) asked Kayla, "What are you, anyway?" Kayla slammed her textbook closed and left the classroom abruptly. When Kayla met with the counselor, she appeared justifiably upset and angry but insisted she just found the interaction funny. The incongruence between Kayla's presentation and her words concerned the counselor, who wanted to provide empathy to Kayla, connect her with students with similar struggles, and assist her in her identity development. Another concern was Kayla's executive functioning skills. Kayla demonstrated substantial difficulty maintaining an adequate level of concentration to complete tasks, noting that she appeared hypervigilant and was easily distracted by external stimuli such as noises and movement. The counselor also recognized Kayla's difficulty with organization, planning, and time management - skills necessary for completing most academic tasks.

The SLP's assessment of Kayla's language skills revealed many similarities. Kayla continues to struggle with comprehension and production of complex vocabulary and complex syntax. She demonstrates social-pragmatic skills that are below that of her same-aged peers. Most noticeably, she exhibits difficulty inferring a speaker's intended message from indirect comments and making logical predictions about others' perspectives. A classroom observation revealed that Kayla appears to approach assignments in a disorganized manner. She seems distracted when reading instructions, often failing to finish doing so. She does not seem to develop a plan for approaching assignments, such as brainstorming ideas, drafting an outline, or using graphic organizers. Instead, she will impulsively begin writing, often without knowing how to complete the sentences she starts. Kayla also seems to exhibit poor awareness of the amount of time and effort needed to complete assignments.

Together, the counselor and SLP recognized that Kayla could make greater progress in her counseling sessions with improved language skills, and she would make greater progress in language intervention with improved social and affective cognitive skills. Additionally, both school professionals acknowledged the need for Kayla, along with members of her IEP team, to develop a plan for her to transition to adulthood. Based on these findings, the SLP and counselor developed complementary treatment plans with IEP goals for improving vocabulary development, complex syntax, social-pragmatic skills, and self-regulation skills. These findings also helped inform the development of Kayla's individualized transition plan.

8.6.2.2 *Interdisciplinary Transition Planning*

Transition planning was initiated through conversations with Kayla about her plans for her future and assessment of her vocational interests and readiness for independent living. Conversations with Kayla revealed that she does not have strong feelings about what she wants to do after graduation, but she did mention that she was not interested in pursuing postsecondary education. She reported that she has a very good relationship with her foster parents and is not looking forward to moving out of their home. Kayla explained that her foster parents' expectations of her are clear, the routine in the home is regular, they are warm and caring, and that they have horses on their property. Kayla enjoys caring for and riding the horses, and her foster parents have been gradually increasing her responsibilities for their care. Results from the Occupational Information Network Interest Profiler (U.S. Department of Labor, 2002) revealed Kayla's preference for professions involving artistic creativity, working outdoors, and/or working with animals. The Casey Life Skills Assessment (Casey Family Programs, 2012) was administered, and of the nine functional areas of independent living, Kayla demonstrated relative strength in daily living (e.g., preparing meals, laundering clothes) and housing, money management, and transportation (e.g., obtaining a driver's license, creating a budget). She exhibited relative weakness in the remaining areas of self-care (e.g., obtaining health insurance, managing mental health), relationships and communication (e.g., self-advocacy, assessing relationships), work and study life (developing a resume, recognizing discriminatory practices), career and education planning (e.g., accessing job training), civic engagement (e.g., registering to vote, joining community groups), navigating the child welfare system (e.g., knowing legal rights), and looking forward (e.g., possessing confidence and pride about one's future). Kayla was also administered the Casey Life Skills Supplemental Assessment for American Indian/Native Alaskan students (Casey Family Programs, 2012), and her responses indicated the need for development in all areas—tribal affiliation (e.g., knowledge of how to become an enrolled tribal member, familiarity with tribal customs), family and community (e.g., feeling connected to one's tribal community), beliefs and traditions (e.g., living in balance and harmony), and living in two worlds (e.g., experiencing respect in non-native environments). These assessment results were discussed with Kayla, and she indicated that she was interested in addressing each of the areas in which her skills were underdeveloped. Communication with Kayla's case manager revealed that Kayla and her foster parents were in favor of extending her foster care. Based on these findings, the IEP team, including Kayla, developed the following transition goals (see Table 8.1).

Student involvement in the transition planning process not only increases their understanding of their own strengths, needs, and interests, as well as how these interests relate to potential careers, it promotes student motivation to participate in goal-directed behavior to attain these goals (Martin & Williams-Diehm, 2013). Additionally, student involvement in this process is in direct alignment with two of the guiding principles of trauma-informed practices. The first, empowerment and choice, is essential for

Table 8.1 Kayla's Individualized Transition Plan Goals

Measurable postsecondary transition goals	
After graduation, Kayla will:	
Postsecondary education/training	• enroll in a training or certification program that will prepare her for working with animals.
Employment	• secure employment working with animals following completion of her training or certificate program.
Independent living and community participation	• determine her eligibility for and access to benefits, such as health insurance and pre-employment training vouchers.
	• manage her mental health through individual and group counseling.
	• increase her connections to her tribal community.

fostering a sense of control and autonomy, and the second, collaboration and mutuality, focuses on shared decision-making. Short-term objectives were created to support Kayla's transition goals as well as her IEP goals. Because students in secondary school are expected to become self-directed, self-regulated learners, interventions will primarily target strategy instruction instead of direct skill instruction. Regardless of the skills or strategies targeted in intervention, the clinicians will continually make explicit to Kayla how they relate to attaining her postsecondary goals.

8.6.2.3 *Interdisciplinary Interventions*

The school counselor and SLP collaborated to provide in-school support for Kayla as well as connect her with additional community resources. Considering Kayla's struggle with her own identity development and exposure to both overt and implicit racism, the school counselor also invited her to the Indigenous Student Association (ISA), an active student-led group whose mission is to bring awareness, acknowledgment, and education of Native Americans and allies through culturally related events and activities. Because the ISA hosts a "healing circle" for members experiencing grief or loss, the counselor encouraged Kayla to consider participating. Healing circles are based on Indigenous traditional belief systems and have long been fundamental to Indigenous healing practices. This suggestion supports two of the primary principles of a trauma-informed approach, viz., peer support and appreciation of cultural practices. It is also aligned with Kayla's postsecondary transition goal of increasing her connection to her tribal community.

Because of the complementary nature of the goals targeting language and cognition, the SLP and counselor elected to frame their interventions around a journaling activity. Journaling is an advantageous approach for a variety of reasons. Writing in therapeutic contexts contributes to identity formation and promotes problem-solving, emotional regulation, and interpersonal effectiveness (DeGangi & Nemiroff, 2010). Many adolescents find journaling less threatening than therapy solely focused on oral communication because it provides therapeutic distance between the individual and their narrative (DeGangi & Nemiroff, 2010). Another advantage of journaling is that it allows the individual to externalize their thoughts and feelings, allowing them to view them in a more objective manner (Bolton et al., 2004). Executive functioning skills can be strengthened through the writing process (e.g., planning, prioritizing, organizing, self-monitoring), as can vocabulary development and use of complex sentence structures.

To ensure that Kayla is invested in her own progress in therapy, the SLP and counselor explained their plan for her to see each school professional once weekly during the school year and requested her feedback. They explained that each session would involve writing in a journal. Early in the week, Kayla would work with the counselor to address social and affective cognitive skills, and later in the week, Kayla would bring her journal to her session with the SLP to address language skills. Kayla admitted that she was apprehensive about this plan because she felt that she was not a "good writer" but felt that this would help her improve and agreed to proceed.

Kayla's counseling session focused on the identification of emotions. The school counselor encouraged Kayla to write about her thoughts, feelings, and experiences on a daily basis. She explained that Kayla should not focus on self-identified "good" or "bad" feelings and instead treat each feeling, positive or negative, with curiosity and acceptance. The school counselor collaborated with Kayla's Photography and Media Art teacher, who suggested adding a visual component to the journal. Each week, Kayla was encouraged to take a photograph that evoked any sort of feeling in her. When the counselor reviewed Kayla's journal entries with her, she noted that she limited her descriptions of her feelings and emotions to either "good" or "bad." As the counselor attempted to explore these good and bad emotions with Kayla, the counselor observed her having trouble replacing these terms with more nuanced descriptions. As such, she presented Kayla with a bank of words used to describe feelings and emotions (e.g., *troubled, content, resentful*). After the counselor discovered that she did not possess a solid understanding of the meanings of most of these words, she communicated this to the SLP.

The SLP used this as an opportunity to address vocabulary, sentence structure, and planning and organization. Before introducing specific interventions, the SLP discussed the importance of using precise vocabulary and complex sentence structure in expressing one's intended message. She linked these abilities to Kayla's transition goals of applying to a postsecondary training program and for a job. Reminders that these skills will benefit her in her future endeavors were helpful in illustrating why these therapeutic tasks were meaningful and in motivating her to fully participate. To begin, the SLP explained that Kayla would need to investigate the meanings of the words presented by the counselor using The Free Thesaurus (www.freethesaurus.com), one of the independent word-learning strategies she has been developing. After researching the meanings of these words, intervention included a discussion about organizing this information. The SLP guided Kayla in critically thinking of the most useful way to organize these words, asking her to think of how she might use these words in her counseling sessions. Kayla indicated that she would use these words to describe how she was feeling, then decided to categorize them as words for "happy," "sad," "surprised," "angry," or "fearful." Next, the SLP directed Kayla to think about the words for "happy," and asked her how words within this category should be organized, again reminding her of the purpose of the activity in which these words would be used. Kayla determined that the words in each category should be arranged hierarchically from "very mild feelings" to "very strong feelings." Determining the "strength" of a feeling was difficult since these words were presented in a decontextualized manner. The SLP instructed Kayla to read the sample sentences in the thesaurus and provided sample sentences of her own to provide context clues, which helped her distinguish the subtle differences between words with similar meanings. To help solidify her vocabulary knowledge while simultaneously addressing complex sentence structures, the SLP then explained to Kayla that they would be constructing sentences containing adverbial clauses in her journal using these words. She reminded Kayla that an adverbial clause is a dependent clause that modifies a verb, adjective, or adverb in a main clause, and provided her with a bank of subordinating conjunctions to use (e.g., *when, until, before, unless, even if, because, since, where*). The SLP explained that they would create sentences that included both a "feeling word" and a subordinating conjunction. She encouraged Kayla to think of sentences that were meaningful to her, although the sentences did not need to be about her. After selecting "ecstatic" from the "happy" category, the SLP noted that this was a "very strong feeling," and prompted Kayla to write, "I feel ecstatic... " in her journal. She then asked Kayla what might make her feel "ecstatic." She indicated that riding her horse, Cookie, at a full gallop would result in this feeling, and the SLP pointed to the conjunction bank and asked, "How could you add this information about riding Cookie to your sentence?" Kayla reviewed the conjunctions and selected "when," creating the sentence, "I feel ecstatic when I'm riding Cookie." Next Kayla selected the "mild feeling" word, "serene," noting the thesaurus indicated it meant "peaceful, calm, not bothered by anything," and wrote "I feel <u>serene</u>... " in her journal. The SLP again prompted Kayla to think of what might cause her to feel calm, peaceful, and not bothered by anything. Kayla noted that she liked sitting outside watching the sunset when the weather was warm. This time the SLP selected a conjunction for her- "unless." She asked Kayla to think about what she just described and how she could use "unless" in this sentence. Kayla first wrote, "I feel <u>serene</u> unless...," but was uncertain how to continue. The SLP prompted her to revise this statement by saying, "What makes you serene?" Kayla erased "unless" and replaced it with "watching the sunset." The SLP asked her to add "unless" and think about the conditions under which watching the sunset made her feel serene. Kayla completed her sentence to read, "I feel <u>serene</u> watching the sunset unless the weather is cold." Writing these journal entries not only provided Kayla with guided experience in formulating sentences containing adverbial clauses, they gave personal meaning to these words of which she only previously had a vague understanding.

Once Kayla improved her ability to identify and label feelings and emotions, the counselor shifted the focus of intervention to social-perceptual skills training to help Kayla learn to monitor, discriminate, and identify cues related to her own emotions and feelings, others' emotions and feelings during interactions, as well as the characteristics and social rules of specific social situations. To support her in this regard, the counselor invited Kayla to a school-based social skills group with peers with similar struggles and goals. In this group, Kayla and her peers learned about the ABC model of Cognitive Behavioral Therapy (Sælid & Nordahl, 2017). Kayla was encouraged to share any **A**ctivating events that happened during the week, her immediate **B**eliefs about the event, and the **C**onsequences of those beliefs, which include behavioral and emotional responses. From there, she would consider if her beliefs were rational or irrational and if the consequences of those beliefs were positive or negative. Group members were also instructed to give their peers feedback, encouragement, and at times, role-play social situations that were causing undue anxiety or stress.

During the first session, Kayla shared how she usually enjoys Visual Art and Photography class but that recently had changed. She then explained the activating event,

> Today, another student kept staring at me as I worked, obviously judging me and thinking my project was awful. She then came up to me and asked why I chose the lens I did. I told her to mind her own business and get away from me!

The counselor expressed empathy for Kayla's situation and then asked if the other group members had any thoughts to share. Bradley, one of Kayla's classmates, spoke up, "I saw your project in class and you are such a good photographer, I think everyone else just wants to know your technique!" The counselor then said "Kayla, it seems like you might have had some beliefs about that interaction that were off base. I wonder if the same thing happened again, what alternative beliefs might be going through your head?" Kayla paused and then said, "I guess I wouldn't assume she was judging me and instead just share my technique with her." After everyone had a chance to share, the group leader instructed everyone to continue to practice throughout the week by writing about interpersonal challenges they encountered and applying the ABC model.

During Kayla's next meeting with her SLP, she shared her journal entries, including her practice with the ABC model. In reviewing her entry about the social skills group, the SLP noticed Kayla's initial reaction to her classmate's inquiry as to why she chose the lens she did and used this as an opportunity to examine some finer points of pragmatics and nonverbal communication. To begin, she asked Kayla what made her take the question as a criticism at first. Kayla admitted to having a habit of negative evaluations of others' actions toward her. The SLP then explained that although "why" questions (e.g., "Why did you use that lens?") are sometimes used as veiled criticisms, these questions are also used to simply gather information. Determining how they are used can usually be deduced by examining the speaker's context, tone, and body language. She instructed Kayla to recall and examine the situation using the following questions: Did the other students like your work? What was the inquiring classmate's facial expression, body language, and tone of voice? Kayla could not recall facial expressions and body language, but she did remember that everyone seemed to appreciate her work and determined that the classmate's tone of voice seemed more curious than reproachful in retrospect. The SLP explained that those cues are good evidence that the question was intended as an authentic inquiry and indicated appreciation for her work.

The school counselor and SLP stressed that interpreting others' perspectives, beliefs, thoughts, and feelings across communication contexts is a critical social learning skill that will benefit Kayla in the school and social and work settings. Explicitly linking these skills to both Kayla's immediate school environment as well as her postsecondary plans helped motivate her to participate fully in these interventions. This level of transparency plays another important role in trauma-informed care; it is essential for building trust and promoting a sense of safety. The school counselor and SLP encouraged Kayla to refer to the ABC framework (e.g., challenging

IEP: Intervention & transition planning

Intervention

Emotion regulation   Complex syntax

Emotional vocabulary   ⟷   Complex vocabulary

Incongruence   Social inferencing/Theory of Mind

Executive functions   Executive functions

Intervention & transition plan

Counselor's intervention   SLP's intervention

Identity development   Syntax

Emotional vocabulary   ⟷   Emotional vocabulary

Journalling   Social inferencing/Theory of Mind

Social-perceptual skills training   Pragmatics, nonverbal communication

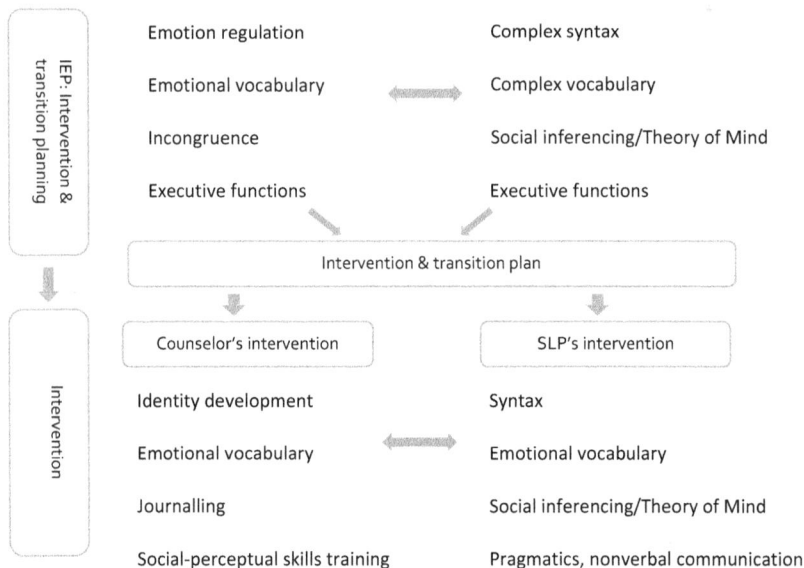

Figure 8.1 Overview of Collaborative Process

beliefs, appraising the situation, evaluating the communication partner) when making inferences. They assured Kayla that misunderstandings occur at all ages and across all communication contexts, but addressing misunderstandings provides an opportunity for both communication partners to better understand each other's perspectives.

Figure 8.1 provides an overview of the collaborative process of the counselor and SLP working together on evaluation, planning, and intervention. In the figure, single arrows denote time (sequential) relationships, while double arrows depict relationships of mutual influence between the counselor's and the SLP's work. As evident from the visual, there are broad, global influences between virtually all the areas each professional assessed and targeted in intervention, which we will now spell out in detail.

Consider, first, the counselor's evaluation results. All four of Kayla's trouble areas are interconnected, of course: emotion regulation benefits from emotional vocabulary and executive functions, and communicative incongruence may be enhanced by the former two. All these areas, in turn, are interconnected with the cognitive-linguistic skills assessed by the SLP. Emotion regulation depends partly on pertinent vocabulary and syntax, as the ability to express emotions appropriately contributes to their modulation (Rimé, 2007). Social inferencing and theory of mind also require complex linguistic skills.

For intervention, the counselor chose to concentrate on those skills in the context of identity development. While the SLP did not directly contribute to this overarching goal, the skills she addressed in her therapy closely aligned with those addressed by the counselor. Emotional vocabulary acquisition was tackled by both professionals simultaneously from different angles: the counselor focused on the accurate labeling of inner states, while the SLP provided the lexical background skills and knowledge to do so. Journaling was facilitated by vocabulary and syntax intervention, and social skills training was closely interlinked with Kayla's growing understanding of pragmatics and nonverbal communication. Executive functioning was addressed by both clinicians throughout.

8.7   Summary

The impact of trauma on adolescent development and well-being has the potential to be devastating. However, when protective factors are in place and policies designed to promote the successful transition to adulthood are utilized, the likelihood of favorable outcomes increases. Though not comprehensive in scope, the sample intervention sessions in this case example illustrate how language skills can be addressed using an interdisciplinary, trauma-informed approach. The skills and strategies described will benefit adolescents such as Kayla in their immediate environments and will promote adaptive behaviors that will benefit them in new environments (e.g., postsecondary training, employment) they encounter as they transition to adulthood. Additionally, including adolescents in transition planning helps make the purpose of therapeutic activities more transparent and fosters involvement, motivation, and trust.

Given the sheer prevalence of childhood trauma and the difficulty accessing remedial services for vast swaths of the population, many individuals reach adolescence with unaddressed or insufficiently addressed traumatic burdens. This makes a challenging time of life even more so. Adolescents experience rapid physiological, neurological, socioemotional, and cognitive changes that require patience and endurance even in otherwise well-adjusted individuals and their families. Children without a supportive family environment who reach adolescence pervasively dysregulated due to trauma exposure are bound to experience amplified struggles, making them vulnerable to further traumatization. Adolescents commonly experience a strong need to belong and often seek peers or other non-familial attachments who provide them with a sense of identity beyond those they have developed in their childhood contexts. However, adolescents who have experienced trauma are likely to embark on this developmental quest with a threefold disadvantage. They may not have developed a stable self-image as a basis for individuation, are often reared in unstable, unsupportive environments without guidance in navigating the typical struggles of adolescence and may lack the interpersonal skills to form attachments outside of their immediate family. All these issues are likely to exacerbate the unhealthy behaviors common to adolescence, such as undue risk-taking, and inhibit one's ability to experience a healthier adolescence, which in turn impedes their growth into fully functioning, mature adults.

The picture becomes even more complicated when considering population-level and historical dynamics that impact the traumatized adolescent. If they belong to historically marginalized populations who are experiencing rejection by the dominant culture, adolescents' intense need for belonging and identity may be further derailed. They may find themselves caught between two worlds, or unmoored from their roots as they attempt to integrate into an "American mainstream," however broadly conceived. And finally, all these problem areas are particularly salient in the lives of foster youth. As seen in our case study, even relatively stable foster environments may present them with significant challenges not faced by other adolescents. And absent such comparably ideal circumstances, foster situations themselves can be sources of trauma, including but not limited to abuse and neglect.

Language and communication skills and socioemotional skills, such as self-regulation and relationship management, are intimately intertwined. While important at any age across the lifespan, those skills are particularly relevant for adolescent identity development, and especially so for adolescents impacted by trauma. Interdisciplinary teams of SLPs and counselors can be invaluable resources to help individuals overcome these obstacles and transition into fulfilling healthy adult lives. Together, they can address all six key areas of trauma-informed practice: safety, trust, peer support, collaboration, empowerment, and consideration of cultural, historical, and gender issues (CDC, 2020). In the case discussed in these pages, the SLP and the counselor provided a safe place for Kayla and gained her trust by never dismissing her experience and by giving her time and space to work through her social-pragmatic and emotional issues in preparation for independence. They provided support for each other and collaborated, while also fostering peer support and mutuality in Kayla's therapy through group sessions. Together, this empowered Kayla to become more open to potentially ambiguous social interactions and to engage more deeply with the wider social world in order to find her place and identity within it. Given her complex cultural background, relevant considerations were woven into therapy throughout to ensure that Kayla would find opportunities for growing into her Indigenous identity.

As we hope to have shown, intervention with youth who have experienced trauma differs somewhat from some interventions with which many SLPs are more familiar, such as those implemented with clients diagnosed with autism or developmental language disorder. For children with communicative disabilities, who are otherwise thriving in a nourishing, supportive environment, SLPs are likely to focus on skill development (i.e., the "how" of communication). These youth who experience healthy interactions daily mainly need the means to emulate them. For adolescents with a history of trauma exposure, clinicians are likely to find themselves working on the "what" and the "why" of communication as well. Having grown up without good models of healthy communication, clients with a history of trauma may need to learn the basics of human interaction from scratch—not because they lacked the skills or capacities to learn them, but because they were deprived of the opportunity to do so. To borrow a phrase from de Botton (2019), youth with a trauma background need "a better map of the terrain of normality" (p. 73). Such a map is inevitably both linguistic and sociopsychological; healthy functioning ("normality") requires congruence between inner states and outward behaviors, as well as a viable interpretation of others' inner states. A collaboration between speech-language and mental health professionals is uniquely positioned to foster both.

References

American Psychiatric Association (2022). *Diagnostic and statistical manual of mental disorders* (5th ed., text rev.). Washington, DC: American Psychiatric Publishing. https://doi.org/10.1176/appi.books.9780890425787

Arain, M., Haque, M., Johal, L., Mathur, P., Nel, W., Rais, A., & Sharma, S. (2013). Maturation of the adolescent brain. *Neuropsychiatric Disease and Treatment, 9*, 449–516. https://doi.org/10.2147/NDT.S39776

Berkowitz, S. J. (2012). Childhood trauma and adverse experience and forensic child psychiatry: The Penn Center for youth and family trauma response and recovery. *Journal of Psychiatry & Law, 40(1)*, 5–22. https://doi.org/10.1177/009318531204000102

Blakemore, S. J., & Choudhury, S. (2006). Development of the adolescent brain: Implications for executive function and social cognition. *Journal of Child Psychology and Psychiatry, 47(3–4)*, 296–312. https://doi.org/10.1111/j.1469-7610.2006.01611.x

Blaustein, M. E., & Kinniburgh, K. M. (2015). Providing the family as a secure base for therapy with children and adolescents. *Intervening Beyond the Child: The Intertwining Nature of Attachment and Trauma*. Retrieved from http://www.traumacenter.org/clients/Intertwining_Nature_of_Attachment_and_Trauma.pdf.

Bolton, G., Howlett, S., Lago, C., & Wright, J. (2004). *Writing cures: An introductory handbook of writing in counseling and psychotherapy*. London: Brunner-Routledge.

Casey Family Programs (2012). *Casey life skills*. Seattle, WA: Author.

Casey, B. J., Jones, R. M., & Hare, T. A. (2008). The adolescent brain. *Annals of the New York Academy of Sciences, 1124,* 111–126. https://doi.org/10.1196/annals.1440.010

Centers for Disease Control and Prevention (2020). *Infographic: 6 guiding principles to a trauma-informed approach.*

Center for Disease Control and Prevention (2022). *Fast facts: Preventing child abuse and neglect*. Retrieved from https://www.cdc.gov/violenceprevention/childabuseandneglect/fastfact.html#:~:text=Child%20abuse%20and%20neglect%20are%20common.,because%20many%20cases%20are%20unreported

Chiarenza, G. A. (1990). Motor-perceptual function in children with developmental reading disorders: Neuropsychophysiological analysis. *Journal of Learning Disabilities, 23,* 375–385. https://doi.org/10.1177/002221949002300609

Clark, C., Classen, C. C., Fourt, A., & Shetty, M. (2015). *Treating the trauma survivor: An essential guide to trauma-informed care*. New York, NY: Routledge.

Copeland, W. E., Keeler, G., Angold, A., & Costello, E. J. (2007). Traumatic events and posttraumatic stress in childhood. *Arch Gen Psychiatry, 64*(5), 577–584. https://doi.org/10.1001/archpsyc.64.5.577

Darnell, D., Flaster, A., Hendricks, K., Kerbrat, A., & Comtois, K. A. (2019). Adolescent clinical populations and associations between trauma and behavioral and emotional problems. *Psychological Trauma, 11*(3), 266–273. https://doi.org/10.1037/tra0000371

Davis, M. (2003). Addressing the needs of youth in transition to adulthood. *Administration and Policy in Mental Health and Mental Health Services Research, 30,* 495–509. https://doi.org/10.1023/A:1025027117827

de Botton, A. (2019). *The school of life: An emotional education*. London: Author.

DeGangi, G. A., & Nemiroff, M. A. (2010). *Kids' club letters: Narrative tools for stimulating process and dialogue in therapy groups for children and adolescents*. New York, NY: Routledge.

De Klerk, V. (2005). Slang and swearing as markers of inclusion and exclusion during adolescence. *Talking Adolescence: Perspectives on Communication in the Teenage Years, 3,* 111.

Delima, J., & Vimpani, G. (2011). The neurobiological effects of childhood maltreatment: An often overlooked narrative related to the long-term effects of early childhood trauma? *Family Matters,* (89), 42–52. Retrieved from https://search.informit.org/doi/10.3316/ielapa.717010661945019

Dumontheil, I., & Blakemore, S. J. (2012). Social cognition and abstract thought in adolescence: The role of structural and functional development in rostral prefrontal cortex. *British Journal of Educational Psychology Monograph Series II, 8,* 99–113. https://doi.org/10.1348/97818543371712X13219598392372

Erikson, E. H. (1980). *Identity and the life cycle*. New York, NY: W. W. Norton & Co.

Felitti, V. J., Anda, R. F., Nordenberg, D., Williamson, D. F., Spitz, A. M., Edwards, V., Koss, M. P., & Marks, J. S. (1998). Relationship of childhood abuse and household dysfunction to many of the leading causes of death in adults: The adverse childhood experiences (ACE) study. *American Journal of Preventive Medicine, 14*(4), 245–258. https://doi.org/10.1016/s0749-3797(98)00017-8

Franke, H. A. (2014). Toxic stress: Effects, prevention and treatment. *Children, 1*(3), 390–402. https://doi.org/10.3390/children1030390

Giano, Z., Wheeler, D. L., & Hubach, R. D. (2020). The frequencies and disparities of adverse childhood experiences in the U.S. *BMC Public Health, 20*, 1327. https://doi.org/10.1186/s12889-020-09411-z

Herd, T., & Kim-Spoon, J. (2021). A systematic review of associations between adverse peer experiences and emotion regulation in adolescence. *Clinical Child and Family Psychology Review, 24*, 141–163. https://doi.org/10.1007/s10567-020-00337-x

Hoppen, T. H., & Chalder, T. (2018). Childhood adversity as a transdiagnostic risk factor for affective disorders in adulthood: A systematic review focusing on biopsychosocial moderating and mediating variables. *Clinical Psychology Review, 65*, 81–151. https://doi.org/10.1016/j.cpr.2018.08.002

Iachini, A. L., Petiwala, A. F., & DeHart, D. D. (2016). Examining adverse childhood experiences among students repeating the ninth grade: Implications for school dropout prevention. *Children & Schools, 38*(4), 218–227. https://doi.org/10.1093/cs/cdw029

Individuals with Disabilities Education Improvement Act of 2004. 20 U.S.C. § 614 *et seq.* (2004). (reauthorization of the Individuals with Disabilities Education Act of 1990).

Johnson, D. R. (2005). Key provisions on transition: A comparison of IDEA 1997 and IDEA 2004. *Career Development for Exceptional Individuals, 28*(1), 60–63. https://doi.org/10.1177/08857288050280010801

Karatekin, C., & Hill, M. (2019). Expanding the original definition of adverse childhood experiences (ACEs). *Journal of Child & Adolescent Trauma, 12*(3), 289–306. https://doi.org/10.1007/s40653-018-0237-5

Lanier, P. (2020). *Racism Is an Adverse Childhood Experience.* Jordan Institute for Families. Retrieved from https://jordaninstituteforfamilies.org/2020/racism-is-an-adverse-childhoodexperience-ace/

Levy, J., Goldstein, A., & Feldman, R. (2019). The neural development of empathy is sensitive to caregiving and early trauma. *Nature Communications, 10*(1905). https://doi.org/10.1038/s41467-019-09927-y

Miller, A. B., Esposito-Smythers, C., Weismoore, J. T., & Renshaw, K. D. (2013). The relationship between child maltreatment and adolescent suicidal behavior: A systematic review and critical examination of the literature. *Clinical Child and Family Psychology Review, 16*(2), 146–172. https://doi.org/10.1007/s10567-013-0131-5

Nemeroff, C. B. (2016). Paradise lost: The neurobiological and clinical consequences of child abuse and neglect. *Neuron, 89*(5), 892–909. https://doi.org/10.1016/j.neuron.2016.01.019

Nippold, M. A. (1993). Developmental markers in adolescent language: Syntax, semantics, and pragmatics. *Language, Speech, and Hearing Services in Schools, 24*(1), 21–28. https://doi.org/10.1044/0161-1461.2401.21

Nippold, M. A. (2017). Reading comprehension deficits in adolescents: Addressing underlying language abilities. *Language, Speech, and Hearing Services in Schools, 48*(2), 125–131. https://doi.org/10.1044/2016_LSHSS-16-0048

Nippold, M. A. (2018). The literate lexicon in adolescents: Monitoring the use and understanding of morphologically complex words. *Perspectives of the ASHA Special Interest Groups, 3*(1), 211–221. https://doi.org/10.1044/persp3.SIG1.211

Nippold, M. A., Hegel, S. L., Sohlberg, M. M., & Schwarz, I. E. (1999). Defining abstract entities: Development in pre-adolescents, adolescents, and young adults. *Journal of Speech, Language, and Hearing Research, 42*(2), 473–481. https://doi.org/10.1044/jslhr.4202.473

Nippold, M. A., Schwarz, I. E., & Undlin, R. A. (1992). Use and understanding of adverbial conjuncts: A developmental study of adolescents and young adults. *Journal of Speech, Language, and Hearing Research, 35*(1), 108–118. https://doi.org/10.1044/jshr.3501.108

Rimé, B. (2007). Interpersonal emotion regulation. In J. J. Gross (Ed.), *Handbook of emotion regulation* (pp. 466–485). The Guilford Press.

Romeo, R. D. (2013). The teenage brain: The stress response and the adolescent brain. *Current Directions in Psychological Science, 22*(2), 140–145. https://doi.org/10.1177/0963721413475445

Sælid, G. A., & Nordahl, H. M. (2017). Rational emotive behaviour therapy in high schools to educate in mental health and empower youth health. A randomized controlled study of a brief intervention. *Cognitive Behaviour Therapy, 46*(3), 196–210. https://doi.org/10.1080/16506073.2016.1233453

Schickedanz, J. A., Schickedanz, D. I., Forsyth, P. D., & Forsyth, G. A. (2001). *Understanding children and adolescents* (4th ed.). Boston, MA: Allyn & Bacon.

Sesma, H. W., Mahone, E. M., Levine, T., Eason, S. H., & Cutting, L. E. (2009). The contribution of executive skills to reading comprehension. *Child Neuropsychology, 15*, 232–246. https://doi.org/10.1080/09297040802220029

Slaughter, V., Dennis, M. J., & Pritchard, M. (2002). Theory of mind and peer acceptance in preschool children. *British Journal of Developmental Psychology, 20*(4), 545–564. https://doi.org/10.1348/026151002760390945

Spann, M. N., Mayes, L. C., Kalmar, J. H., Guiney, J., Womer, F. Y., Pittman, B., ... & Blumberg, H. P. (2012). Childhood abuse and neglect and cognitive flexibility in adolescents. *Child Neuropsychology, 18*(2), 182–189. https://doi.org/10.1080/09297049.2011.595400

Stein, B. D., Zima, B. T., Elliott, M. N., Burnam, M. A., Shahinfar, A., Fox, N. A., & Leavitt, L. A. (2001). Violence exposure among school-age children in foster care: Relationship to distress symptoms. *Journal of the American Academy of Child & Adolescent Psychiatry, 40*(5), 588–594. https://doi.org/10.1097/00004583-200105000-00019

Substance Abuse and Mental Health Services Administration (2015). *Trauma-informed care in behavioral health services [KAP keys for clinicians, based on*

TIP 57]. HHS Publication No. (SMA) 15–4420. Rockville, MD: Substance Abuse and Mental Health Services Administration. Retrieved from https://store.samhsa.gov/sites/default/files/d7/priv/sma15-4420.pdf

Sun, L., & Nippold, M. A. (2012). Narrative writing in children and adolescents: Examining the literate lexicon. *Language, Speech, and Hearing Services in Schools, 43*, 2–13. https://doi.org/10.1044/0161-1461(2011/10-0099)

Swanson, H. L. (2003). Age-related differences in learning disabled and skilled readers' working memory. *Journal of Abnormal Child Psychology, 85*, 1–31. https://doi.org/10.1016/s0022-0965(03)00043-2

Udry, J. R., Li, R. M., & Hendrickson-Smith, J. (2003). Health and behavior risks of adolescents with mixed-race identity. *American Journal of Public Health, 93*(11), 1865–1870. https://doi.org/10.2105/ajph.93.11.1865

U.S. Department of Labor (2002). *O*Net career interest inventory*. St. Paul, MN: JIST Works.

9 Attachment-based Narrative Speech Styles in Adults with Post-Traumatic Stress

Karin Riber and Emma Beck

9.1 Background

After decades of academic discussion, posttraumatic stress disorder (PTSD) was included in DSM-III as an official diagnosis for the first time in 1980. Although it was useful to finally have a diagnosis that validated patients' reactions to traumatic events, clinicians and researchers have since then been critically arguing for and pointing out the need for a diagnosis that captures the more complex trauma reactions and posttraumatic phenomena, which has been observed repeatedly in the past century in both children and adults subjected to complex trauma (Friedman, 2010; Herman, 1997). Recently, the WHO decided to include complex posttraumatic stress disorder (CPTSD, 6B41) along with PTSD in ICD-11, under Disorders specifically associated with stress (WHO, 2022). Consequently, the basic PTSD diagnosis is now clearly defined as comprising three core symptoms: *re-experiencing*, *avoidance of traumatic reminders*, and *hypervigilance* following exposure to an extremely threatening event. The symptoms persist for several weeks and cause significant functional impairment. In addition to the requirements of PTSD, CPTSD contains three features describing trauma's severe and persisting impacts on the organization of self, namely pervasive disturbances in *affective*, *self-concept*, and *relational* domains. CPTSD develops following exposure to one or repetitive extremely horrific events from which escape is difficult or impossible, for example, prolonged childhood sexual or physical abuse, ongoing domestic violence, slavery, torture, or genocide (Cloitre et al., 2013; WHO, 2022). Accordingly, studies involved in the diagnostic process for ICD-11 revealed important differences between ordinary and complex PTSD, finding single traumatic events a stronger predictor of ordinary PTSD, whereas being subjected to chronic traumatic events is a stronger predictor of complex PTSD. Traumatic events during childhood have also been found to increase the likelihood of developing CPTSD. Finally, people with CPTSD display higher

DOI: 10.4324/9781003225270-11

personal, familial, social, educational, and occupational functional impairment than those with PTSD (Cloitre et al., 2013; Karatzias et al., 2017).

To enhance our understanding of adults with (C)PTSD, this chapter aims to describe narrative speech styles, especially from an attachment-informed point of view and explore the relationship between attachment patterns and certain characteristics of (C)PTSD, i.e., how they may interact and mutually affect one another. Besides the theoretical framework of attachment theory, the chapter presents perspectives from mentalization-based theory to demonstrate how disruptions from complex trauma types, posttraumatic stress, and insecure and disorganized attachment patterns may impact mental health, level of language functioning, and well-being in traumatized adults. Finally, elements from narrative therapy and therapeutic approaches using exposure are briefly discussed.

9.2   Attachment Patterns and Posttraumatic Stress Disorder

Attachment theory has been applied in different traditions within psychology. In terms of the terminology in this chapter, "attachment patterns" refer to studies that measure attachment as a category, using observer-rated interviews/experiments; whereas "attachment styles" refer to studies that measure attachment as dimensions, using self-rating questionnaires (Ravitz et al., 2010).

Attachment theory plays a steadily growing role in the fields of PTSD, loss, trauma, and adult psychotherapy. Attachment patterns originate in the early interactions with a primary caregiver, and they establish as cognitive, affective, and behavioral mental models that serve as a basis for later interpersonal strategies. There is increasing evidence that adult attachment patterns play an important role the development of PTSD, maintenance of PTSD, and response to PTSD, but the relationships between the attachment patterns, trauma types, and symptoms are less clear. On the one hand, results from a meta-analysis of PTSD and attachment style found an association between secure attachment style and lower PTSD symptom levels, as well as an association between insecure attachment styles and higher PTSD symptom levels, thus confirming the theory that secure attachment style can function as a protection against psychopathology (Woodhouse et al., 2015). However, a prospective, controlled study re-examining veterans 18 and 30 years after war, found that those veterans who had been prisoners of war, deteriorated in both PTSD symptoms *and* insecure attachment styles over time, displaying both more attachment insecurity as well as worse PTSD symptoms, decades after imprisonment. They also found that the PTSD symptoms predicted the deterioration in attachment status, and not vice versa (Solomon et al., 2008). In opposition to community samples, clinical samples contain many individuals with insecure adult attachment patterns (73%), and up to 43% classified as Unresolved-Disorganized with respect to loss and trauma. Accordingly, meta-analytic studies have demonstrated the impact of trauma on attachment, finding strong correlations between PTSD and attachment disorganization in adults and pointing out that unresolved-disorganized attachment patterns are especially characteristic or even overrepresented in adults with trauma reactions such as PTSD (Bakermans-Kranenburg & van Ijzendoorn, 2009). Being classified with unresolved trauma on the Adult Attachment Interview (AAI) has been found to increase the likelihood of being diagnosed with PTSD 7.5-fold among adult women with a history of childhood sexual abuse (Stovall-McClough & Cloitre, 2006). Among this group, insecure attachment and general psychiatric impairment was associated (Cloitre et al., 2008). Finally, secure and fearful attachment style has been found significantly associated with the disturbances of self-organization, seen in the three added symptom clusters in CPTSD (Karatzias et al., 2021). In conclusion, attachment and traumatic stress seem to mutually influence one another in complex ways, positively or negatively.

Adult attachment patterns can be defined as cognitive, affective, and behavioral mental models that unfold in close relationships, and involve affect-regulating strategies. Table 9.1 shows how adult states of mind with respect to attachment are categorized according to the AAI classification system (Hesse, 2008; Main et al., 2003).

9.3   Attachment Patterns and Attachment-based Narrative Speech Styles

The attachment system is a motivational system distinct from yet connected to the fight-flight-freeze system. It becomes activated when facing distress, danger, threats to one's life and in the case of separation, loss, and trauma (Bowlby, 1969, 1973, 1980; Mikulincer & Florian, 1998). It can also become activated in the therapist-client relationship in response to working with difficult or traumatic experiences and when unconscious thoughts, feelings, and behavioral tendencies related to personal experience with care, rejection, and abandonment become more accessible (Daniel, 2015).

Attachment patterns originate in the early interactions with primary caregivers and establish as cognitive, affective, and behavioral mental models that serve as a basis for later interpersonal strategies. In adults, they can be defined as individual patterns of expectations, attention-, affect-regulating-, and behavioral strategies that unfold in close, intimate relationships (George et al., 1996; Main et al., 2003) and thus describe an individual's characteristic way of viewing, relating to, and interacting

Table 9.1 Adult Attachment Patterns

Adult attachment patterns			
Organized categories		Secure-autonomous	Open, balanced, explorative speech patterns and adaptive affect-regulation
	Insecure attachment patterns	Dismissing attachment	Distancing speech patterns, minimizing relational needs, and deactivating affect-regulation
		Preoccupied attachment	Overinvolved speech patterns, maximizing relational needs and hyperactivating affect-regulation
Disorganized categories		Unresolved – Disorganized with respect to loss, abuse and other trauma	Local, temporary narrative breakdowns in speech style, when narrating events related to loss, abuse, or other trauma, during the Adult Attachment Interview
		Cannot classify	Global narrative breakdowns in speech style, displaying an inability to use one single narrative strategy when describing ones childhood experiences with caregivers, during the Adult Attachment Interview

with close significant others, such as parents, children, and romantic partners (Levy et al., 2019). In children, attachment patterns are observed as certain behavioral strategies that regulate distance and closeness to their attachment figure, whereas in adults, attachment patterns are displayed as different narrative speech styles or discourses, that unconsciously, reflect distance and closeness in the adult's state of mind with respect to attachment (Broberg et al., 2010).

Adult attachment patterns can be assessed using *The Adult Attachment Interview* (AAI), a quasi-qualitative interview, exploring the relationship with primary caregivers in childhood, as well as separation, loss, trauma, and how these experiences are currently understood. The interview is transcribed and coded based on discourse characteristics and coherence, i.e., rather from the narrative style and way of narrating experiences, than the actual narrative content. A certified AAI-coder classifies the interview as either Secure-Autonomous or into one of the two insecure categories, the Dismissing or the Preoccupied attachment category. The AAI can also be classified as Unresolved-Disorganized with respect to loss, abuse, or other trauma, for example if the interviewee's speech temporarily breaks down in local parts of the interview while discussing these events. Finally, it can be assigned as Cannot Classify, if the speech style is characterized by global narrative breakdowns, displaying how the interviewee is unable to use one single narrative strategy when telling her or his story (Hesse, 2008).

On the AAI, adults with insecure attachment patterns display a lack of coherence and balance in their autobiographic stories of childhood experiences with caregivers. The adult speaker thus narrates the relationship with parents in ways that become untruthful, irrelevant, unclear, too long and overly detailed, or too short and terse (Hesse, 2008; Main et al., 2003). In addition, adults categorized as Unresolved-Disorganized, have particular difficulties narrating their experiences of loss and trauma in a coherent manner, displaying disturbed responses and momentary fractures in speech and thinking. These linguistic signs reflect confusion, unresolved traumatic elements and poor adaptation to loss and trauma (Jacobvitz & Reisz, 2019; Mikulincer & Shaver, 2013). Attachment insecurity have also been found to influence the narrative processes in both psychoanalytic and cognitive-behavioral therapy, where clients with preoccupied attachment patterns talk more and have longer speaking turns compared to clients with dismissing attachment patterns who generate more pauses (Daniel, 2011).

Generally, adults with insecure attachment patterns are characterized by distrust in others' intentions and are either very cautious of entering close relations or have very high needs for closeness and affirmation from others. When activated, insecure adult attachment patterns trigger defensive affect-regulation strategies. Adults with a dismissing attachment pattern apply deactivating strategies whereby they suppress emotional distress, minimize their personal needs and distance themselves in close relations. They either have a negative or an idealized view of close others, that seem to serve as maintaining a positive self-image, and they often describe themselves as strong and independent of others. In opposition, adults with a preoccupied attachment pattern apply hyperactivating strategies whereby they increase emotional distress, maximize their personal needs, and insatiably seek out contact in close relations. They have a positive and often idealized, dependent view of others and a negative view of self as not being able to cope autonomously (Mikulincer et al., 2003; Stroebe et al., 2010). These characteristics make it more difficult for clients with insecure adult attachment patterns to build and maintain a therapeutic relation, as well as coming to agreement on the goals and tasks of therapy, compared to clients with secure attachment patterns who create better alliances and have more successful outcomes of therapy (Bernecker et al., 2014; Diener & Monroe, 2011). Because these two insecure attachment patterns both apply one specific strategy to obtain a feeling of safety, they constitute so-called organized attachment (Hesse, 2008; Main et al., 2003). Adults with unresolved-disorganized attachment patterns have a negative view of self as well as a negative view of others. They long for closeness although it feels uncomfortable, and at the same time they fear rejection, and so their affect-regulation fluctuates between the two insecure strategies, deactivation versus hyperactivation (Hesse, 2008; Stroebe et al., 2010). At first glance, clients with a preoccupied attachment pattern seem easy to treat because they appear relationally engaged and willing to talk about their concerns. However, evidence-based research in psychotherapy relationships point out that longer and more complicated treatments generally should be expected with these clients (Levy et al., 2019).

Finally, attachment theory understands the formation of attachment patterns as a universal phenomenon that establishes in any culture (Bowlby, 1969, 1973, 1980). Accordingly, attachment studies have found the three primary attachment patterns across African, Chinese, Israeli, Japanese, and Indonesian cultural settings (van Ijzendoorn & Sagi-Schwartz, 2008), as well as in samples of asylum-seekers and refugees with different European and Mideastern backgrounds (De Haene et al., 2010; Riber, 2016). Meta-analytic results point out that adult attachment patterns are independent of gender, cultural background, and diagnosis (Bakermans-Kranenburg & van Ijzendoorn, 2009).

9.4 Narrative Style and Trauma Reactions in Unresolved-Disorganized Adult Attachment

The disorganized adult attachment pattern is a complex pattern in which fear plays a central role. Seen from an intrapersonal AAI-level, a classification as Unresolved-Disorganized is a distinct aspect of state of mind which is always assigned in conjunction with the best-fitting alternative or organized adult attachment category, i.e., secure-autonomous, dismissing, or preoccupied. Besides the basic attachment pattern, adults can thus be disorganized with respect to certain single loss, abuse or other trauma experiences. These adults often present with incoherent, chaotic narratives and display difficulties creating an overall meaning of their trauma experience (Jacobvitz & Reisz, 2019; Main et al., 2003). A disorganized state of mind appears as unintegrated elements in the speaker's cognitive, affective, and behavioral mental model, and is displayed "locally" when the interviewee narrates these events, as opposed to a "global" disorganization throughout the entire interview (Hesse, 2008). The narrative style observed on the AAI in responses to loss, abuse, and other trauma is characterized by unconscious speech errors, abrupt holes, or collapses in the reasoning and monitoring of discourse, or reports of extreme behavioral reactions during the discussion of these loss- or trauma-related events. When talking about trauma experience such as abuse, the speaker may for example mix up self and other, i.e., victim and perpetrator, mix up past and present tense, as though the present moment is invaded by the past event, or talk about a deceased attachment figure as though he or she was still alive. Another example is the presence of markedly long pauses of silence while describing the death of a close relative, or a traumatic episode involving a parent, apparently without noticing (not commenting on) this very long pause in the middle of a story. Such linguistic lapses in attention, affect, and cognition may reflect traits of posttraumatic intrusion or re-experiencing, as though the trauma is actualized in the speaker and re-experienced during the retelling of the event, which then activates psychological defense mechanisms such as displacement, denial, or dissociative responses during narration (Broberg et al., 2010; Main et al., 2003). According to Main et al. (2003), speakers with abuse experiences can react with resolution, dismissal, or disorganization, and the latter responses, for example, appear in a failure to speak about abuse without denying the abusive aspects, in oscillations between reporting and denying abuse, in confused and irrational thought processes and speech patterns surrounding the event, such as on the one hand describing being hit very hard, while also saying that it was never really that bad, or admitting sexual assaults while saying that the self was the one who led the abusive parent on, or displaying incoherent, disoriented speech with extraordinary long pauses or inability to finish sentences and meaning-making (Main et al., 2003). Unresolved loss, abuse, and other trauma are thought to originate from fear associated with memories connected to different types of trauma experience. With respect to the affected speech styles, researchers assume that the breakdown of language occurs because the trauma memories are poorly integrated and therefore intrude into the coherent thought and speech processes in normal consciousness (Broberg et al., 2010, s. 201; Jacobvitz & Reisz, 2019; Juen et al., 2013).

With respect to unresolved loss, the death of a parent can have been so devastating, or the relation so complex, that the loss is difficult to integrate into the bereaved speaker's autobiographical narrative and memory. This can lead to continuing problems acknowledging the reality of the loss, or the loss continuously being permeated by "unrealness" (Boelen, 2006, 2010). According to Main et al. (2003), such loss responses originate in frightening experiences after a loss, or frightening ideas about the way the loss occurred or frightening thoughts regarding the relationship with the lost person. Feeling sadness and distress do not in itself reflect unresolved loss. Rather, discussing the death of a close one with so extreme attention to detail that the speech falls apart and the listener does not understand, or, if a speaker linguistically reveals that he thinks a dead parent is still alive, or reacts with an extreme response, such as a suicide attempt, such instances indicate disorganization or disorientation in thinking, discourse or behavior (Broberg et al., 2010; Main et al., 2003). Unresolved loss has been found easier to resolve, compared to unresolved trauma (Jacobvitz & Reisz, 2019).

Seen from an interpersonal level, adult clients with disorganized patterns have fundamental problems regulating fear and often display breakdowns in this affect-regulation. Clinically, they often present a relational style that shifts between denying their need for help versus showing intensive crisis, based on complicated inner working models of others' help as being both extremely risky and necessary at the same time. Therefore, these clients constitute a great therapeutic challenge (Daniel, 2015; Jacobvitz & Reisz, 2019). These adult clients' disorganized states of mind reflect an unresolved emotional reaction in relation to loss, abuse, or other trauma. Besides traumatic experiences such as childhood abuse, disorganizing experiences might also be the result of overwhelmed caregivers' overwhelming reactions to the client as a child due to, for example, personal anxiety, mental illness, trauma, death, or because the caregiver felt too helpless to be able to serve as a secure base and safe haven for the child (Broberg et al., 2010; Cyr et al., 2010; Lyons-Ruth & Jacobvitz, 2008). Finally, evidence-based research in psychotherapy relationships and therapist responsiveness point out that beneficial therapy outcome varies highly among adults with disorganized attachment patterns, emphasizing the general importance of being especially attentive to the structure of the inner working model in these clients (Levy et al., 2019).

9.5 Two Case Stories

Case story 1: Nordic woman with complex childhood trauma, complex PTSD, and borderline personality disorder – an example a of dismissing and disorganized attachment pattern.

Anne was a Northern European woman in her forties who was referred to psychiatry after her father's death had triggered various symptoms and a significant decrease in her level of functioning. She was brought up in a dysfunctional family and had been vulnerable throughout her life. As a child, Anne was bullied, and she spent most of her spare time hiding in a small loft room alone, but at nighttime, she was exposed to alcoholic strangers who were drinking with her father in their flat. Throughout her childhood, Anne had been subjected to persistent and repeated maltreatment such as physical abuse (primarily the father, but also older brothers), probably sexual abuse (the alcoholic strangers), and emotional abuse and neglect (both parents). She had lived with her father's atrocities, protected by the fantasy that her mother was more caring. After he died, her mother blamed Anne for his death. This triggered Anne's mental condition. In the psychiatric clinic, her most characteristic feature was extremely high anxiety and fundamental affect-regulation disturbances, displayed in angry frustration and ongoing outbursts of rage. During the diagnostic assessment, she described frightening nightmares and flashbacks with daunting fragments that implied her being sexually abused by men in a dark place. She feared that an exploration of these memories would onset an uncontrollable avalanche and therefore dismissed doing so. She had high levels of distress and pervasive distrust in others (the health care providers, psychiatrist, psychologist, case managers, extended family, neighbors etc.), evident chronic arousal and hypervigilance, and an inability to leave her home. She avoided ordinary places such as the local supermarket, she avoided other people, and merely thinking about exposure to either her mother, her brothers, or her childhood experience, could trigger panic attacks. At the time, Anne was diagnostically assessed with posttraumatic stress disorder and comorbid borderline personality disorder according to ICD-10; and had the ICD-11 criteria been available, she would likewise have fulfilled the diagnostic criteria for complex PTSD because of the disturbances in the organization of self, seen in all three domains (affective, self-concept, relational). When Anne cautiously entered psychological treatment, she displayed fast and furious shifting strategies of denying emotional needs and distancing herself while in the next moment increasing her emotional distress whenever she felt some kind of insecurity or fear of rejection. Anne viewed herself as a fundamentally bad person, and while a part of her longed for care, affirmation, and understanding, she generally held a distrusting and negative view of others based on traumatic experiences in the ongoing chaotic attachment relationship during her upbringing. Seen from an attachment perspective, Anne's attachment pattern was disorganized, with features of unresolved loss and trauma and shifting insecure affect-regulation strategies. Obviously, Annes experience and symptomatology colored the course and processes of therapy, as well as the therapeutic relationship.

If Anne had been asked questions about her childhood experiences with her parents in a context of the AAI, her speech style could have looked like this (interviewer in bold):

Could you describe the relationship with your parents, starting as far back as you remember?.. I.. I don't really remember anything. My dad was all discipline, and my mom generally more protective, but.. uhm. **Okay. Which parent did you feel closest to and why?** Uhm.. in my childhood, there was not mu.. well, my mom. **Okay, and why her?** I guess, I think, she was she was more there than he was.. I don't know.. my dad he was a tough one, he.. you know, I took care of myself you know. So really.. no comments. **Have you ever felt rejected as a child?** Oh my god. All the time. Every time something went wrong, they all blamed it on me. All the time. **And how did you feel about that?** Bad. I felt really, really.. like trash. This was all the time. 'What have you done? What did you do now? You are always messing around! We should send you away to go live somewhere else!' This.. I felt bad.. but.. I just became immune. I hid in the loft room. **Did they realize how this made you feel?** No. I don't know.. I don't think he she.. but then.. I don't think she knew I was.... cause she was more being protective.... **Why do you think they did as they did?** No idea. I was a.. very bad child.. they they.. that's what they said. I don't know.

Case story 2: Middle eastern man with complex childhood trauma, decades of war trauma and complex PTSD symptoms – an example of preoccupied attachment pattern with unresolved-disorganized traumatic losses.

Amir was a 44 year-old man from a small village in a Middle Eastern country. His father worked as a soldier in the military for thirty-three years and was absent from their home in long periods, with ten days off every three months. His mother was a housewife and worked in farming. The family was poor. Amir grew up with eight siblings, two elder sisters, four elder brothers, one younger sister and one younger brother. Amir's mother had given birth to other children that only lived shortly, and Amir was named after an older deceased brother. When Amir was eight years old, he lost an older brother in an accident, and many years later, he lost an older brother, who had taken care of him in his early childhood. Amir grew up in a context of constant civil war and shifting wars, during his upbringing.

Amir described his father as cold, hard, neglecting, and acted like a general who disciplined his children as though they were soldiers. Amir had memories of him commanding the group of children out of bed, to stand in line, to always be quiet, and they were punished with beatings with a stick for even small misdemeanors. According to their traditions, Amir and his siblings washed his fathers' feet, a common cultural practice to pay respects, but there was something utterly humiliating, in the manner his father carried out this performance. Although beatings were not uncommon in families in their village, his fathers' violence was well-known in the village and regarded as out of line. Amir felt fatherless and could not think of any positive experiences with him. He recalled him as a self-absorbed stranger. Amir's mother was loving, sad and silent. She was never angry, but hid her thoughts, feelings, and losses inside herself. She was always dressed in black and he slept in her arm until he was fifteen years old. This felt safe, and Amir said they had a very close and strong relation. Later, Amir was forced to work in the military. He then fled and came to a Nordic country, where he was referred to a psychiatric trauma clinic. Amir presented with symptoms corresponding to CPTSD. He lived a very isolated existence, barely leaving his small apartment and his hypervigilance bordered the paranoid, making him oppose the use of an interpreter, although he struggled with the local Nordic language. He had severe nightmares and flashbacks of the traumatic losses and torture experiences. Upon mentioning traumatic war events, Amir got up from the chair, showed his scars, became very talkative in an automatic manner, concretely demonstrated what had happened, mimicked gunshots, and was cut off from emotional resonance. Yet, sometimes when exploring his losses and family relations, he reacted moved, tears welled up, he breathed deeply, and would either just stop speaking trying to find the right words, ask for a short break, or simply get up and leave the therapy session. He often sat there with a bowed head, expressing deep shame and guilt. He generally had a positive view of others, valued his relations, slightly idealized his mother, and conveyed a negative view of self, describing an alienation, shamefulness, and a fundamental insecurity of self, affecting his ability to make even small decisions in his everyday life or accomplishing small tasks. Seen from an attachment perspective, Amir presented with an insecure, preoccupied attachment pattern with unresolved-disorganized traumatic losses and other trauma (war).

The following presents linguistic examples of how Amir's unresolvedness with respect to loss and trauma looked like, in the context of the AAI. Based on Amir's speech style, it seems evident that his memories of his mother's reactions are associated with fear, and that his language breaks down and becomes incoherent many places, probably because the trauma memory intrudes into his coherent normal consciousness while he thinks about and narrates his story.

When asked if he had lost any close relatives (a parent or sibling) as a child, Amir first paused and said no. Then, when probing for other losses, it turns out that Amir had lost a brother in his childhood, and also a brother in his adult life:

> ... {{3 seconds}} I don't think she reacted very.. *(okay)*. Because what what I saw with my ahm bigbrother *(mm)*.. so much has happened and mentally she too has had.. *(mm)* she started during the funeral, she will not even come backe home *(mm)*.. and she she she she hits herself, she wants to commit suicide *(aha, okay)*. There were much pain for her, because I stil remember ssss well still while we grew up, we couldn't say my bigbrothers name *(mm)* because if we did, she would get very sad

and cry *(mm)*. I did not understand what death was, but it was shocking to see my mother slapping herself.. her eye bled, she dresses in black and cries for five, six years until she gets...... {{5 seconds.}} because at nights she is walking to his grave site and she sits there with him. **How old were you at the time?** I think I was 8 years old.. no one explains anything to you and if you ask, they hit you *(okay)*. **Do you think this has affected your personality?** I don't... {{3 seconds}} but but but my other big brother who died.. I had a close contact, especially to this brother *(aha, okay)* I could call him and speak for a long time, I miss him.. very, very.. sometimes I think he is not dead *(mm)* I dream many times that he is back, it it always becomes a nightmare *(mm)*. It is two days since I saw him.. I hear him coming and I am really happy. Th.. then suddenly he looks at me and his face is all wrong, his eyes are missing, and this.. {{Amir breathes heavily}} *(mm)*. I was on the phone with them in the hospital next to his machine, that bip bip.. Suddenly I hear screaming and I know he is dead. I got so angry and I threw my phone across the room...... {{6 seconds}}. It is good my children were not at home *(yeah)*.. {{Amir breathes heavily}}.

When Amir was asked if he had other traumatic experiences in his life, he first replied no after a pause. When further probed, he answered:

.... {{4 seconds}}. Traumatic? It when when it gets dark *(mm)*.. I I get panic and yes I dont know why *(okay)*. **Have you experienced any concrete events that were scary or very overwhelming?/** I felt very unplea.. when they took me to the military in my youth *(mm)*.. around 17–18–19... {{3 seconds}}. I collected dead people *(okay, yes)*. I collected heads, legs, arms, so so the helicopter kills people, and so we walk right after them, we/ **you were on the ground?** Yes *(yes)*. I collect those that are not dead and I have to kill them. **You had to shoot them? This sounds gruesome?** It it it was like normal for me then *(mm)*. **How did you react?** In the beginning I was scared *(mm)*. When I see a face and I look at it *(yeah)*.. I just, I I.. finally I started looking at faces and then.. and then started to cuddle them... **-you cuddled them?** Yes *(yes)* and my shirt and my whole face became full of blood *(mm)* blood blood *(mm)* all over. **You got blood all over.** Yes. When when when I dream, I dream of this face *(mm)*. When I hold this head it is like the head says to me: put me back *(mm)*, I can live, I can live, and I say: No, you cannot live anymore *(mm)*. And children and women and.. tiny little babies, we have killed very.. but people were............... {{15 seconds}}. **How did you react to these experiences?** I was, it was like, not voluntary, so in the beginning I got very scared when I saw dead people *(mm)*. I wanted to run away *(mm)*. But someone is behind me with a Kalasnikof.. and.. I always remember him.. It it its no use *(mm)*. they know me, they know my family, that was the problem in this country, if they can't find you, they would take your mother or your father, too *(right)*.

9.6   An Attachment-Informed Mentalization-based, Approach to Treating Complex Trauma

As demonstrated above, both Anne and Amir were subjected to complex childhood trauma, i.e., prolonged, repeated traumatic experiences in ongoing chaotic relationships with their caregivers. In addition, Amir grew up in the extremely stressing context of poverty, war, imprisonment, torture, and traumatic losses. During their psychological development, they were trapped in the caregiving relation they depended on for survival, and normal development.

Mentalization-based treatment (MBT) relies heavily upon attachment theory as it presents a developmental psychopathology model in which the quality of early attachment relationships plays an important role for the development of the capacity to mentalize.

Mentalization has been defined as our capacity to understand and interpret – implicitly and explicitly – one's own and others' behavior as an expression of mental states such as feelings, thoughts, fantasies, beliefs, and desires (Fonagy et al., 2002). Mentalizing is sometimes referred to as "thinking about thinking" and, in its controlled, explicit form, involves relatively slow, executive functioning and prefrontal activity optimized by mild to moderate levels of arousal. When extreme, fear-driven levels of arousal are triggered, mentalizing is compromised by a "neuro-chemical switch" (Mayes, 2000) to more rapid, automatic, fight/flight mode of thinking needed for finding safety.

The theory postulates that attachment security is the developmental context through which mentalization develops: A sensitive, mentalizing caregiver stimulates attachment bonding and promotes secure attachment, through his/her affect regulating responses to the child's communication of needs. The child, in turn, internalizes these responses which ultimately becomes representations of the affective states of the self, from which a coherent sense of self as a mental agent develops (Sharp & Fonagy, 2008). When the caregiver is sensitive, the child feels safe to explore mental states in oneself and others, i.e., to mentalize and learns to affect regulate.

In general, MBT aims to facilitate proper affect-regulation in patients vulnerable to non-mentalizing modes of thinking by training the patients' awareness of when a switch to non-mentalizing modes occurs and by deploying specific therapeutic techniques to help patients regain adequate mentalizing. To illustrate how mentalizing versus non-mentalizing is expressed verbally, an example of high mentalizing would be

I think that me getting this job actually, maybe, mattered to him, and the disappointing news overwhelmed him and he needed some space to regroup, before talking to me about it. But to me, when he left the room, it felt like he left me, and I felt rejected by both him and the company that did not hire me.

The sentence demonstrates that the person saying it is aware that she is expressing her mental state and that she can't be certain about her own assumptions (*I think*), which she uses to attribute meaning to his actions. A demonstration of low mentalization of the same situation would be "He *just walked away, because that how he is*". In that sentence there is no sign of awareness that she is thinking about mental states, but rather a focus on the physical concreteness of actions (walked away) instead of the mental state leading to them.

The mentalizing approach to treating trauma focuses on complex trauma, defined as "*types of trauma that occur repeatedly and cumulatively and typically in the context of close relationships, often caregivers*" and therefore "*often used interchangeably with the notion of attachment trauma*" (Luyten & Fonagy, 2019). Experiencing attachment trauma in critical developmental periods is related to both dysfunction in the human stress system at the biological level and to decreased capacity for mentalizing often triggered by complex feelings of shame, anger, and guilt. Importantly, repetitive caregiver maltreatment and neglect tends to trap the child in an insoluble approach-avoidance conflict that consequently may decrease the capacity for seeking help in others and become a hard-to-reach patient for health professionals.

9.6.1   Clinical Implications for Health Professionals' Communication with Adults with Attachment Trauma

Several clinicians have pointed out that clients with complex trauma difficulties put high demands on therapists and are challenging to form sustainable therapeutic relationships and positive alliances with because of their mistrust and emotional complexity. Their paths of recovery are lengthy and unclear, involving recurrent periods of crisis and personal chaos (Chu, 2011; Herman, 1997). Thus, integrating attachment-informed approaches and models of trauma that capture the disturbances from the developmental and relational contexts in which they appear is suggested, with interventions designed to increase coherence of mind, and mentalizing capacities toward establishing stable, balanced inner working models and attachment security.

In MBT, the concept of epistemic trust is introduced to explain why not only the information delivered in treatment but also how it is conveyed is of particular importance in the case of complex trauma. Epistemic trust is defined as a person's *"confidence in the authenticity and personal relevance of interpersonally transmitted knowledge"* (Bateman et al., 2018) and the capacity to be open to social learning opportunities when offered. Epistemic mistrust develops as an adaptive response to neglect, early attachment trauma and insecurity, and the mind *"become closed to processing new information, particularly when it is offered by other who claim that they can be trusted"* (Luyten & Fonagy, 2019, p. 90) and is not perceived as personally relevant information.

MBT of trauma aims to re-open *"the epistemic highway"* (Luyten & Fonagy 2019) with a number of strategies and interventions, including (1) presenting a convincing model for understanding the client's mind that increases feelings of agency and control and makes the client feel validated, (2) conveying to the patient that the therapist can tolerate and mentalize feelings, and memories intolerable to the client. As this leads to more trust and robust client mentalizing, narratives become more coherent. Slowly this development generalizes to contexts outside therapy in which the client also opens up to social communication and becomes more epistemically trustful. It is suggested that these mechanisms of therapeutic change are not specific to MBT, but rather at play in all effective psychotherapeutic treatments for complex and/or attachment trauma.

9.7   Concluding Remarks

9.7.1   *Exposure based and Constructivist Approaches to Treating Trauma*

While the evidence-base for CPTSD psychotherapeutic programs is still limited (Dorrepaal et al., 2014), a number of treatments for PTSD have shown to be effective. These treatments apply exposure as a central curative element, and generally focus on and emphasize aspects of trauma that involve memory, cognitions, and behavior, and aim to reduce anxiety and enhance control. Such treatments include Prolonged Exposure Therapy (PE) (Powers et al., 2010), Trauma-focused Cognitive Behavior Therapy (TF-CBT) (Seidler & Wagner, 2006), Eye Movement Desensitization and Reprocessing (EMDR) (Watts et al., 2013), and Narrative Exposure Therapy (NET) (Siehl et al., 2021). Further, evidence-based research in psychotherapy relations, point out that psychologists should concurrently use evidence-based relationships and evidence-based treatment methods, adapted to the whole client, because the client, the psychologist, and the therapy relationship, substantially and consistently contribute to and account for effective vs ineffective psychological treatment, independent of treatment methods (Norcross & Lambert, 2019; Norcross & Wampold, 2019).

Finally, narrative processes and a constructivist, meaning-making approach to loss and trauma could be important when developing interventions. In both loss and trauma, it can be hard to "find meaning," especially when the circumstances are scary, violent, or if the client's safety and development of autonomy and identity depended on the person who inflicted the trauma or the person they lost. Existential crisis, loss, or traumatic events can lead to breakdowns in those narratives through which humans construct and define themselves and make meaning out of experience. Adapting to complex relational trauma or loss by confirming or reconstructing meaning could take place, partly, through narrating the event and partly, by constructing the meaning of the events to the client, to create balanced inner working models and restore or build up attachment security. Hence, the meaning of the trauma or loss can be explored and revisited many times during the course of psychotherapy, aiming at integrating these experiences into a coherent narrative, reflecting a coherent mind (Neimeyer, 2012; Riber & Lindvig, 2011).

9.7.2 Cultural Sensitivity

Clinical psychologists and clients alike, are rooted in their own cultural perspectives, perceptions, and preferences. Culture is crucial in mental health treatments; therefore, it is important for professionals to be aware of our own cultural worldviews, and take an open, not-knowing, and curious position when working with adult clients with other ethnic backgrounds and experiences than oneself. What we do not ask about, we cannot know, and hence we cannot adapt treatment. Handling cultural issues in a sensitive, respectful, and humble way, is strongly related to client outcome (Soto et al., 2019). In Amir's case, for example, the therapist could get caught up in a judgment about his mother's mourning behavior when his younger brother died. If relevant, one could ask Amir, if her reaction exceeded what was considered typical in their culture. However, what seems more clinically important is that Amir was a small boy who did not understand what dying meant, and because no one was able to or found it important to help him understand what had happened, and what was going on in his mother's mind, and in his mind, this memory seems fragmented and immediately merges with the loss of his older brother (see an in-depth discussion about culture in mental health treatment by Soto et al., 2019).

9.7.3 On the Interplay between the Threat System and Attachment System in Psychotherapy

When treating trauma, both the threat system and the attachment system activates during therapeutic processes and affect clients' capacity for affect-regulation and mentalizing as well as their (C)PTSD symptoms.

Furthermore, CPTSD and insecure attachment patterns contain overlapping characteristics that may interact and mutually affect one another. CPTSD symptoms contain components of avoidance behavior, arousal, disturbances in affect-regulation, self-concept, and interpersonal problems (Cloitre et al., 2013), and likewise the insecure and disorganized attachment patterns contain affect-regulation strategies with components of avoidance and arousal that appear in close relations and treatment relationships, and their inner working model of self and others can cause interpersonal problems (Green et al., 2012; Mallinckrodt, 2010). These overlapping characteristics and symptoms may appear simultaneously and affect both intrapersonal and social functioning. In trauma therapy it could be useful to assess or evaluate what is at play and distinguish between trauma-related avoidance (of events, places, or people due to stimuli that reminds of the original trauma) versus attachment-related avoidance (based on fear of closeness and intimacy), and trauma-related arousal (anxiety e.g. caused by intrusion) versus attachment-related arousal (based on dependency and fear of relational rejection or unavailability) and let psychotherapy approaches be based on both trauma-, and attachment information.

References

Bakermans-Kranenburg, M. J., & van Ijzendoorn, M. H. (2009). The first 10,000 adult attachment interviews: Distributions of adult attachment representations in clinical and non-clinical groups. *Attachment & Human Development, 11*(3), Art. 3. https://doi.org/10.1080/14616730902814762

Bateman, A., Campbell, C., Luyten, P., & Fonagy, P. (2018). A mentalization-based approach to common factors in the treatment of borderline personality disorder. *Current Opinion in Psychology, 21*, 44–49. https://doi.org/10.1016/j.copsyc.2017.09.005

Bernecker, S. L., Levy, K. N., & Ellison, W. D. (2014). A meta-analysis of the relation between patient adult attachment style and the working alliance. *Psychother Res, 24*(1), Art. 1. https://doi.org/10.1080/10503307.2013.809561

Boelen, P. A. (2006). Cognitive-behavioral therapy for complicated grief: Theoretical underpinnings and case descriptions. *Journal of Loss and Trauma, 11*(1), 1–30. https://doi.org/10.1080/15325020500193655

Boelen, P. A. (2010). A Sense of "Unrealness" about the death of a loved-one: An exploratory study of its role in emotional complications among bereaved individuals. *Applied Cognitive Psychology, 24*, 238–251. https://doi.org/10.1002/acp.1557

Bowlby, J. (1969). *Attachment and loss: Attachment* (Bd. 1). Basic Books.

Bowlby, J. (1973). *Attachment and loss: Separation, anxiety and anger* (Bd. 2). Basic Books.

Bowlby, J. (1980). *Attachment and loss: Sadness and depression* (Bd. 3). Basic Books.

Broberg, A., Mothander, P. R., Grandquist, P., & Ivarsson, T. (2010). *Tilknytning i praksis—Tilknytningsteoriens anvendelse i forskning og klinisk arbejde.* Hans Reitzels Forlag.

Chu, J. A. (2011). *Rebuilding shattered lives: Treating complex PTSD and dissociative disorders* (Version 2, 2. udg.) [Computer software]. Wiley.

Cloitre, M., Garvert, D. W., Brewin, C. R., Bryant, R. A., & Maercker, A. (2013). Evidence for proposed ICD-11 PTSD and complex PTSD: A latent profile analysis. *European Journal Psychotraumatol, 4.* https://doi.org/10.3402/ejpt.v4i0.20706

Cloitre, M., Stovall-McClough, C., Zorbas, P., & Charuvastra, A. (2008). Attachment organization, emotion regulation, and expectations of support in a clinical sample of women with childhood abuse histories. *Journal of Traumatic Stress, 21*(3), Art. 3. https://doi.org/10.1002/jts.20339

Cyr, C., Euser, E. M., Bakermans-Kranenburg, M. J., & Van Ijzendoorn, M. H. (2010). Attachment security and disorganization in maltreating and high-risk families: A series of meta-analyses. *Development and Psychopathology, 22*(01), Art. 01. https://doi.org/10.1017/S0954579409990289

Daniel, S. I. F. (2011). Adult attachment insecurity and narrative processes in psychotherapy: An exploratory study. *Clinical Psychology & Psychotherapy, 18*(6), 498–511.

Daniel, S. I. F. (2015). *Adult attachment patterns in a treatment context, relationship and narrative* (First Edition, First Edition) [Computer software]. Routledge.

De Haene, L., Grietens, H., & Verschueren, K. (2010). Adult attachment in the context of refugee traumatisation: The impact of organized violence and forced separation on parental states of mind regarding attachment. *Attachment & Human Development, 12*(3), Art. 3. PsycINFO. https://doi.org/10.1080/14616731003759732

Diener, M. J., & Monroe, J. M. (2011). The relationship between adult attachment style and therapeutic alliance in individual psychotherapy: A meta-analytic review. *Psychotherapy, 48*(3), Art. 3. https://doi.org/10.1037/a0022425

Dorrepaal, E., Thomaes, K., Hoogendoorn, A. W., Veltman, D. J., Draijer, N., & van Balkom, A. J. L. M. (2014). Evidence-based treatment for adult women with child abuse-related complex PTSD: A quantitative review. *European Journal of Psychotraumatology, 5*(1), 23613. https://doi.org/10.3402/ejpt.v5.23613

Fonagy, P., Gergely, G., Jurist, E. L., & Target, M. (2002). *Affect regulation, mentalization and the development of the self.* New York: Other Press.

Friedman, M. J. (Red.). (2010). *Handbook of PTSD: Science and practice.* Guilford.

George, C., Kaplan, N., & Main, M. (1996). *The Adult attachment interview. Unpublished manuscript,* Berkeley:, University of California.

Green, B. L., Kaltman, S. I., Chung, J. Y., Holt, M. P., Jackson, S., & Dozier, M. (2012). Attachment and health care relationships in low-income women with trauma histories: A qualitative study. *Journal of Trauma & Dissociation, 13*(2), Art. 2. https://doi.org/10.1080/15299732.2012.642761

Herman, J. L. (1997). *Trauma and recovery. The aftermath of violence—From domestic abuse to political terror.* Basic Books.

Hesse, E. (2008). The adult attachment interview—Protocol, method of analysis, and empirical studies. In J. Cassidy & P. R. Shaver (Red.), *Handbook of attachment—Theory, research, and clinical application* (s. 552–598). The Guildford Press.

Jacobvitz, D., & Reisz, S. (2019). Disorganized and unresolved states in adulthood. *Current Opinion in Psychology, 25*, 172–176. https://doi.org/10.1016/j.copsyc.2018.06.006

Juen, F., Arnold, L., Meissner, D., Nolte, T., & Buchheim, A. (2013). Attachment disorganization in different clinical groups: What underpins unresolved attachment? *Psihologija, 46*(2), 127–141. https://doi.org/10.2298/PSI1302127J

Karatzias, T., Shevlin, M., Ford, J. D., Fyvie, C., Grandison, G., Hyland, P., & Cloitre, M. (2021). Childhood trauma, attachment orientation, and complex PTSD (CPTSD) symptoms in a clinical sample: Implications for treatment. *Development and Psychopathology*, 1–6. https://doi.org/10.1017/S0954579420001509

Karatzias, T., Shevlin, M., Fyvie, C., Hyland, P., Efthymiadou, E., Wilson, D., Roberts, N., Bisson, J. I., Brewin, C. R., & Cloitre, M. (2017). Evidence of distinct profiles of posttraumatic stress disorder (PTSD) and complex posttraumatic stress disorder (CPTSD) based on the new ICD-11 trauma questionnaire (ICD-TQ). *Journal of Affective Disorders, 207*, 181–187. https://doi.org/10.1016/j.jad.2016.09.032

Levy, K. N., Johnson, B. N., Gooch, C. V., & Kivity, Y. (2019). Attachment style In: Norcross, J. C., & Wampold, B. E., (Eds.) *Psychotherapy Relationships that Work: Vol. 2. Evidence-Based Therapist Responsiveness*. 3rd ed (pp. 15–55). Oxford: Oxford University Press.

Luyten, P., & Fonagy, P. (2019) Mentalizing and trauma. In: Bateman, A and Fonagy, P. (Eds.) *Handbook of mentalizing in mental health practice*. American Psychiatric Association Publishing: Washington DC, USA.

Lyons-Ruth, K., & Jacobvitz, D. (2008). Attachment disorganization: Genetic factors, parenting contexts, and developmental transformation from infancy to adulthood. In J. C. P. R. Shaver (Red.), *Handbook of attachment: Theory, research, and clinical applications (2nd ed.)* (s. 666–697). Guilford Press.

Main, M., Goldwyn, R., & Hesse, E. (2003). *Adult attachment scoring and classification systems* [Unpublished manuscript, version 7.2].

Mallinckrodt, B. (2010). The psychotherapy relationship as attachment: Evidence and implications. *Journal of Social and Personal Relationships, 27*(2), Art. 2. https://doi.org/10.1177/0265407509360905

Mayes, L. C. (2000). A developmental perspective on the regulation of arousal states. *Seminars in Perinatology, 24*(4), 267–279. https://doi.org/10.1053/sper.2000.9121

Mikulincer, M., & Florian, V. (1998). The relationship between adult attachment styles and emotional and cognitive reactions to stressful events. In J. A. Simpson & W. S. Rholes (Red.), *Attachment theory and close relationships* (s. 143–165). NY: Guildford.

Mikulincer, M., & Shaver, P. R. (2013). Attachment insecurities and disordered patterns of grief. I *Complicated Grief: Scientific Foundations for Health Care Professionalsa*. Routledge.

Mikulincer, M., Shaver, P. R., & Pereg, D. (2003). Attachment theory and affect regulation: The dynamics, development, and cognitive consequences of attachment-related strategies. *Motivation and Emotion, 27*, 77–102.

Neimeyer, R. A. Retelling the narrative of the death. In: Neimeyer R. A, (Ed.). *Techniques of grief therapy: Creative practices for counselling the bereavement. Series in death, dying, and bereavement.* New York: Routledge, Taylor & Francis; 2012. pp. 86–90.

Norcross, J. C., & Lambert, M. J. (2019). *Psychotherapy relationships that work: Evidence-based therapist contributions* (3. udg., Bd. 1). Oxford University Press.

Norcross, J. C., & Wampold, B. E. (Red.). (2019). *Psychotherapy relationships that work: Evidense-based therapist responsiveness* (3. udg., Bd. 2). Oxford University Press.

Powers, M. B., Halpern, J. M., Ferenschak, M. P., Gillihan, S. J., & Foa, E. B. (2010). A meta-analytic review of prolonged exposure for posttraumatic stress disorder. *Clinical Psychology Review, 30*(6), 635–641. https://doi.org/10.1016/j.cpr.2010.04.007

Ravitz, P., Maunder, R., Hunter, J., Sthankiya, B., & Lancee, W. (2010). Adult attachment measures: A 25-year review. *Journal of Psychosomatic Research, 69*(4), Art. 4. https://doi.org/10.1016/j.jpsychores.2009.08.006

Riber, K. (2016). Attachment organization in Arabic-speaking refugees with post traumatic stress disorder. *Attachment & Human Development, 18*(2), Art. 2. https://doi.org/10.1080/14616734.2015.1124442

Riber, K., & Lindvig, D. (2011). Narrativ og evidensbaseret behandling af komplekst traumatiserede mennesker. *Psyke & Logos, 32*(2), Art. 2.

Seidler, G. H., & Wagner, F. E. (2006). Comparing the efficacy of EMDR and trauma-focused cognitive-behavioral therapy in the treatment of PTSD: A meta-analytic study. *Psychological Medicine, 36*(11), 1515–1522. https://doi.org/10.1017/S0033291706007963

Sharp, C., & Fonagy, P. (2008). The parent's capacity to treat the child as a psychological agent: Constructs, measures and implications for developmental psychopathology. *Social Development, 17*(3), 737–754. https://doi.org/10.1111/j.1467-9507.2007.00457.x

Siehl, S., Robjant, K., & Crombach, A. (2021). Systematic review and meta-analyses of the long-term efficacy of narrative exposure therapy for adults, children and perpetrators. *Psychotherapy Research, 31*(6), 695–710. https://doi.org/10.1080/10503307.2020.1847345

Solomon, Z., Dekel, R., & Mikulincer, M. (2008). Complex trauma of war captivity: A prospective study of attachment and post-traumatic stress disorder. *Psychology Medicine, 38*(10), Art. 10. https://doi.org/10.1017/S0033291708002808

Soto, A., Smith, T. B., Griner, D., Rodriguez, M. D., & Bernal, G. (2019). Cultural adaptations and multicultural competence. In: Norcross, J. C., & Wampold, B. E., (Eds.).*Psychotherapy Relationships that Work: Vol. 2. Evidence-Based Therapist Responsiveness.* 3rd ed. Oxford: Oxford University Press; (2019). pp. 86–132.

Stovall-McClough, K. C., & Cloitre, M. (2006). Unresolved attachment, PTSD, and dissociation in women with childhood abuse histories. *Journal of Consulting and Clinical Psychology, 74*(2), Art. 2. https://doi.org/10.1037/0022-006X.74.2.219

Stroebe, M. S., Schut, H., & Boerner, K. (2010). Continuing bonds in adaptation to bereavement: Toward theoretical integration. *Clinical Psychology Review, 30,* 259–268. https://doi.org/10.1016/j.cpr.2009.11.007

van Ijzendoorn, M. H., & Sagi-Schwartz, A. (2008). Cross-cultural patterns of attachment: Universal and contextual dimensions. In J. Cassidy & P. R. Shaver (Red.), *Handbook of attachment: Theory, research, and clinical applications (2nd ed.)* (s. 880–905). Guilford Press.

Watts, B. V., Schnurr, P. P., Mayo, L., Young-Xu, Y., Weeks, W. B., & Friedman, M. J. (2013). Meta-analysis of the efficacy of treatments for posttraumatic stress disorder. *The Journal of Clinical Psychiatry,* 74(06), e541–e550. https://doi.org/10.4088/JCP.12r08225

WHO (2022, februar). *6B41 Complex post traumatic stress disorder in ICD-11 for Mortality and Morbidity Statistics.* https://icd.who.int/browse11/l-m/en#/http://id.who.int/icd/entity/585833559. https://icd.who.int/browse11/l-m/en#/http://id.who.int/icd/entity/585833559

Woodhouse, S., Ayers, S., & Field, A. P. (2015). The relationship between adult attachment style and post-traumatic stress symptoms: A meta-analysis. *Journal of Anxiety Disorders, 35,* 103–117. https://doi.org/10.1016/j.janxdis.2015.07.002

10 Post-Traumatic Stress Disorder and Cognitive Communication Effects

Linda Carozza

10.1 Introduction

This chapter will address cognitive-communicative changes associated with posttraumatic stress disorder (PTSD), with focus on populations suffering from PTSD associated with war-related injury and other catastrophic etiologies. Veterans, are, as a group, a highly vulnerable population who may suffer many cognitive-communication impairments including, but not limited to attention deficits, memory loss, poor recall, poor social appropriateness, and direct and indirect executive function deficits; all of which may impact communication in daily interactions and higher order domains, such as making career and life decisions, politics or business, and involvement in a family structure. In this chapter, the author will emphasize the vulnerability of the human communication system when global or subtle deficits arise secondary to PTSD. For these and similar populations, the focus is to bring to the forefront underlying etiologies, related symptomatology with the purpose of informing treatment modalities, long-term recovery, and quality of life adjustment.

As stated in the U.S. World News Report by Elaine Howley in her 2019 report on Statistics of PTSD in Veterans,

> PTSD is often thought of as a problem only for certain people who've been to war or who've lived through a massive trauma, Ken Yeager, director of the Stress, Trauma and Resilience (STAR) Program at The Ohio State University Wexner Medical Center, notes that in 2013 – as part of a larger update to its diagnostic manual for psychological disorders called the DSM – the American Psychological Association expanded the definition of PTSD to include people who have witnessed events. The DSM-5 "changed the definition of PTSD to include vicarious traumatization, which means that previous editions suggested that you had to be traumatized and it had to include life-threatening risks to you. The current revised DSM acknowledges that you don't have to be

DOI: 10.4324/9781003225270-12

the person who's threatened. You can witness (a trauma) – you can see it or you can hear about it and be traumatized by what you're hearing." This change in the diagnostic criteria reflects an improved understanding of what PTSD is and the many ways it can manifest in different individuals.

(Howley, 2019)

This report necessarily broadens who and how an individual may be affected by posttraumatic stress disorder. Firstly, in addition to a host of various individual and group characteristics in such a large population as the military, there are many different locations and kinds of deployment, which result in differing experiences and diagnostic profiles. These, in addition to multiple re-enlistments, complicate the picture of PTSD in veterans. Therefore, for purposes of this report and due to the breadth of this topic, the discussion will focus on several broad topics with a description and analysis of PTSD of active members of the military and veterans, and more specifically, how cognitive-communication changes may impact related diagnostic and treatment considerations.

10.2   Relevant Background Data

PTSD is a condition with more than 3 million new cases per year in the United States. alone (Todorov et al., 2020). It is estimated that PTSD affects 6.8% of adults in the United States. Veterans have a higher prevalence of PTSD than other civilians. The rate of PTSD in Vietnam veterans is estimated at 30.9% for males and 26.9% for females. Gulf War veterans have an estimated rate of 12.1%, and Iraq veterans have an estimated rate of 13.8% (Gradus, 2007).

An important consideration in the discussion of PTSD is that the term is a broad diagnostic "umbrella" which subsumes a variety of subtypes with differing nomenclature, description, and course. Subtype analysis is essential in the understanding of the complexity of disabilities subsumed under "PTSD." In the research reported by Dalenberg and colleagues (2012), there are three major PTSD subtypes: namely complex PTSD, externalizing/internalizing PTSD, and dissociative/non-dissociative PTSD. Their work suggests methodology for subtype evaluation, for the purposes of clarity of diagnosis and understanding of the underlying etiologies and hence, clinical management. However, the report indicates that current understanding of the pathways of PTSD are not agreed upon in research and further analysis is necessary to determine practical courses of assessment and treatment. This information is vital for researchers and clinicians in the allied health professions so we can contribute to the current state of knowledge. They apply effective recommendations to the current understanding of the onset and mechanism of PTSD and communication-cognitive changes encountered in patients.

Human communication may be highly impacted by PTSD. Communication is the highest neuro-biological function in the living species, and as such, is the foundation for individual and group adjustment in society, education, and social function. A disorder in communication affecting any domain of receptive and expressive language, speech production or secondary language skills, such as reading and writing, will impact personal-social adjustment, educational attainment, and livelihood to name but a few of the many interconnecting systems that depend on intact higher order human interaction in modern society.

According to the International Classification of Disease (ICD) model, there are two main divisions by which disease domains may be conceptualized. Part 1 of the model deals with functioning and disability and Part 2 governs contextual factors. Each domain has its subpart; functioning and disability deals with body functions and structures, and Part 2, Activities and Participation, which include contextual factors such as the environmental (climate and terrain) and personal factors (race, gender, educational level, etc.). Further, the International Classification of Functioning, Disability, and Health (ICF) model categorizes disability into four major areas: physical, developmental, behavioral, or emotional, and sensory impairments. The ability to communicate effectively in one's peer environment is essential to human connectivity, life satisfaction and participating fully as an engaged member of society. Changes and difficulties in speech patterns can be very upsetting and life changing. Those with PTSD may note changes in speech regulation, language comprehension, verbal expression, reasoning, abstractions, and as such may impact adjustment to disability as per the ICF model.

10.3   Research on Language Change Patterns Associated with PTSD

The reporting of incidence and specific disorders in veterans with PTSD is confounded by many significant methodological variables and is further complicated that assessments may be based on clinical observation or self-report, with the possibility of under and over-reporting in both instances. According to Marmer and colleagues in 2019, their study reported a method, which was to obtain speech samples from warzone-exposed veterans, using the Clinician-Administered PTSD Scale (Weathers et al., 2013). They obtained over 40,000 speech features which were analyzed for markers of speech rate, monotony, and tonal variety. The researchers demonstrated that a speech-based algorithm can objectively differentiate PTSD cases from controls based on objective speech-marker features that indicate PTSD. This is significant for the goal of increasing reliable assessment for interventions of speech and cognitive-mediated disabilities that may occur secondary to PTSD in veteran populations. Additionally, the specific findings of this study may be useful as indicators for the development of much-needed future assessment and treatment paradigms. This is especially important given the current paucity of relevant diagnostic data for service planning and will contribute significantly to the issue of differential diagnosis with related symptoms such as depression and other disorders that may affect speech presentation.

Additional studies report acquired dysfluency, interrupted flow of speech and ease of communication, as a comorbid speech finding in PTSD. A study conducted by Norman and colleagues (2018) demonstrated that acquired stuttering may be a comorbidity of both traumatic brain injury and PTSD. These are complex issues of comorbidity that require skilled analysis and history. Effects of dual diagnoses as well as use of medications that affect speech fluency such as antidepressants, anxiolytics, and antiepileptics should be considered in developing a clinical impression given history and complexity of presenting behaviors as either primary or secondary to trauma and/or effects of medication.

Yoder and Norman (2015) report findings over the last ten years on co-occurring PTSD and neurocognitive disorders (NCD). The overlap between symptom presentation obscure conclusive data; however, they make the point that "dementia" is no longer used as an umbrella term and is replaced in the DSM-5 by the classification of NCD which is preferable since it considers dementias, which are not degenerative in nature and are typically caused by secondary injuries including brain trauma such as may be suffered by individuals who have faced combat. Importantly, a deficit in the cognitive domain may include issues of attention, executive function, learning and memory, language skills, perceptual motor functioning and social pragmatic communication. The National Center for PTSD under the U.S. Department of Veterans Affairs publishes material, which is useful for clinicians to understand the comprehensive nature of PTSD, contained in various resources published by the Veterans Affairs Mental Health websites.

The study of speech and cognitive disorder secondary to PTSD in veterans requires ongoing longitudinal and cross-sectional study given the complexity of symptom presentation and overlap, which may obscure definitive diagnostic and treatment planning for veterans. Continued research, especially in clinical differential diagnosis, to evaluate individual client presentation and co-existing findings is essential in careful treatment planning for cognitive-communication and related life adjustment. It is important to bear in mind the foundational report by Yehuda and colleagues

(1998) that PTSD may be facilitated by an inherent pre -existing atypical biological response in the immediate aftermath of a traumatic event, which in turn leads to a maladaptive psychological state. Therefore, clinicians must be aware of possible predictors of disorder and utilize pre-screening for individuals with a history and pre-existing inherent biological states that may render them more susceptible to PTSD symptomatology. This can be facilitated by a team approach with other medical professionals which is a cornerstone of care in the work with PTSD patients.

Current research regarding PTSD focuses on comorbidities, speech-based biomarkers, behavioral changes, psychiatric changes, and cognitive changes (Marmar et al., 2019). These studies utilize speech-based biomarkers to aid in the diagnosis of PTSD. This team analyzed recorded interviews to determine markers specific to PTSD. These interviews were conducted through NYU School of Medicine on veterans who fought in Afghanistan/Iraq with the ultimate purpose of differential diagnosis. As mentioned earlier, speech segments consistent with the diagnosis of PTSD included monotonous tone, slow speech segments, and extended words/ vowels such as "uh" (Marmar et al., 2019). Additional research supporting similar findings also suggest that subjects with PTSD have consistent findings especially in parameters such as reduced tonality during vowel sounds (Low et al., 2020). Further research reports that objective speech markers useful in assessing PTSD are indicated in the work of Scherer et al. (2013). This body of research is fruitful given laboratory methodology in voicing detection and formant tracking for vowel space assessment that is more consistently available for speech analysis and may become more available as technology develops in speech analysis outside of the laboratory setting.

Comorbidities also play a role in language and speech patterns for those with PTSD and bear careful analysis in assessment and treatment. Common comorbid conditions include TBI and Depression. While studying veterans in the VA hospitals, Norman et al. (2018) found that those with Comorbid PTSD and TBI have the following prevalence of acquired stuttering: of 309,675 U.S. veterans from the Iraq and Afghanistan wars, 235 were diagnosed with adult-onset stuttering (Norman et al., 2018). It is important to recognize that comorbid disorders have a likelihood of affecting speech patterns independent of the PTSD diagnosis and should be included in treatment planning as will be continued to be discussed in this report.

Speech-language complications following PTSD are a primary finding. Common speech disturbances included in brain injury and stress related conditions in addition to stuttering as discussed earlier, include difficulty producing speech, poor word articulation, and possibly vocabulary challenges (Ben-Aharon, 2022). When patients suffer a traumatic brain injury, which may be complicated by PTSD, they may exhibit loss of expressive vocabulary, as well as secondary language impairment in skills such as reading, writing, and paralinguistic communication. Combined, the effects of these linguistic sequelae serve to impede independent social function and may have significant deleterious effects on ability to effectively engage in interpersonal communication within family as well as in civilian life, while seeking post-military employment and within home-life-community adjustment in general.

Surrounding the issues of cognitive-communication injury is the overriding factor of emotional overlay, appearing either pre-morbidly, post-morbidly, or both. Research has been done on the linguistic properties of trauma narratives. In fact, the interrelated qualities of reduced linguistic function and acquired cognitive changes complicate diagnoses of acquired communication disabilities secondary to PTSD. The use of language sampling, role play, modeling, and creative problem-solution scenarios, especially those involving implicit communication strategies, may be helpful once a patient is adjusted to seeking speech-language rehabilitation for daily living.

Overall, identifying PTSD early is essential to effectively treat and prevent PTSD. Kleim and colleagues (2018) used a computerized analysis of trauma narratives and found that these narratives included distress, arousal, and reduced introspective ability in addition to meaningless elaboration in speech, and an increase in the number of words regarding death. The researchers conclude that those who exhibited these symptoms were more likely to demonstrate PTSD symptoms within 6 months. Therefore, utilizing language-based processing to predict PTSD may be highly useful in predicting adjustment to civilian life.

The close assessment of individuals suffering trauma- related linguistic and cognitive change continues to be a topic of intense scrutiny, especially in today's current international arena where many types of conflict situations may be encountered than ever before. Trauma may be due to many etiologies and language changes may not be fully evident until the victim has had time to heal from the original injury. Nevertheless, the full range of cognitive function and alertness may be affected on a vast continuum and the evolution of a brain-based language disability requires a great degree of training and specialization in acquired neurogenic communication disorders. The research below continues to describe some of the many efforts aimed at understanding the depth and scope of injury-related communication changes.

It is established that accurate and timely diagnosis of PTSD is essential to assure treatment and recovery for the individual. Unfortunately, the complex symptomology of PTSD complicates the timely evaluation process. Previous studies reveal language patterns are an excellent tool in recognizing complex mental disorders. Analyzing language patterns as opposed to what the patient states may be a beneficial methodology to avoid bias in analysis of self-reports. Word usage patterns were assessed as well, which varies based on the person and content of the conversation (Todorov et al., 2020). Tools may be developed using this information to assist in PTSD diagnosis, leading to more efficient treatment modalities, although methodological constraints exist such as subject matching and related experimental confounds. Nevertheless, clinical, and laboratory-based models are essential to develop an efficacious methodology, although elusive, due to the ongoing issue of disparate nature of the PTSD populations.

In terms of speech communication, related to receptive and expressive language dysfunction are disabilities of intelligibility secondary to neurological injury. The specific characteristics may vary depending on whether an injury is "closed head" or "penetrating" and the site of lesion as well as characteristics of the injury site and surrounding anatomical areas, along with individual differences. Neurologically damaged speech and vegetative functions come under the diagnostic category of dysarthria and may, in some cases, be a very significant part of communication challenges faced.

Scherer and colleagues (2015) studied specific vowel changes in individuals with psychological and neurological disabilities. These include reduced frequency range, commonly seen in affective disabilities such as depression and posttraumatic stress disorder since motor control is affected. Assessment and vowel space (the frequency range spanned by the first and second formant of the vowels with respect to the reference population, according to Scherer), however, often are based on subjective assessments or on analysis of speech using controlled tasks such as paragraph reading. The authors investigated an automatic unsupervised technique to assess vowel space in recordings of 253 individuals. Results demonstrated reduced vowel space in subjects that scored positively on the questionnaires of depression and PTSD. Findings were attributed to psychomotor slowing of articulation and motor control. Findings such as these may shed further light on the physical nature of speech disturbance in PTSD and may be useful in the experimental description of speech sound characteristics, and hence, therapeutic planning.

Dysarthria following TBI was reported by Samuel et al. (1998). In addition, neurogenic stuttering/disfluency may occur as several reports contained within this manuscript describe. Dysarthria will affect speech intelligibility and potentially eating function, while stuttering affects flow of speech and ease of communication. It can be psychogenic or neurogenic (or a combined etiology) and has been known as difficult to treat due to the rate of recidivism when stressors re-emerge. Of note, however, is that when studying veterans, it is noted that 80% of those with TBI also have underlying psychiatric comorbidity. Outcomes for these patients may be affected including cognitive/ somatic issues, social abilities, and overall quality of life. Since the rate of PTSD as a common comorbidity with TBI is 43.9%, the discussion of correlated symptoms is appropriate to consider. Typical complaints by those with PTSD include concerns with concentration, attention, learning, and memory. All these issues serve to complicate the assessment and prognosis of these disabilities in language, speech, fluency, and cognitive communication abilities.

Etiologically, the core features of PTSD and related cognitive-communication disabilities are in large part attributable to the disruption in cognitive systems including changes in memory, judgment, attention, and perception. It is unfortunate, but of note that retained automatic processing makes trauma-related memories more accessible to those with PTSD (Bomyea et al., 2016). These thoughts are often spontaneously accessed, causing distress for the individual. The cumulative result of this behavior is that those with PTSD often respond in a more volatile threatening manner (such as?) than those who do not have PTSD. According to Bomyea (2016), this volatile response occurs since those with PTSD have been reported to have a longer gaze duration when presented with a threat, thus making threats more impactful to them (Bomyea et al., 2016).

Related to the discussion of the cognitive underpinnings of language-communication dysfunction and proposed underlying factors, is the all-important discussion of cause and effect. While human language in and of itself, is nature's most complex phenomenon, the basic understanding of human perception underling the complexity of communication must be underscored, in that there is an interplay between the physical act of speech and the underlying mental representation of speech, which is an ongoing topic in neurolinguistic study of typical as well as impaired populations. In this vein, research has focused on a concept called Theory of Mind (ToM) to understand how humans perceive and relate to each other. ToM occurs within adult communicators but has its origins in developmental psychology and has been related to language dysfunction in populations such as individuals with autism, and now also has been related to PTSD phenomena.

Trauma is not limited to veterans, and trauma throughout various populations may appear differently but have similar effects on the individual. As an example, adverse childhood experiences such as abuse, or neglect may lead to cognitive dissociation - a common and debilitating symptom that may occur secondary to PTSD. Emotional and physical dysregulation, poor self-esteem, difficulty concentrating, avoidance, social withdrawal, and reduced emotional expression may occur (Westby, 2018). Trauma effects brain development and there are many imaging studies performed to understand how PTSD may affect the brain structures such as the amygdala and surrounding areas where emotional regulation is known to occur. Early stress has been shown to decrease hippocampal volume, which affects memory as well as reduced volume in the orbital frontal cortex which in turn affects emotional and social regulation. In some cases, involving deprivation, there is a lack of environmental simulation, resulting in abnormal synaptic pruning (Westby, 2018). Synaptic pruning is related to speech and language development. It bears further mention that although this finding has been related to adverse childhood experiences, soldiers, and other victims of psychological and physical threats, can be thought to suffer similarly due to adverse environmental trauma. Subjects who have been diagnosed with PTSD, have been assessed as having similar brain-level synaptic deficits, which contribute to extensive and complex symptomatology (Krystal et al., 2017). Further, onset of cognitive-communication impairment in veterans may have co-existing factors of pre-existing etiology of brain difference, biological-chemical predisposition and life experiences that predispose some individuals to sustained effects of stress.

10.3.1   The Course of PTSD

Associations between PTSD symptoms and the evolution of related symptoms have been assessed by Segal et al. (2019). Subjects were 925 newly recruited Israel Defense Force soldiers, all male, between 18 and 24 years old, all healthy both physically and mentally (Segal et al., 2019). Patients were assessed at 6 months after completing training (pre-deployment) and reassessed six months after infantry combat. It was hypothesized that "network-strength psychopathology" is stronger post combat than pre-combat. This means some clinical symptoms of PTSD may be more loosely related during pre-deployment (training) compared to direct symptom correlation post combat. Participants rated PTSD symptoms six months into training, and six months after combat. Increase in stress post - combat was evaluated using the combat experience scale. The combat experience scale is a tool used in the Deployment Risk and Resilience Inventory to measure effects of exposure to combat-related experiences (Weathers et al., 2013). This is an objective measurement and does not include the persons interpretation to exposures, it is directly related to events that occurred (Weathers et al., 2013). Pre-deployment training was controlled and did not include actual combat. Sixteen percent of the sample of 645 soldiers reported more than a single combative event pre-deployment, 45% of soldiers reported serious exposure to combative events post deployment. Three percent of mentally healthy individuals resulted in reporting PTSD symptoms post deployment (Segal et al., 2019). When diagnosing PTSD using the DSM-5 criteria, there is an outline of required symptomology. This symptomology includes direct or indirect exposure to the trauma.

Intrusion symptomology is associated with the traumatic event. Avoidance symptomology includes tireless avoidance of any stimuli related to the trauma. Additionally, negative alterations in mood/cognition will occur related to the event, as well changes in arousal and reactivity in relationship to the event. The disturbance will continue for at least one month, and may cause significant distress on social impairment, and daily functioning, which will not be related to substance use (U.S. Department of Health and Human Services, Substance Abuse and Mental Health Services Administration, Center for Substance Abuse Treatment, 2014). In the study being evaluated, the intrusion symptom cluster had the highest prevalence following combat (Segal et al., 2019). Avoidance symptoms were also prevalent post combat, which was judged to be most likely due to high reactivity to triggers of conflict related trauma. Hence, avoidant behavior may be demonstrated, which means the individual would have no opportunity to modify negative perceptions and beliefs related to the trauma. Furthermore, the article reported significant changes in the soldiers' sleep patterns, increased irritability, and poor concentration (Segal et al., 2019).

Therefore, the underpinnings of cognitive – communication changes secondary to trauma have elements of homogeneity as well as heterogeneity. The work in this area necessarily crosses over many disciplines. This is further necessarily complicated by the fact that the various traumas endured are unique to the individual/s who suffered them, are therefore immensely complicated both diagnostically and prognostically. The following research elucidates the complexity of analyzing the effects of psycho-traumatic experiences.

Understanding psychological trauma is an experimental challenge within research, challenging psychology, neurobiology, sociology, anthropology, and other fields of scientific inquiry. Although there are strides in understanding PTSD, it is still a disability that may be mis-diagnosed for various significant reasons. Many patients with PTSD exhibit symptoms that are reflected by a pattern of dissociative language functioning. Etiology for dissociative language may result from damage to areas of the brain responsible for affecting language and memory, storage, retrieval, and assembly. Examples include repetition, unexpected pauses, incorrect words, unusual pronunciation, loss of thought placement, lack of or excess use of words, and slow or absent word processing (Gillette, 2022). All these characteristics may serve to obscure diagnosis. Based on advanced computational linguistic methodology, which included analysis of transcribed traumatic event narratives for disfluencies, coherence, word repetitions, incomplete words, and other salient features. Based on this study, there is hope for increased understanding of the methodology to reliably assess traumatic linguistic syndromes (Gayraud & Auxéméry, 2021).

10.3.2 Major Theoretical Frameworks

Judith Herman (1992) hypothesized a triphasic model regarding PTSD, and continued research has been done to create a bond between Herman's model as well as modern neuroscience. Protagonists of the triphasic model argue that trauma survivors have common threads in their clinical symptoms (Zaleski et al., 2016). Herman states that PTSD symptoms and trauma can be characterized by three concepts: hyperarousal, intrusion, and constriction. Each of these concepts is described below:

Hyperarousal: The hyper-arousable subtype is defined as having a high startle response. The patient may have high responses of anger to what might be perceived by others to be minimal provocation. Therefore, a hypothesis may be that veterans may suffer from this; as Herman found they have "chronic simulation of the sympathetic nervous system and those traumatic events seem to recondition the human nervous system." (Herman, 1992 as cited in Zaleski et al., 2016, p. 379).

Intrusion: "… the reliving of events with the same vividness and emotional force as if they were happening in the present and are potentially caused by seemingly insignificant reminders." (Herman, 1992 as cited in Zaleski et al., 2016, p. 379). Herman stated that intrusions are the brain's futile attempt to make sense of, or master, the memory, despite being unwelcomed and causing additional stress and rage to the individual.

Constriction: This state sometimes begins at the time of trauma, through dissociation or numbing, to separate oneself from the pain and fear caused by a traumatic event. Constriction is "demonstrated by attempts to withdraw from others, a narrowing of perception, and an impoverished life" (Herman, 1992 as cited in Zaleski et al., 2016, p. 379).

PTSD is also heavily impacted by the correlated activity in the amygdala (Weston, 2014). The amygdala drives hyperactivity, likely creating a hyper-arousable state/ hyper-arousable symptoms. "Grounded" cognition occurs in the amygdala. It is often suggested the amygdala drives the development of PTSD symptoms as it interconnects with numerous cortical areas. These symptoms include re-experiencing trauma, avoiding trauma, and negative alterations in mood/cognition. Hippocampal activity is also affected causing memory impairments. Major potential social consequences of the hyper-arousable subtype that may occur in the general as well as veteran population include divorce, economic challenges, social challenges, isolation, homelessness, unemployment, and imprisonment. Comorbidities also often include depression, anxiety, alcohol, and other types of substance abuse (Weston, 2014). Hyper-arousable PTSD is more common than dissociative. Dissociative PTSD accounts for about 6–30% of cases as per research by Bailey and Brand (2017).

Both aforementioned subtypes, hyper-arousable and dissociative PTSD, may occur in veterans who go on to suffer war-related catastrophe. Dissociative PTSD is typically associated with those who underwent extensive childhood trauma, has a higher probability to affect males and highly impacts social function with related impairments and suicidal ideations reported (Bailey & Brand, 2017). The development of dissociation is related to factors such as neurobiological functioning, cognitive functioning, and cultural barriers. Since trauma and stress may be processed through the brain differently, it is thought that those with dissociative PTSD have increased connectivity between the amygdala and prefrontal cortex beyond the typical range. Attachment disorganization is found to be related to cases with increased amygdala reactivity (Bailey & Brand, 2017). All these factors underscore the direct association between PTSD experiences and neurological change.

10.4 Cultural Responsiveness

Cultural competence is a necessary component in creating a treatment plan for those with PTSD as it maximizes outcomes. The American Speech-Language and Hearing Association defines cultural competence as the understanding and appropriate responding to the unique combination of cultural variables and full range of dimensions of diversity that the professional and clients bring to interactions (ASHA, n.d.). Culture sensitive psychotherapy involves understanding the patient's life, and cultural components of a patient's illness (Schnyder et al., 2016). Understanding the culture of one's clinical patients is essential to the success of treatment and to afford treatment to all veterans reduces health disparities in delineating a client's triggers, and flashbacks (Schnyder et al., 2016). Trauma is not independent of cultural influence, sometimes cultural influence may lead to trauma (Ranjbar et al., 2020). For example, trauma can be caused by the race-based stress of hate crimes, microaggressions (brief everyday exchanges that send denigrating messages to someone as they are part of a racialized group), and macroaggressions (systemic forms of oppression toward people of a certain race, gender, or group) such workplace incidents, and systemic racism (Ranjbar et al., 2020). Healthcare disparities are at the forefront of society, as well as clinical medicine and rehabilitation. Cultural beliefs and lack of opportunity may greatly impact access to appropriate healthcare services and hence recovery from trauma. Patients' own recognition of culture will also play a role in the patient's specific response to trauma (Schnyder et al., 2016). Both in the United States and elsewhere, such as other high population countries, there may not be access to current technologies and latest research concepts about mental health, knowledge bases such as in psychotherapy, or access to providers and medical interventions that may help mental illness (Schnyder et al., 2016). Across high population countries, there are generally large gaps in access to health care and disparities in availability for necessary treatment. Access is dependent on economic status and social or cultural acceptance of disabilities where knowledge of disability varies. It is an unfortunate situation that accessibility of advanced methodologies is reduced in current political and economic climates and must be addressed in the ever-shrinking world we live in for universal health and co- existence for the present and generations to come.

Therefore, one of the most important takeaways regarding cultural competence, is for providers to make it their mission to educate themselves regarding beliefs and attitudes that may underlie cultural stereotyping within their practices (internal and external belief systems). Additionally, clinicians must educate themselves in biases both conscious and subconscious which may affect treatment planning. Research emphasizes that professionals must always assume a non-judgmental attitude while trying to understand others' cultural background (Schnyder et al., 2016). This is essential to healthcare ethics and part of the deep understanding of cultures that underlies best practice in evidence-based medical care in all disciplines. Self-knowledge of unconscious biases that may affect public awareness of needs of the PTSD population is an ongoing socio-cultural public health issue.

10.4.1   Case Examples

There are many case reports supporting data that PTSD may impair cognitive communication skills and speech related functions as well as data implying beneficial treatment modalities. Additionally, there are treatment modalities that work best depending on the patient's culture. When treating those from any setting, it is essential to consider their underlying cultural beliefs. As an example, some trauma patients such as rape victims may perceive themselves as bringing shame to their families for exhibiting symptoms of PTSD, or for even going through the trauma all together. When managing these patients after a trauma, they may benefit from providers of similar cultural values, beliefs, and assumptions (Schnyder et al., 2016).

Effective modalities may include accessing the trauma through painting, writing, dancing, singing, utilizing an instrument and other specific creative modalities (Schnyder et al., 2016). These alternative approaches, nonpharmacological in nature, have been in recent news reports of re-integration of individuals who have suffered psychological and other trauma. Following are case examples demonstrating the cross – universality of PTSD as a symptom cluster from world-wide reports in the literature, including the United States and other regions. Selected examples from published literature follow below.

According to Schnyder et al. (2016), there is variation of patient and clinician perspectives related to how society views trauma treatment and recovery. A review of the literature indicates that there are similarities, as well as differences, on perspectives related to PTSD cross-culturally. In some cases, a patient may not recognize the diagnosis for themselves, but defer to a clinician to assume their needs. Other cultural perspectives may include shame, responsibility, and reluctance to reveal the trauma, while others do not focus on the individual, but more on the individual's ability to readjust to society in terms of work and social function in a community. In some places, approach to therapy varies considerably, especially where there are multicultural perspectives within the same region that conflict with each other. Furthermore, certain countries have high levels of violence and expectations of treatment support, prosecution, and governmental support are reflected in how PTSD is viewed. There are countless approaches to PTSD, which are dependent on socio-cultural attitudes specific to different regions, as per Schynder et al. (2016).

As an example, some data collected regarding PTSD and the United States is based in the state of Pennsylvania. Pennsylvania is a cross-cultural area where cultural treatments disseminate into each other (Schnyder et al., 2016). Prolonged exposure therapy was developed in Philadelphia, PA. The therapy mainly involved individuals of African American, Latino, Asian, and Caucasian descent were all investigated while developing the treatment. Among all ethnic groups the outcomes of this therapy were consistent and successful. To determine which symptoms are the priority to treat, providers must examine similarities and differences between patient symptoms. Typical symptoms after a traumatic event, regardless of cultural background include avoidance and safety behaviors. It is not uncommon that an individual would view the world as a dangerous place after trauma. Focused conversations help providers guide the treatment plan accordingly, as part of the dissemination process (Schnyder et al., 2016).

Another U.S. case study report (Boyd et al., 2016) involves a veteran with cognitive symptoms including poor verbal recall, stuttering, slowed speech, and poor writing ability. Additional symptoms included anxiety, depression, poor concentration, memory disturbance, insomnia, noise sensitivity, disturbing dreams, and decreased energy. Five months following TBI, his pre-morbid speech was categorized as halting, dysfluent, and slow paced. The primary treatment in this case was CPT-C (cognitive processing therapy) without pharmacologic assistance. CPT-C focuses on content of thoughts. Daily worksheets were assigned to help the patient recognize errors in thought processes; skills are taught, and emphasis is placed on enforcing balanced thinking. At the first session, the patient presented with soft, slow speech, a severe stutter, and limited eye contact. He had difficulty retaining information. Weekly meetings exhibited improvements in speech fluency. When addressing measurable outcomes, the patient had a 26-point reduction in self-reported PTSD symptoms. Patient had a 17-point reduction in self-reported depressive symptoms. The patient also showed improvements in processing speed. The patient's stutter was unremarkable by the end of treatment. The patient also had a dramatic improvement in speech from therapy although there was no formal speech involvement in treatment. The authors concluded that cognitive rehab may be a beneficial plan for this patient, and by extension, hopefully others.

A further treatment case study involves a neurolinguistic analysis that has been published on a 57-year-old male involved in a car accident (Bijleveld, 2015). Primary symptoms resulting from the car accident included stuttering and word finding. This patient suffered a TBI after the accident, with comorbid PTSD. Immediately after the accident the patient suffered high levels of anxiety, speech hesitations, and slowed speech. Stuttering began to develop about 3 weeks following the accident. It was expected that those with comorbid TBI and PTSD may not exhibit symptoms until a few weeks later:

> It is known that mild TBI and PTSD are associated with mild axonal injury in brainstem, frontal, prefrontal and temporal regions, with subcortical involvement (hypothalamus, amygdala, BG and thalamus); injury of the cortico-striatal- pallidal-thalamic pathway that plays a role in the manifestation of emotions, stress, learning and stuttering." (Bijleveld, 2015, p. 41). This report confirms changes in mood, personality, behavior, and emotional instability as indicated by the author.

10.5   Practical Treatment/Intervention Considerations

From an immediate standpoint of self-knowledge for veterans suffering from PTSD, it is essential to note that self-education, awareness, and acceptance within a supportive community are essential for human growth and resilience during any high challenge set of experience. Therefore, the Make the Connection web resource published by the U.S. Department of Veterans Affairs is a primary resource for effected individuals as well as professional providers and can be found at the U.S. Department of Veteran Affairs website. There is also a comprehensive Continuing Education program through the Veterans Affairs website, with free resources for professionals who work with populations affected by PTSD. Notably, there is a one-hour course regarding the relationship between PTSD and dementia, and the association between PTSD, cognitive impairment, and behavioral problems (Vasterling & Thorp, 2022).

It is from this standpoint that the following treatment options are described. Treatment options proven to be successful in PTSD include cognitive behavioral therapy (CBT; Friedman, 2015). CBT may include prolonged exposure therapy and cognitive processing therapy (Friedman, 2015). Additional therapies may include, eye-movement desensitization therapy and reprocessing, stress induction therapy, and group therapy (Friedman, 2015, p. 40).

Music therapy has also been recognized as a treatment for wounded soldiers since WWII (Bronson et al., 2018). Reports suggest that using music as treatment for wounded veterans helped promote healing and recovery. Currently, new-onset PTSD is a prevalent issue. Between 2000 and 2014, 149,000 active-duty service members have been recently diagnosed with PTSD (Bronson et al., 2018). Typical symptom presentation in these patients have inhibited the quality of their daily functioning. Music therapy aims to encourage multidisciplinary collaboration with co-treatment. Music therapy is used to support speech and language, cognition, motor coordination, socialization, and familial support. Music therapy uses a similar planning and implementation process as other therapies such as referrals, eligibility, and goals. Music-based neurologic interventions are established set to improve cognition, motor response, speech/language comprehension, and execution, as well as behavioral issues (Bronson et al., 2018). Common issues that arise during a TBI (which commonly may co-exist with PTSD), include difficulty with memory/concentration, problems with conversational language, disorganized expression, dysfluent speech, word retrieval issues, difficulty problem- solving, poor judgment, and reduced socio-behavioral engagement; all of which may affect communication and interpersonal adjustment. Additionally, those with PTSD may experience intrusive hypervigilance, sleep disturbances, and social isolation. Music therapy utilizes the concept of neuroplasticity and is reported to affect the rebuilding of neuronal connections within the brain, specifically as it recruits right hemisphere functions, such as emotions, imagination, visual, and auditory awareness, to assist in responsivity and neural interconnectedness. These functions are also targeted as byproducts of speech, language, and hearing services, and there is an intersection between restoring right hemisphere function and speech. Neuroimaging data has lent support to the theory that music plays a role in increasing neuroplasticity (Bronson et al., 2018).

Dance/movement therapy (DMT) has also been a successful treatment for those with dissociative PTSD (Pierce, 2014). The aim of this therapy is psychological and physiologic integration. Dance therapy recruits the right side of the brain with the aim of re- establishing of neural networks that may have been impaired due to an underlying dissociative disorder by developing safety and security through repeated use of beneficial/effective dance/movement therapy practices, per Pierce. Dissociation alters consciousness, memory, personal information/identity, and may cause amnesia, derealization, and depersonalization. This research indicates that dissociation occurs in the vertical axis of the right brain; brain imaging studies support this theory of right hemisphere dominance during traumatic recall. Imaging also indicates smaller hippocampus and amygdala volume. Dance/ movement therapy has been reported to have a positive psychological effect on subjects, increasing trust and a sense of control. Dance therapy is also reported as effective in causing a spike in neural networks which carry information along the axis that connects subcortical, limbic- brainstem, and cortical brain areas. Reports indicate that this integration improves memory regulation, narrative state, and overall interpersonal relationships, and helps create a sense of self. All these actions help in the resolution of symptoms of dissociative PTSD. Therapy is described as occurring in three phases of therapy: phase 1- developing safety and security through mirroring the work of early attachment, "where clients gain the basic, implicit, and often nonverbal capacities for emotional bonding and self-regulation," phase 2- integrating traumatic memories, through eye-movement desensitization and reprocessing (EMDR), sensorimotor psychotherapy, and somatic experiencing and phase 3- developing relational self and rehabilitation through reconnection with their community outside of the therapy room and coming to terms with their trauma. DMT addresses brain regions and connections that are also used for speech functions and new learning or adjusting. SLPs can use these interventions or collaborate with a specialist for the benefit and progress of their patients. Furthermore, dance therapy is a nonverbal activity for the most part, which may be beneficial to those with speech challenges related to PTSD (Pierce, 2014).

In contrast, however, it is reported that two thirds of veterans treated for PTSD retain their diagnosis despite treatment (Levi et al., 2021). A study was performed to examine treatment modalities and address effectiveness in treating PTSD. Researchers used a diagnostic procedure pretreatment to identify candidates for the study, the same questionnaire was performed at the end of treatment to measure outcomes. Researchers utilized symptom clusters to determine which treatment would be advised. The patient was also allowed to give their input on the case. Twenty-seven percent (27%) of patients received CBT, 42% received psychodynamic therapy, and 31% received pharmacotherapy, while 94% of patients agreed to the treatment plan assigned to them. Group treatment was not utilized or offered during this study. CBT consisted of 20 weekly sessions of trauma focused interventions, and utilized prolonged exposure therapy, as well as CPT. There were five stages to treatment beginning with education on the trauma, narrative reconstruction, identification of thoughts, in vivo exposure, such as loud noises or abrupt environmental changes, and termination of the trauma. Psychodynamic psychotherapy lasted one year. The treatment was comprised of three stages including, establishment of therapeutic alliance, exploration of unconscious conflicts, and termination of loss made through trauma/ rebuilding relationships. The goal was to identify how the trauma affected their personality. Pharmacotherapy typically consisted of medications such as Selective Serotonin Reuptake Inhibitors (SSRIs), followed by Serotonin Norepinephrine Reuptake Inhibitors (SNRIs). the dosage was started low and titrated up based on therapeutic response. Therapy included 12 weeks of treatment with six-month continuation to assure symptoms did not relapse. Remission rates were calculated based on diagnostic criteria for each symptom cluster. Results were calculated in a dimensional analysis conducted by an in-house Israeli Defense Force (IDF) professional clinic, based on mean reductions in symptom severity of intrusion, avoidance, and hyperarousal on a PTSD severity scale. In addition to calculating remission, the rates of patients who remain symptomatic for one cluster but not others were calculated. Researchers also calculated patients who have a negative response compared to pretreatment. Overall remission rate was 39.4%. Intrusion had a 15.8% remission rate, avoidance had a 31.7% remission rate, and hyper-arousable had a 22.7% remission rate. Of the 39.4% of those in remission, 27.2% of patients had remission from all three symptom clusters, 7.6% of patients had remission from both intrusion, and avoidance,16.5% from avoidance, and hyperarousal, 5.3% from intrusion alone, 29.4% from avoidance only, and 14% from hyperarousal only, 0% of patients remitted from intrusion and hyperarousal. Of those who remitted, 78.2% continued to meet diagnostic criteria for at least one symptom cluster. A dimensional analysis revealed a reduction in overall symptom severity. Intrusion had a lower reduction in symptom severity, 6.2% of patients revealed a negative response to treatment. Overall remission rates for the three treatments had minimal variation. Treatments did have varying remission rates per symptoms cluster. In the intrusion cluster, higher remission rates were noted for CBT, and psychodynamic therapy, compared to pharmacotherapy. The hyper-arousable symptom cluster, as well as avoidance symptom cluster did not vary based on treatment. Overall, it was noted that intrusion symptoms responded most poorly to treatment, and some direct symptoms such as flashbacks, and poor recall had no response to treatment. Currently, additional therapeutics are being simultaneously developed, including targeted psychological counseling approaches such as Dialectical Behavior Therapy (Lynch et al., 2006).

An additional technique, reported by Souza et al. (2019) reported that "vagus nerve stimulation (VNS) enhances extinction of conditioned fear and reduces anxiety in rat models of PTSD using moderate stress." These and similar studies support neurophysiological treatment as a primary long-term strategy in humans as animal trials continue and effectiveness determined.

Taken as a whole, the future technologies, both online, off-line, and combined, and laboratory-based, hold promise for future medical and psychotherapeutic research and interventions for the sequelae of long-term PTSD.

10.6 Existing Policies and Supports for PTSD

An example of current and future trends is the increased use of technology for both the patients and providers. In today's technological world, online resources are key to many veterans' link to the latest information and supports. Currently there is a new app released by the National Center for Telehealth and Technology. This app is called "Provider Resilience." This is a unique resource in that it accounts for the secondary fatigue that service providers many encounters which in turn may affect the quality of care to patients. It is important to recognize the providers treating those with PTSD may suffer from burnout, and secondary PTSD (PTSD symptoms developed due to exposure to a traumatized individual). This app helps benefit providers which in turn will benefit patients. The app provides psychoeducation and self-assessments for the provider. The home screen to the application will give a snapshot of the providers' resilience rating, as well as compassion fatigue, burnout, secondary trauma ratings. This allows the provider to self-reflect on themselves before treating patients. The app also provides mindful and meditation techniques, to help providers manage daily stress. The app provides users with a self-assessment to rank their risk for burnout and suggests materials and coping mechanisms accordingly.

10.6.1 *Policies that are Needed to Eliminate PTSD*

Currently research is limited on overall PTSD prevention. There are attempts made to help decrease stressors/prevent PTSD before it occurs. These include treatment of potential PTSD in military and veteran personnel by identifying markers. Currently, there are mandated protocols published by the Department of Defense that describe ongoing efforts and practices for early identification of potential PTSD aligned with the type of conflict personnel are exposed to as well as other salient characteristics, as documented in Treatment for Posttraumatic Stress Disorder in Military and Veteran Populations: Initial Assessment. Washington (DC): National Academies Press (U.S.); 2012 Jul 13. PMID: 24830058 Bookshelf ID: NBK201098 DOI: 10.17226/13364, which is a U.S. government publication.

Additional programs are currently preparing those enrolled in active duty for stressors they may face while serving (Institute of Medicine of the National Academies, 2014). Programs aim to use interventions that focus military members on avoidance of exposure to trauma while serving, as well as providing them with techniques that may be used as a proper response to the trauma. Some efforts made are aimed at detecting and treating symptoms while the patient is in "Acute Stress Disorder," as opposed to when the patient has progressed to PTSD. Current studies find that those who were prepared for stressors responded more realistically, as opposed to those who found low-level combat to be traumatic (Institute of Medicine of the National Academies, 2014).

It has been established that there are precursors and "warning" signs to those at high risk of developing PTSD. Increased understanding of these risks may assist in preventing PTSD prior to enlisting in the military. There are known neuroendocrine, neurochemical, and neuroanatomic factors that affect the brain and may increase the patient's susceptibility for developing PTSD. Neurochemical features regulate fear response, neuroanatomic features affect adaptation to stress and fear conditioning, which in turn render every individual's response to stressors vary based on pre-existing factors (Sherin & Nemeroff, 2011).

As indicated, authors Sherin and Nemeroff (2011) further provide a comprehensive review of literature pertaining to the understanding of PTSD, describing the neurobiological factors that impact the development of PTSD in biologically and experientially pre-disposed individuals, to explain the different effects of trauma on certain individuals. These authors indicate that evidence to date points to individual differences in the dysregulation of the nervous system responsible for reflexive survival behaviors is responsible for the array of reactions encountered by different individuals to similar events. They further state that there is a pathology of PTSD that interacts with an individual's pre-existing biological and experiential determinants. Although Sherin and Nemeroff (2011) emphasize a relative paucity of data due to methodological constraints such as subject matching of pre-morbid neurobiological and historical factors, available evidence suggests the presence of certain predicative factors such as chemical brain difference between the genders, which in turn, help explain the differential brain activity and individual cascade of effects within the autonomic nervous system (i.e. heart rate and blood pressure) found between males and females in laboratory studies. It therefore appears that a combination of genetic and epigenetic factors accounts for differential findings. What is still pending investigation are factors such as whether the observed changes are a result of pre-conditioning or an effect of the traumatizing event and other exogenous factors such as timing of occurrence and etiology the traumatizing event itself.

Other risk factors that may contribute to PTSD that have been outlined in this report warrant further investigation as well. Women more often than men suffer from PTSD. Exposure to stress early in life is another risk factor to developing PTSD. When assessing Vietnam veterans, those with childhood adversity had a higher risk of developing PTSD post combat. TBI and other physical injuries also increased the risk of PTSD when assessing Vietnam veterans, Iraq veterans, and Afghanistan veterans. Other less investigated concomitant factors require research attention to this important national and international matter.

10.6.2   Unsolved Problems/Research Still Needed

When assessing the deployment cycle, there is need for further investigation of what more can be done during each phase to help prevent and properly care for those with combat-related PTSD. Pre-deployment, deployment, and post deployment are the three phases under investigation. Pre-deployment includes basic military training and preparation for combat. Deployment is the actual service. Post deployment is when the service member returns from combat and must act as an active member in their community (Riggs & Sermanian, 2012).

During pre-deployment there are a few approaches to assist in preventing PTSD prior to combat. Currently there is no standardized screening tool being used prior to enlisting or being deployed. There are individual risk factors such as previous trauma, biological conditions, family history of psychiatric conditions that should be included in the screening tool (Riggs & Sermanian, 2012). There are many educational opportunities pre-deployment that may assist in preventing PTSD. Currently, the Marine Corps combat Operational Stress Control and Army's Battlemind Program uses social support systems as a method to assist in trauma recovery. "Battlemind training augments... by building upon the Warrior's proven combat skills and mental fortitude--for truly we cannot send their bodies where we have not prepared their minds to go" (Orsingher et al., 2008). Operation Stress Control "embeds mental health personnel within the Marine Corps units and extends their reach by training officers and noncommissioned officers to recognize Marines showing signs of stress and intervene early" (Vaughan et al., 2015). The Army Battlemind Program focuses on three cycles of military life: life-cycle training, deployment-cycle training, and soldier support training.

> The objectives of Battlemind training are to mentally prepare our Warriors for the rigors of combat and other military deployments; to assist our Warriors in their successful transition back home; to provide our Warriors with the skills to assist their Battle Buddy* to transition home; and, finally, to prepare our Warriors to deploy again in support of all types of military operations, including additional combat tours.
>
> (Orsingher et al., 2008)

Additional research should be performed to determine the efficacy of these programs. Other programs that may be considered are exposure-based therapies, educating those at combat about the consequences of avoidance, and cognitive therapies may all serve as a benefit. Research needs to be performed to assess if stress/anxiety management skills training would be beneficial to those prior to combat, as opposed to after combat. Additionally, research should assist providers in choosing a prevention program based on the person's unique personality, using a screening tool (Riggs & Sermanian, 2012).

Current data states that military environments play a role on the emotional aspect of combat based on the leadership and unit cohesion (Riggs & Sermanian, 2012). Specific techniques are still under investigation and there currently is scant research regarding whether the training process for military members is involved in the risk for PTSD (Riggs & Sermanian, 2012). Further research should emphasize proper education and techniques for military leadership to help aid in cohesiveness while the member is based in their unit.

Digital health research appears to suggest that those with health conditions that carry a stigma are drawn to online support groups. Online support groups are utilized to assist in management of a myriad of conditions. However, currently, sufficient research is lacking regarding the interaction between the user and the technology, specifically what draws the user to the technology and how it helps (Yeshua-Katz, 2021). The authors report a study that was performed to assess how Facebook and WhatsApp support groups can be utilized to help veterans diagnosed with PTSD. Some results of the study revealed that members found quite a few aspects helped symptomology with technology. The users revealed that the visibility, availability, multimodality, surveillance, and synchrony of the online support groups were beneficial for coping with PTSD. More studies like this one would be beneficial to better understand how online communication can be used to maximize health outcomes, and to can assist digital intervention designers regarding directions to maximize communication in those with PTSD (Yeshua-Katz, 2021).

Further, Dana S. Dunn addressed how disability and personhood are important to be addressed in the future. Dunn remarks that, The American Psychological Association (APA) emphasizes the importance of using person-first language, as opposed to identity- first language, when referring to people with disabilities to reduce bias in psychologic writing (Dunn & Andrews, 2015). For example, saying "people with disabilities" instead of "disabled people" is beneficial. This allows the person to be identified first as opposed to being identified by their disability. The rationale behind person-first language is linked to many current models. Treating psychologists and all providers should be actively aware of avoiding identity-first language to enhance cultural competence regarding disability issues and communications (Dunn & Andrews, 2015). This is a concept that is currently debated among different populations of people with disabilities.

Overall, this philosophy is explored within the work of Yvette D. Hyter and Marlene B. Salas-Provance (2023) and Schnyder, U. et al. (2016) who are focused on the social model of disability. It is essential that individuals who suffer PTSD must be dealt with using the most appropriate and culturally competent practices in communication sciences and disorders to provide strategies more meaningfully for long-term quality of life enhancement in individuals affected by PTSD and all related conditions (see Hyter & Salas-Provance, 2023, Schnyder et al., 2016).

10.6.3 A Final Note Re: Existing Policies that Support Work with PTSD and Future Directions

The U.S. government has specialized resources to support ongoing work with individuals suffering from PTSD due to military service. These include: www.specialneedsalliance.org and resources via the Wounded Warriors Project (https://www.woundedwarriorproject.org/).

However, based on the research in the current chapter,

1 policies in need of further development include pre-screening for characteristics that may indicate a predisposition to vulnerability to PTSD.
2 earlier detection assessment conducted via objective measurement as opposed to self-report,
3 development of formal protocols to examine precipitating history and events during service, and
4 improved diagnostic tools to differentiate between PTSD subtypes such as hyper-arousable vs. dissociative characteristics.

These necessary research topics are in addition to ongoing need for improved tools for differential diagnosis and co-existing conditions such as traumatic brain injuries. Furthermore, the office of Diversity Management and Equal Opportunity (https://diversity.defense.gov/) is a resource for the advancement of culturally sensitive services for all personnel in the military. Support for PTSD services which are diversified can reduce fear of revealing diagnoses and related loss of opportunity and support; and lastly, but likely most importantly, family, and social support for the "invisible injuries" endured by military personnel facing posttraumatic stress disorder.

10.7   A Call to Action

The call to action for speech-language pathologists and audiologists is underscored in this most recent article describing the fact that psychological trauma such as occurs in posttraumatic stress disorder may be a hidden primary and secondary etiology. Pre-morbid factors and individual history along with many still to be analyzed factors affect how individuals may respond differently to similar traumas. There may be subtle changes in addition to significant individual biological and environmental factors that predispose certain individuals to sustained reactivity to catastrophic events that may be unaccounted for in clinical settings. It behooves the profession of communication sciences and disorders to recognize "the relentless hurt of trauma" and acknowledge "Trauma is often hidden. But recognizing it and understanding its triggers can help us appropriately shift treatment of adult patients" (LaGrange, 2022).

References

American Speech-Language-Hearing Association (n.d.). *Cultural Competence*, American Speech-Language-Hearing Association. Retrieved August 5, 2022 from https://www.asha.org/practice-portal/professional-issues/cultural-responsiveness/

Bailey, T. D., & Brand, B. L. (2017). Traumatic dissociation: Theory, research, and treatment. *Clinical Psychology: Science and Practice, 24*(2), 170–185. https://doi.org/10.1111/cpsp.12195

Ben-Aharon, A. (2022, January 2). *Does mild brain injury affect your speech? Symptoms.* Great Speech. Retrieved January 10, 2022 from https://greatspeech.com/how-does-mild-traumatic-brain-injury-affect-your-speech/

Bijleveld, H.-A. (2015). Post-traumatic stress disorder and stuttering: A diagnostic challenge in a case study. *Procedia - Social and Behavioral Sciences, 193*, 37–43. https://doi.org/10.1016/j.sbspro.2015.03.242

Bomyea, J., Johnson, A., & Lang, A. J. (2016). Information processing in PTSD: Evidence for biased attentional, interpretation, and memory processes. *Psychopathology Review, a4*(3), 218–243. https://doi.org/10.5127/pr.037214

Boyd, B., Rodgers, C., Aupperle, R., & Jak, A. (2016). Case report on the effects of cognitive processing therapy on psychological, neuropsychological, and speech symptoms in comorbid PTSD and TBI. *Cognitive and Behavioral Practice, 23*(2), 173–183. https://doi.org/10.1016/j.cbpra.2015.10.001

Bronson, H., Vaudreuil, R., & Bradt, J. (2018). Music therapy treatment of active duty military: An overview of intensive outpatient and longitudinal care programs. *Music Therapy Perspectives, 36*(2), 195–206. https://doi.org/10.1093/mtp/miy006

Committee on the Assessment of Ongoing Efforts in the Treatment of Posttraumatic Stress Disorder, Board on the Health of Select Populations, & Institute of Medicine (2014). *Treatment for posttraumatic stress disorder in military and veteran populations: Final assessment.* National Academies Press (US).

Center for Substance Abuse Treatment (US) (2014). *Trauma-informed care in behavioral health services.* Substance Abuse and Mental Health Services Administration (US).

Dalenberg, C., Glaser, D., & Alhassan, O. (2012). Statistical support for subtypes in posttraumatic stress disorder: The how and why of subtype analysis. *Depression and Anxiety, 29*(8), 667–747. https://doi.org/10.1002/da.21926

Dunn, D. S., & Andrews, E. E. (2015). Person-first and identity-first language: Developing psychologists' cultural competence using disability language. *The American Psychologist, 70*(3), 255–264. https://doi.org/10.1037/a0038636

Friedman, M. J. (2015). *Posttraumatic and acute stress disorders.* Springer.

Gayraud, F., & Auxéméry, Y. (2021). Identification of the marks of psychic trauma in spoken language: Definition of the "Split-10" diagnostic scale. *Annales Médico-Psychologiques, Revue Psychiatrique.* https://doi.org/10.1016/j.amp.2021.09.016

Gillette, H. (2022, February 11). *The signs and causes of disorganized speech.* Psych Central. Retrieved September 29, 2022 from https://psychcentral.com/schizophrenia/disorganized-speech

Gradus, J. (2007, January 31). *Va.gov: Veterans affairs.* Epidemiology of PTSD. Retrieved October 18, 2021, from https://www.ptsd.va.gov/professional/treat/essentials/epidemiology.asp#three

Herman, J. (1992). Complex PTSD: A syndrome in survivors of prolonged and repeat trauma. *Journal of Traumatic Stress, 5*(1), 377–391. https://doi.org/10.1002/jts.2490050305

Howley, E. K. (2019, June 18). *Statistics on PTSD in Veterans | US News.* U.S. News and World Report. Retrieved October 6, 2022 from https://health.usnews.com/conditions/mental-health/ptsd/articles/ptsd-veterans-statistics

Hyter, Y., & Salas-Provance, M. (2023). *Culturally responsive practices in speech, language and hearing sciences* (2nd ed.). Plural Publishing, Inc.

Kleim, B., Horn, A. B., Kraehenmann, R., Mehl, M. R., & Ehlers, A. (2018). Early linguistic markers of trauma-specific processing predict post-trauma adjustment. *Frontiers in Psychiatry, 9*, 645. https://doi.org/10.3389/fpsyt.2018.00645

Krystal, J. H., Abdallah, C. G., Averill, L. A., Kelmendi, B., Harpaz-Rotem, I., Sanacora, G., Southwick, S. M., & Duman, R. S. (2017). Synaptic loss and the pathophysiology of PTSD: Implications for ketamine as a prototype novel therapeutic. *Current Psychiatry Reports, 19*(10). https://doi.org/10.1007/s11920-017-0829-z

LaGrange, E. (May/June 2022). The relentless hurt of trauma. *The ASHA Leader Live.* Retrieved from https://leader.pubs.asha.org/do/10.1044/leader.FTR3.27052022.trauma-informed-care.24/full/

Levi, O., Ben Yehuda, A., Pine, D. S., & Bar-Haim, Y. (2021). A sobering look at treatment effectiveness of military-related posttraumatic stress disorder. *Clinical Psychological Science*. https://doi.org/10.1177/21677026211051314

Low, D. M., Bentley, K. H., & Ghosh, S. S. (2020). Automated assessment of psychiatric disorders using speech: A systematic review. *Laryngoscope Investigative Otolaryngology, 5*(1), 96–116. https://doi.org/10.1002/lio2.354

Lynch, T. R., Chapman, A. L., Rosenthal, M. Z., Kuo, J. R., & Linehan, M. M. (2006). Mechanisms of change in dialectical behavior therapy: Theoretical and empirical observations. *Journal of Clinical Psychology, 62*(4), 459–480. https://doi.org/10.1002/jclp.20243

Marmar, C. R., Brown, A. D., Qian, M., Laska, E., Siegel, C., Li, M., Abu-Amara, D., Tsiartas, A., Richey, C., Smith, J., Knoth, B., & Vergyri, D. (2019). Speech-based markers for posttraumatic stress disorder in US veterans. *Depression and Anxiety, 36*(7), 607–616. https://doi.org/10.1002/da.22890

Norman, R. S., Jaramillo, C. A., Eapen, B. C., Amuan, M. E., & Pugh, M. J. (2018). Acquired stuttering in veterans of the wars in Iraq and Afghanistan: The role of traumatic brain injury, post-traumatic stress disorder, and medications. *Military Medicine, 183*(11–12). https://doi.org/10.1093/milmed/usy067

Office for Diversity, Equity, and Inclusion – Department of Defense (n.d.). Retrieved from https://diversity.defense.gov/

Orsingher, J. M., Lopez, A. T., & Rinehart, M. E. (2008). Battlemind training system: "Armor for your mind". *U.S. Army Medical Department Journal, 66*. Retrieved from https://pubmed.ncbi.nlm.nih.gov/20088068/

Pierce, L. (2014). The integrative power of dance/movement therapy: Implications for the treatment of dissociation and developmental trauma. *The Arts in Psychotherapy, 41*(1), 7–15. https://doi.org/10.1016/j.aip.2013.10.002

Ranjbar, N., Erb, M., Mohammad, O., & Moreno, F. A. (2020). Trauma-informed care and cultural humility in the mental health care of people FROM minoritized communities. *Focus, 18*(1), 8–15. https://doi.org/10.1176/appi.focus.20190027

Riggs, D. S., & Sermanian, D. (2012). Prevention and care of combat-related PTSD: Directions for future explorations. *Military Medicine, 177*(8S), 14–20. https://doi.org/10.7205/milmed-d-12-00140

Samuel, C., Louis-Dreyfus, A., Couillet, J., Roubeau, B., Bakchine, S., Bussel, B. & Azouvi, P. (1998, April). Dysprosody after severe closed head injury: An acoustical analysis. *Journal of Neurology Neurosurgery, and Psychiatry*. Retrieved July 7, 2022 from https://www.ncbi.nlm.nih,gov/pmc/articles/PMC2170057/

Scherer, S., Stratou, G., Gratch, J., & Morency, L.-P. (2013). Investigating voice quality as a speaker-independent indicator of depression and PTSD. *Interspeech 2013*. https://doi.org/10.21437/interspeech.2013-240

Scherer, S., Lucas, G., Gratch, J., Rizzo, A., & Morency, L. (2015). Reduced vowel space is a robust indicator of psychological distress: A cross-corpus analysis. Conference: ICASSP 2015-2015 IEEE International Conference on Acoustics, Speech and Signal Processing (ICASSP). https://doi.org/10.1109/ICASSP.2015.7178880

Schnyder, U., Bryant, R. A., Ehlers, A., Foa, E. B., Hasan, A., Mwiti, G., Kristensen, C. H., Neuner, N., Oe, M. and Yule, W. (2016) Culture-sensitive psychotraumatology. *European Journal of Psychotraumatology, 7*(1). https://doi.org/10.3402/ejpt.v7.31179

Segal, A., Wald, I., Lubin, G., Fruchter, E., Ginat, K., Ben Yehuda, A., Pine, D. S., & Bar-Haim, Y. (2019). Changes in the dynamic network structure of PTSD symptoms pre-to-post combat. *Psychological Medicine, 50*(5), 746–753. https://doi.org/10.1017/s0033291719000539

Sherin, J. E., & Nemeroff, C. B. (2011). Post-traumatic stress disorder: The neuro-biological impact of psychological trauma. *Dialogues in Clinical Neuroscience, 13*(3), 263–278.

Souza, R. R., Robertson, N. M., Pruitt, D. T., Gonzales, P. A., Hays, S. A., Rennaker, R. L., Kilgard, M. P., & McIntyre, C. K. (2019). Vagus nerve stimulation reverses the extinction impairments in a model of PTSD with prolonged and repeated trauma. *Stress (Amsterdam, Netherlands), 22*(4), 509–520. https://doi.org/10.1080/10253890.2019.1602604

Todorov, G., Mayilvahanan, K., Cain, C., & Cunha, C. (2020). Context- and subgroup-specific language changes in individuals who develop PTSD after trauma. *Frontiers in Psychology, 11.* https://doi.org/10.3389/fpsyg.2020.00989

U.S. Department of Veteran Affairs (2011). *PTSD: Symptoms & treatment: Military veterans: Make the connection.* Symptoms & Treatment | Military Veterans | Make the Connection. Retrieved October 19, 2022 from https://www.maketheconnection.net/conditions/ptsd?gclid=EAIaIQobChMIh-Gn0s-6-QIVDLLICh0MaQDuEAMYASAAEgJsTvD_BwE

Vasterling, J. J., & Thorp, S. R. (2022, June 24). *Continuing Education: PTSD and Dementia.* U.S. Department of Veteran Affairs. Retrieved October 19, 2022, from https://ptsd.va.gov/professional/continuing_ed/dementia_ptsd.asp

Vaughan, C. A., Farmer, C. M., Breslau, J., & Burnette C. (2015). *Evaluation of the operational stress control and readiness (OSCAR) program.* Santa Monica, CA: RAND Corporation. Retrieved from https://www.rand.org/pubs/research_reports/RR562.html. Also available in print form.

Veterans Charity - Non Profit Organization for veterans: WWP. Wounded Warrior Project. (n.d.). Retrieved from https://www.woundedwarriorproject.org/

Weathers, F. W., Blake, D. D., Schnurr, P. P., Kaloupek, D. G., Marx, B. P., & Keane, T. M. (2013). *The Clinician-Administered PTSD Scale for DSM-5 (CAPS-5).* [Assessment] Retrieved from www.ptsd.va.gov

Westby, C. (2018). Adverse childhood experiences: What speech-language pathologists need to know. *Word of Mouth, 30*(1), 1–4. https://doi.org/10.1177/1048395018796520

Weston, C. S. (2014). Posttraumatic stress disorder: A theoretical model of the hyperarousal subtype. *Frontiers in Psychiatry, 5,* 37. https://doi.org/10.3389/fpsyt.2014.00037

World Health Organization (2022, January). *World Health Organization.* Retrieved from https://icd.who.int/en

Yehuda, R., McFarlane, A. C., & Shalev, A. Y. (1998). Predicting the development of post traumatic stress disorder from the acute response to a traumatic event. *Biological Psychiatry, 44,* 56–63.

Yeshua-Katz, D. (2021). The role of communication affordances in post-traumatic stress disorder Facebook and WhatsApp support groups. *International Journal of Environmental Research and Public Health, 18*(9), 4576. https://doi.org/10.3390/ijerph18094576

Yoder, M., & Norman, S. (2015, September 10). *Va.gov: Veterans Affairs.* Co-occurring PTSD and Neurocognitive Disorder (NCD). Retrieved from https://www.ptsd.va.gov/professional/treat/cooccurring/ncd_cooccurring.asp

Zaleski, K. L., Johnson, D. K., & Klein, J. T. (2016). Grounding Judith Herman's trauma theory within interpersonal neuroscience and evidence-based practice modalities for trauma treatment. *Smith College Studies in Social Work, 86*(4), 377–393. https://doi.org/10.1080/00377317.2016.1222110

With gratitude to Ms. Bianca DiSomma and Ms. Grace Ramey, Graduate Research Assistants, Pace University, NY.

11 Language Research in Post-Traumatic Stress

Where Do We Go from Here?

Yvette D. Hyter

Trauma-informed care is about understanding the pervasive nature of trauma and promotes practices of healing and recovery rather than practice in ways that might be retraumatizing (ITTIC, 2021). Trauma-responsive care "requires activity and engagement, not just knowledge" (Daniels, 2022, p. 41), and this activity and engagement should be integrated, interdisciplinary, and culturally responsive. In a search of the articles published in journals of the American Speech-Language-Hearing Association, only 18 manuscripts mention trauma-informed care, the first of which was published in 2012. Of these 18 manuscripts, only three mention trauma-informed in the article's title or abstract. There are no publications in this database that even mention trauma-responsive.

This text, *Language Research in Post-Traumatic Stress*, is one of the very few texts that focus on the impact of trauma on language. In addition to social workers and counselors, speech-language clinicians, as well as educators, are among the first professionals who interface with children who have had traumatic experiences because of the impact that post-traumatic stress can have on communication, language, and literacy. Children with these histories are frequently on the caseloads of speech-language clinicians, whether they come with a formal diagnosis. Therefore, it is imperative that clinicians, educators, and scholars focused on language and communication development and function become more aware of and engage in trauma-informed and trauma-responsive practices. This chapter summarizes the main points raised in the previous chapters and poses some questions for exploration, education, research, practice, and policy development in the future.

11.1 What We Know

Archibald and Archibald (Chapter 2 this volume) help us understand that racial inequities negatively affect the mental health of Black, Indigenous, and other People of Color (BIPOC) individuals and families, and these issues

DOI: 10.4324/9781003225270-13

must be accounted for in our engagement with families and individuals. In Chapter 3, Westby writes that migrants and refugees often experience trauma before they move, during their travels to another country, and while gaining access to their new host country. It is important for speech-language educators, clinicians, and scholars to be more familiar with the effects of being dispossessed of one's homeland or the impact that forcible displacement has on relationships and development. Trauma often affects language structure and meaning, but there is a particular concern about social pragmatic communication – the interdependent relationship among social cognition, cognition, and pragmatics. In Chapter 4, Hyter writes that social pragmatic communication is instrumental in establishing and maintaining relationships, reading social situations, and recounting past experiences, and is important for academic success. We learned from Suarez and Masselink (Chapter 5) that post-traumatic stress significantly impacts regulation, which can be supported by tactile, proprioceptive, visual, and auditory sensory input. Caregivers can act as co-regulators of the child's sensory inputs. Collaborations between speech-language clinicians and occupational therapists in the care of individuals and families with post-traumatic stress is important. Telford Rose and Myers (in Chapter 6) remind us that trauma also affects individuals who are multilingual and requires culturally and linguistically responsive practices and more research in this area. Yehuda (in Chapter 7) discusses the impact of post-traumatic stress on language structure and content in children. Knowledge about how trauma affects language development and functioning must be incorporated into academic and clinical coursework and practice. We also know now that post-traumatic stress can affect adolescent language and identity development, as argued by Collins et al. in Chapter 8. School-based interventions for adolescents with trauma histories are different than traditional practices with which speech-language clinicians might be familiar. Riber and Beck (Chapter 9) show us how attachment insecurity is reflected in narrative produced by adults. They discussed the attachment-informed mentalization approach for supporting adults with complex trauma experiences. Finally, Carozza (in Chapter 10) helped us realize the impact of post-traumatic stress in veterans and adults. She indicated the importance of interdisciplinary and interprofessional assessments and interventions in providing effective care. Knowing what comprises and how professionals can support resilience is also important.

11.1.1   Resilience

Over the last three years, the world has experienced the COVID-19 pandemic and numerous wars and political unrest. As a result of this global event, the landscape of speech, language, and hearing practice has changed. The change was dramatic in some ways and not always in ways we would have chosen. We hope to emerge from this collective experience by rebuilding our own resiliency and supporting the resiliency of care partners – the children, families, adults, communities, and organizations with whom we collaborate in their care.

Resilience is the ability to heal from a traumatic experience (Prince-Embury & Saklofske, 2013). Yehuda (2016) defines it as "the strength born of facing, knowing, processing, and growing beyond" pain (pp. 223–224). The American Psychological Association (2020) defines it as adapting after adversity, which involves personal growth. Resilience is also a process we see occurring in nature. The Baobab Tree, native to West Africa, is a perfect example of natural resilience. It survives thousands of years in challenging climates. They prevent soil erosion and provide food and shelter for animals. They retain water and survive in droughts. In Senegal, these trees are often central locations within a community, where community members see collective wisdom and engage in democratic decision-making.

Resilience is a complex concept for Black, Indigenous, and Other People of Color. Some question whether the concept of resilience is a positive one or an insult. Dr. Lourdes Dolores Follins, in an NPR interview, states that "resiliency is left over from slavery, colonization, and indentured servitude" (Dutes et al., 2022). She is concerned that focusing on someone's physical capacities has been confused with resilience. Others indicate that resilience will not mean the same for White communities as for communities of color (Bahl, 2021). For others, suffering has propelled and made them stronger (Thakur, 2023).

There are different ways to be resilient or different sources of resilience. Resisting economic, political, technological, and ecological status quo and promoting resilience through resistance. Often, children with complex histories appear as young, curious children engaging in playful behaviors and simply living their daily lives. Resilience can emerge from living. Other abilities that support resilience are regulation, relationships, self-efficacy, and a sense of one's own story or history.

Regulation is controlling one's thinking, emotions, and behavior. Regulating one's emotions is important in developing resilience (Artuch-Garde et al., 2017). Relationships within and outside of one's family are essential for intellectual, emotional, and cognitive growth. Safe and caring relationships can have co-regulating properties. Self-efficacy is the belief that we have the power to change our own circumstances and to support the change in others' circumstances. This characteristic supports the development of resilience in the face of adverse situations (Schwarzer & Warner, 2013). A history of one's life story is essential for understanding the past – it helps us know who we are and how to make sense of our experiences. Narratives facilitate the transition of fragmented memories into integrated ones (Schauer et al., 2017; Westby, 2020).

11.2   What Is Next?

In speech, language, and hearing sciences, we need to continue to explore the impact of post-traumatic stress on language and communication. Most importantly, we must develop and publish evidence-based interventions supporting language and communication across the ages. Below are some questions and ideas that could serve as a starting point in developing a research and educational agenda in the future.

Some Future Directions and Research Questions

1   What is the current standard of care for providing culturally and trauma-responsive care across the lifespan?
2   How can culturally and trauma-responsive care be conceptualized differently than how practice is currently devised? Are these newly conceptualized care processes effective?
3   Are trauma-informed and trauma-responsive training effective in changing/improving speech-language clinicians' practice with individuals who have experienced trauma?
4   What components of trauma-informed and trauma-responsive education are most impactful for changing/improving the skills of speech-language clinicians and educators?
5   How well do trauma interventions specifically developed by speech-language clinicians improve the language, communication, and literacy of children who have experienced trauma?
6   How much trauma training/education is required for clinicians to feel competent in engaging in trauma-informed and trauma-responsive practices?
7   How well do established interventions, such as *Trust Based Relationship Intervention* (TBRI, Purvis et al., 2013), improve the language and communication skills of individuals with a history of traumatization?
8   What are the outcomes of intervention studies when participatory action research is utilized? Participatory action research includes families experiencing trauma partners in developing, implementing, and interpreting the research questions and findings (Rupert & Bartlett, 2022).

11.2.1   *Curriculum and Education*

Given the current world context of increasing intra- and international conflicts and wars, natural disasters, mass shootings, the rise of racial, ethnic, and religious hatred, the increase of impoverishment and economic insecurity, trauma and its effects are not going away anytime soon. Trauma and the impact of trauma on child development, communication, hearing, language, learning, and literacy as required content in speech-language-hearing curricula is imperative for clinicians to be prepared to meet the growing need for trauma-informed and trauma-responsive practices.

Interdisciplinary or transdisciplinary curriculum content could include such topics as:

- Theoretical frameworks for understanding trauma and for conceptualizing trauma-informed and trauma-responsive care. Learning about frameworks would include understanding the related concepts.
- Definitions of trauma, trauma-informed, trauma-responsive, post-traumatic stress, post-traumatic stress disorder, culturally responsive, resilience
- Causes of trauma, e.g., acute, chronic, complex, systemic events, and experiences
- Current data on the prevalence and incidence of trauma across the age, gender, ability level, ethnicity, racial, economic strata
- Impact of trauma on the brain and body physiology
- Impact of trauma on development, e.g., language, literacy, communication, sensory and emotional and sensory development, cognition (executive functions, memory), social cognition (theory of mind, perspective taking, intention reading, inter- and intrapersonal), social pragmatic communication
- Culturally and trauma-responsive assessment and intervention strategies across settings and age groups

11.2.2   *Clinical Practice: Assessment and Intervention*

Interdisciplinary or transdisciplinary internships could include such assignments as:

- Clinical *observations* in a setting that specializes in assessing and supporting individuals with trauma histories using strength-based and relationship-based strategies that support resilience through relationship building, self-efficacy, and one's ability to remember, tell, and construct their own stories.
- Clinical *practice opportunities* in a transdisciplinary (or interdisciplinary) clinic that provides comprehensive trauma-informed and trauma-responsive assessments and evidence-based interventions. These clinical practice opportunities would ideally be offered to individuals across the age span and in various contexts, such as in clinics, hospitals, and school-based settings.
- Caregiver coaching – following the lead of occupational therapists, speech-language clinicians should engage in more of this practice to ensure client-centered care. Partnering with an occupational therapist can

support caregiver co-regulation and support caregivers in supporting communication, language, and literacy simultaneously (see Suarez, 2023).
* Incorporating expressive therapies (art, music, movement) into speech-language interventions and determining their effectiveness in improving language, communication, literacy, and resilience as measured by self-efficacy, relationships, sense of one's story/history, and regulation (Malchiodi, 2020).

11.2.3 Systemic Issues

As with any practice, reality often needs to lend itself better to what is needed. For example, engaging in transdisciplinary and/or interdisciplinary practice is challenging due to how insurance companies reimburse services. Nevertheless, due to the complex nature of concerns presented by individuals with trauma histories, an interdisciplinary approach at the minimum and ideally a transdisciplinary approach is required for best practices (Collins et al., 2023; Menschner & Maul, 2016). Graduate programs in speech-language-hearing sciences, occupational therapy, education, and social work should be constructed to facilitate interdisciplinary and interprofessional courses and clinical practice opportunities. Pre-service professionals who learn alongside each other will likely continue and seek such opportunities post-graduation. Professional associations with a lobbying voice, such as the American Speech-Language-Hearing Association, should include in their agenda to lobby for a change in how services are delivered and reimbursed so that best practices can be implemented with individuals with histories of trauma. Similarly, caregiver coaching is not traditionally covered by insurance, but being able to systematically support families who have histories of trauma, is a necessary reimbursement.

References

Artuch-Garde, R., Gonzalez-Torres, M. D. C., de la Fuente, J., Vera, M. M., Fernandez-Cabezas, M., & Lopez-Garcia, M. (2017). Relationship between resilience and self-regulation: A study of Spanish youth at risk of social exclusion. *Frontiers in Psychology, 8*, 612. https://doi.org/10.3389/fpsyg.2017.00612

Bahl, R. (2021, July 1). *Resilience educator Komal Minhas is redefining what it means to be resilient and helping People of Colour reclaim their power.* [Interview] The Lovepost. Retrieved from https://www.thelovepost.global/decolonise-your-mind/articles/resilience-educator-komal-minhas-redefining-what-it-means-be-resilient

Daniels, E. (2022). *Building a trauma-responsive educational practice: Lessons from a corrections classroom.* Routledge.

Dutes, K., Hanzhang Jin, C., Nguyen, A., & Handy, V. (2022, August 25). *Why you should stop complimenting people for being resilient* [Radio broadcast]. NPR. Retrieved from https://www.npr.org/2022/08/16/1117725653/why-being-resilient-might-matter-less-than-you-think

Malchiodi, C. A. (2020). *Trauma and expressive arts therapy: Brain, body, and imagination in the healing process.* Guilford Press.

Menschner, C., & Maul, A. (2016). *Issue brief: Key ingredients for successful trauma-informed care implementation.* Retrieved from https://www.samhsa.gov/sites/default/files/programs_campaigns/childrens_mental_health/atc-whitepaper-040616.pdf

Purvis, K. B., Cross, D. R., Dansereau, D. F., & Parris, S. R. (2013). Trust-based relational intervention (TBRI): A systemic approach to complex developmental trauma. *Child & Youth Services, 34*(4), 360–386. https://doi.org/10.1080/0145935X.2013.859906

Rupert, A. C., & Bartlett, D. E. (2022). The childhood trauma and attachment gap in speech-language pathology: Practitioners' knowledge, practice, and needs. *American Journal of Speech-Language Pathology, 31*(1), 287–302. https://doi.org/10.1044/2021_AJSLP-21-00110

Schauer, M., Neuner, F., & Elbert, T. (2017). Narrative exposure therapy for children and adolescents (KIDNET). In M. A. Landolt, M. Cloitre, & U. Schnyder (Eds.), *Evidence-based treatments for trauma related disorders in children and adolescents* (pp. 227–249). https://doi.org/10.1007/978-3-319-46138-0_11

Schwarzer, R., & Warner, L. M. (2013). Perceived self-efficacy and its relationship to resilience. In S. Prince-Embury, & D. Saklofske (Eds.), *Resilience in children, adolescents, and adults* (pp. 139–150). Springer.

Suarez, M. (2023). *Caregiver co-regulation coaching.* Retrieved from https://wmich.edu/resiliencycenter/coaching

Thakur, A. (2023, February 28). *UK Man who couldn't read or write until the age of 18 becomes Cambridge University Professor.* NDTV. Retrieved from https://www.ndtv.com/feature/uk-man-who-couldnt-read-or-write-until-age-18-becomes-cambridge-university-professor-3820378

The Institute on Trauma and Trauma-Informed Care (ITTIC, 2021). *What is trauma-informed care?* Retrieved from http://socialwork.buffalo.edu/social-research/institutes-centers/institute-on-trauma-and-trauma-informed-care/what-is-trauma-informed-care.html

Westby, C. E. (2020). Narrative Exposure Therapy (KIDNET). *Word of Mouth, 32*(1), 13–15. https://doi.org/10.1177/1048395020949087d

Index

ABC model of attitudinal and behavioral racism 14
acculturation stress 122
Adult Attachment Interview (AAI) 209
adverse cultural experiences 20
adverse experiences 19, 166; ACES 18; adolescence 181; childhood 19, 180; cognitive development 181; community 19; cultural 20; language development 183; trauma and 185
aims of the book 3
Area Deprivation Index (ADI) 25
assessment 80, 170, 171; analog 80; assessment frameworks 54; asylum seekers 38; attachment 207; based narrative speech styles 208; informed mentalization-based approach 218; patterns 208; system and threat system 221; theory 207
autobiographical memory 40; culture and 43; effects of trauma/PTSD on 40

behavioral and adaptive functioning 102
bimodal bilingualism 120
brain 71; amygdala 71; hippocampus 72; HPA Axis 71; hypothalamus 71; limbic system 71; locus coeruleus 72; prefrontal cortex 72

cases 26–29, 71, 115–116, 189–199, 213–218, 239–241
child maltreatment 91
code-switching 124

cognitive communication 227–228
cognitive functioning 98
collaborative process 198
complex posttraumatic stress disorder 206–207
constructivist approaches 220; eye movement desensitization and reprocessing (EMDR) 220; meaning making approach 221; narrative exposure therapy 220; prolonged exposure therapy 220; TF-CBT 220
COVID-19 11
cultural considerations in understanding trauma 43, 221; cultural context 80; cultural dimensions 44; cultural humility 102; cultural, historical, intergenerational, and gender issues 23, 187; culturally responsive 127, 255–256, 258; and emotions 46; emotion regulation 47; emotional preferences 46; influences of 45; and perception 46; responsiveness 238; sensitivity 221

Developmental Trauma Disorder 92
Distressed Communities Index (DCI) 25
drivers of racial inequities 18
DSM5 17, 230; DSM-V-TR 180
dysarthria 233

evaluation of trauma 98

Foster Care Independence Act of 1999 (PL 106-169) 188

Fostering Connections to Success and Increasing Adoptions Act of 2008 (PL110-351) 188

gene-environment-culture interactions 48; emotion regulation 49; focus of attention/perception 49; gene-culture 49; gene-environment 48; mood disorders 49; support seeking 50

H. U. M. B. L. E. 30

International Classification of Disease (ICD) 229; ICD10 17; ICD-11 206, 214
International Classification of Functioning, Disability, and Health (ICF) 229; comorbidities 231; neurocognitive disorders (NCD) 230; PTSD and 229; speech markers 231
individual education plan (IEP) 188
individual transition plan (ITP) 188
Individuals with Disabilities Education Act (IDEA, 2004) 188
implications of culture and trauma effects for the asylum process 50; cultural misinterpretations 52; interview process 51
interdisciplinary 190; interventions 193; intervention planning 190; transition planning 191
intergenerational trauma 120
interventions 55, 82, 102, 170, 171; caregiver coaching 260; cognitive behavioral therapy 242; cognitive processing therapy 240; dance/movement therapy 242; expressive therapies 260; KIDNET 56; Music Therapy 242; narrative exposure therapy 56; Neurosequential Model of Therapeutics 105; pharmacotherapy 243; Trauma-Focused Cognitive Behavioral Treatment 106; trauma-focused interventions 55, 187, 193; Trust Based Relational Intervention 103; vagus nerve stimulation (VNS) 245

Jim Crow Laws 15

language: change patterns 229; development 160; learning 158; morphology and syntax 169; phonology and phonological awareness 168; structure 168
life experiences 98
linguistic profiling 121

major theoretical frameworks 213; triphasic model 237
mental health 102
mentalization-based treatment (MBT) 218
memory 76; executive Functions 78
microaggressions 20, 24, 121
middle passage 14
migrant/refugee trauma 38
multilingual 117

narrative styles 208; unresolved-disorganized adult attachment 221
neurodevelopment 101
non-verbal communication 157

Pediatric ACEs and Related Life-Events Screener (PEARLS) 23
phenomenon of language independence 124
policies 245; existing 245; needed 245
post traumatic slave syndrome (PTSS) 16
post-traumatic stress 1, 2, 116
post-traumatic stress disorder 1, 2, 39, 116; DSM5 definition of 2
post-traumatic stress syndrome 117
pragmatics 79
Primary Care PTSD Screen for DSM5 (PC-PTSD-5) 24

racial trauma 16
raciolinguistics 121
racism 11, 12, 13, 14; internalized 16; racism's relationship with stress and trauma 14
refugee 120
regulation 93; emotional 95; executive functions 96; higher level pre-frontal cortex skills 96; sensory processing 94
resilience 256

sensory regulation 78; interpersonal
74; intrapersonal 74; perspective
taking 74; theory of mind 73
sequence 167
social cognition 73
social pragmatic communication 73
stress 69; positive 70; tolerable 70;
toxic 70
Stress, Trauma and Resilience (STAR)
228
survivor syndrome 15
Substance Abuse and Mental Health
Services Agency (SAMHSA) 187

theory of mind 234
translanguaging 115
trauma 39, 68; acute 68; and the
Brain 9; chronic 68; complex 69;
disruptions 163; and language 116,
159; migration traumas 39; and

multilingualism 117; parenting
challenges 40; sources of 39;
systemic 69
trauma-informed culturally responsive
care 170
Trauma Symptoms Discrimination
Scale (TSDS) 24
traumatic brain injury 230; closed
Head 233; penetrating 233
triple ACEs effect 19, 20

UConn Racial/Ethnic Stress and
Trauma Survey (UnRESTS) 24
unsolved problems/research needed 247

verbal communication 157
vocabulary/meaning 160; body state
164; cause and effect 166; emotive
164; literal, ambiguous, and
symbolic meaning 168